HANDBOOK OF
VETERINARY ANESTHESIA

HANDBOOK OF
VETERINARY ANESTHESIA

WILLIAM W. MUIR, III
D.V.M., Ph.D.
Diplomate A.C.V.A.
Chairman, Department of Veterinary Clinical Sciences
The Ohio State University
College of Veterinary Medicine
Columbus, Ohio

JOHN A.E. HUBBELL
D.V.M., M.S.
Diplomate A.C.V.A.
Professor, Department of Veterinary Clinical Sciences
The Ohio State University
College of Veterinary Medicine
Columbus, Ohio

Special acknowledgment to Dr. Roman Skarda for his
contribution on local anesthetic drugs and techniques

with 84 illustrations
illustrations by **Felecia Paras**

The C. V. Mosby Company
ST. LOUIS • WASHINGTON, D.C. • TORONTO   1989

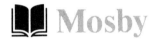

Publisher: Thomas A. Manning
Editor: Robert W. Reinhardt
Developmental editor: Cracom Corporation
Editing and production: Publication Services
Design: Liz Fett

Library of Congress Cataloging-in-Publication Data

Muir, William, 1946–
    Handbook of veterinary anesthesia / William W. Muir III, John A.E.
    Hubbell ; illustrations by Felecia Paras.
        p. cm.
    Includes index.
    ISBN 0-8016-3583-7
    1. Veterinary anesthesia—Handbooks, manuals, etc. I. Hubbell,
John A. E. II. Title.
    [DNLM: 1. Anesthesia—veterinary—handbooks.
SF 914 M953h]
SF914.M85 1989
636.089'796—dc19
DNLM/DLC   88-13136
for Library of Congress   CIP

Printed in the United States of America

The C.V. Mosby Company
11830 Westline Industrial Drive, St. Louis, Missouri 63146

PS/MV/MV 9 8 7 6 5 4 3 2 1

CONTRIBUTORS

RICHARD M. BEDNARSKI, D.V.M., M.S.
Diplomate A.C.V.A.
Department of Veterinary Clinical
   Sciences
The Ohio State University
College of Veterinary Medicine
Columbus, Ohio

ROMAN SKARDA, Dr. med. vet., Ph.D.
Diplomate A.C.V.A.
Department of Veterinary Clinical
   Sciences
The Ohio State University
College of Veterinary Medicine
Columbus, Ohio

CLIFFORD SWANSON, D.V.M., M.S.
Diplomate A.C.V.A.
Department of Anatomy, Physiology
   and Radiology
North Carolina State University
School of Veterinary Medicine
Raleigh, North Carolina

DIANE MASON, D.V.M., M.S.
Department of Surgical Sciences
University of Wisconsin–Madison
School of Veterinary Medicine
Madison, Wisconsin

PETER W. HELLYER
Department of Anatomy, Physiology
   and Radiology
North Carolina State University
School of Veterinary Medicine
Raleigh, North Carolina

PREFACE

The purpose of this preface is to serve as a dedication, prologue, and means of expressing gratitude. Briefly, this handbook of veterinary anesthesiology is dedicated to the veterinary student and practicing veterinarian. It was designed to be used by veterinary students, residents, and veterinary practitioners requiring an immediate source of information relating to the practice of veterinary anesthesia, cardiopulmonary emergencies, and euthanasia. Recent versions have been completely rethought, rewritten, and expanded.

The present edition is the result of the labors of the Section of Anesthesiology of the Department of Veterinary Clinical Sciences at The Ohio State University.

The material contained within this handbook is based upon the collective clinical experiences, research, and teaching activities of each of the contributors. Technical advice and suggestions were offered by Mary Ferguson, Sarah Flaherty, Earl Harrison, William Sheehan, Tom Sherman, Peter Hellyer, and Mark Leonard. Ideas and contributions to earlier versions of this final document were provided by Elaine Robinson, Cheryl Buchanan, and Karen Rosenberry Spenser. The final version is principally due to the concentrated and combined efforts of myself, Richard Bednarski, John Hubbell, Roman Skarda, Clifford Swanson, and Diane Mason. Our individual interests and dedication to teaching have made this work enjoyable. We have attempted to summarize and simplify what has become a very large and oftentimes confusing topic. It is not our intent to have this handbook replace more comprehensive textbooks of veterinary anesthesia, but to supplement them.

William W. Muir, III
John A.E. Hubbell

"To look back is to relax one's vigil"
BETTE DAVIS

"It's what you learn after
you know it all that counts"
ANONYMOUS

CONTENTS

CHAPTER ONE

Introduction to Anesthesia

"There are no safe anesthetic agents; there are no safe anesthetic procedures; there are only safe anesthetists."

ROBERT SMITH

OVERVIEW

The art of anesthesia, anesthetic principles, and anesthetic techniques is based on a general understanding of (1) the terms used to describe the effects of drugs used to produce chemical restraint and anesthesia, (2) the pharmacology of anesthetic drugs, and (3) the correct methods of anesthetic drug administration. This section outlines commonly used terms, uses, and routes of administration of drugs used to produce chemical restraint and anesthesia in animals.

GENERAL CONSIDERATIONS

I. Anesthesia is a reversible process. The purpose of anesthesia is to produce a convenient, safe, and inexpensive means of restraint so that clinical procedures may be expedited with a minimum of pain, discomfort, and toxic side effects to the patient and to the anesthetist

II. Selection of drugs and techniques will depend on
   A. Species, breed, age, and relative size of the patient
   B. Physical status and specific disease processes of the patient and concurrent medication
   C. Demeanor of the patient and the presence of pain
   D. Personal knowledge and experience
   E. Available assistants and their training

1

F. Familiarity with the equipment available

G. Length and type of operation or procedure to be performed

III. Variation in response can be expected because doses and techniques are based on the "average" animal. Thus the ability to modify anesthetic techniques is essential

GLOSSARY

Akinesia: Loss of motor response (movement) due to paralysis of motor nerves

Analgesia: Loss of sensitivity to pain

Anesthesia: Total loss of sensation in a body part or in the whole body, generally induced by the administration of a drug that depresses the activity of nervous tissue either locally (peripherally) or generally (centrally)

Local anesthesia: Anesthesia limited to a local area

Regional anesthesia: Anesthesia limited to a local area

General anesthesia: Loss of consciousness in addition to loss of sensation. Ideally, includes *hypnosis*, *hyporeflexia*, *analgesia*, and *muscle relaxation*. General anesthesia can be produced with a single drug or by a combination of drugs

Surgical anesthesia: Loss of consciousness and sensation with sufficient muscle relaxation and analgesia to allow surgery to be performed without pain to or movement of the patient

Balanced anesthesia: Surgical anesthesia produced by a combination of two or more drugs or anesthetic techniques, each contributing its own pharmacological effects. The agents used generally include tranquilizers, narcotics, nitrous oxide, and muscle relaxants

Dissociative anesthesia: A central nervous system state characterized by catalepsy, profound peripheral analgesia, and altered consciousness produced by the cyclohexamine drugs (e.g., ketamine)

Catalepsy: A state in which there is malleable rigidity of the limbs. The patient is generally unresponsive to aural, visual, or minor painful stimuli

Hypnosis: Artificially induced sleep or a trance resembling sleep from which the patient can be aroused by stimuli

Narcosis: Drug-induced stupor or sedation in which the patient is oblivious to pain, with or without hypnosis

Neuroleptanalgesia: Hypnosis and analgesia produced by a combination of a neuroleptic drug and an analgesic drug

Sedation: A mild degree of central depression in which the patient is awake but calm; a term often used interchangeably with *tranquilization.* With sufficient stimuli, the patient may be aroused. Sedatives act by a dose-dependent depression of the cerebral cortex

Tranquilization, ataraxia, neurolepsis: A state of tranquility and calmness in which the patient is relaxed, awake, and unconcerned with its surroundings and potentially indifferent to minor pain. Sufficient stimulation will arouse the patient. Tranquilizers act by depressing the hypothalamus and the reticular activating system

USE OF ANESTHETICS

I. Restraint
   A. Radiography
   B. Cleaning, grooming, dentals
   C. Bandaging, splinting, plaster casting
   D. Capture of exotic and wild animals
   E. Transportation
II. Examination
   A. Palpation
   B. Endoscopy
   C. Radiography
   D. Diagnosis of lameness
   E. Diagnostic ultrasound
   F. Computerized axial tomography
III. Manipulation
   A. Catheterization
   B. Closed reduction of luxations or fractures
   C. Wound care
   D. Obstetrics
IV. Surgery
V. Control of convulsions
VI. Euthanasia

TYPES OF ANESTHESIA (According to route of administration)

Acupuncture	Inhalation*	Oral*
Controlled hypothermia	Intramuscular*	Rectal
Electroanesthesia	Intraperitoneal	Regional nerve block*
Field block*	Intratesticular	Subcutaneous
Hypnosis	Intrathoracic	Topical*
Infiltration*	Intravascular*	

EFFECT OF ROUTE AND METHOD OF ADMINISTRATION OF ANESTHETIC DRUG

I. Given intravenously (Fig. 1-1): Onset of action is immediate, but peak effect may take minutes. Duration of action is shorter and effects are generally more intense than for other routes
II. Given intramuscularly or subcutaneously: Onset of action may take 10 to 15 minutes; peak effect may not be obtained for many minutes to hours and will depend on the blood supply to the tissues at the site of injection, drug absorption, and the rate of metabolism of the drug

*Routes commonly used in veterinary medicine

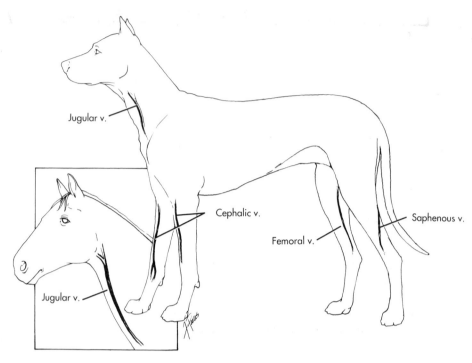

FIG.1-1 The jugular, cephalic, femoral, and saphenous veins are used in the dog (illustrated) and cat for intravenous administration of fluids and drugs. The jugular vein is the most frequently used vein in horses, cattle, sheep, and goats.

III. Rapidity of injection: Faster injections generally cause more intense effects due to decreased mixing of drug with blood

IV. Concentration of solutions
  A. Increasing drug concentrations may increase intensity of immediate effect
  B. Increasing concentrations may increase vascular irritation

V. Onset of action of inhalation drugs requires absorption of gas from alveoli into the blood, then diffusion of anesthetic into the central nervous system

CHAPTER TWO

Patient Evaluation and Preparation

*"For every mistake that is made for not knowing,
a hundred are made for not looking."*

ANONYMOUS

OVERVIEW

Anesthesia involves more than just the delivery of anesthetic drugs to the patient. Safe anesthesia implies proper selection of drugs based on the procedure to be performed as well as the physical status of the patient. This section outlines the essentials of preoperative evaluation with regard to subsequent anesthetic management.

GENERAL CONSIDERATIONS

   I. Information obtained from the preanesthetic evaluation is used in determining the choice and the dose of anesthetics to be used
  II. The history and physical examination are the basis of patient evaluation. The need for further workup is indicated by abnormalities found during physical examination or history information that suggests altered bodily functions
 III. No laboratory test can replace a thorough physical examination
 IV. Maintain patent intravenous routes for all high-risk patients
  V. Maintain an open airway in every patient
 VI. Be prepared for unexpected events

PATIENT EVALUATION

   I. Patient identification
     A. Case number or identification

    B. Signalment
       1. Species
       2. Breed
       3. Age
       4. Sex
    C. Body weight
  II. Client complaint and anamnesis (history)
    A. Duration and nature of illness
    B. Concurrent disease
       1. Diarrhea
       2. Vomiting
       3. Hemorrhage
       4. Epilepsy
       5. Heart failure
       6. Renal failure
    C. Level of activity
    D. Previous and current administration of drugs (see Chapter 13: Anesthesia toxicity, waste gas scavenging, and anesthetic-drug interactions)
       1. Organophosphates
       2. Insecticides
       3. Sulfonamides
       4. Chloramphenicol
       5. Streptomycin, neomycin, polymyxin B
       6. Digitalis glycosides
       7. β-blockers
    E. Previous anesthetic history and reactions
    F. Recent feeding

CURRENT PHYSICAL EXAMINATION

  I. General body condition
    A. Obesity
    B. Cachexia
    C. Pregnancy
    D. Dehydration
  II. Cardiovascular
    A. Heart rate and rhythm (see Table 2-1)
    B. Arterial pulse
    C. Capillary refill time
    D. Auscultation (cardiac murmurs)
 III. Pulmonary
    A. Respiratory rate and depth
       1. Usually 15-25 for small animals, 8-20 for large animals
       2. Tidal volume is approximately 14 ml/kg
    B. Mucous membranes
       1. Pallor (anemia)

TABLE 2-1

NORMAL HEART RATE VALUE RANGES

Animal	Value range
Dog	70-80
Cat	145-200
Cow	60-80
Horse	30-45
Colt	50-80
Sheep, goat	60-90
Pig	60-90

    2. Cyanosis (>5 g/dl of unoxygenated Hb)
  C. Auscultation (breath sounds)
  D. Upper airway obstruction
  E. Percussion
IV. Hepatic
  A. Jaundice
  B. Failure of blood to clot
V. Renal
  A. Anuria
  B. Polyuria/polydipsia
VI. Gastrointestinal
  A. Diarrhea
  B. Vomiting
  C. Parasites
  D. Distention
VII. Nervous system and special senses
  A. Seizures
  B. Coma
  C. Glaucoma
VIII. Metabolic and endocrine
  A. Temperature
  B. Hyperthyroid
  C. Hypothyroid
  D. Diabetes
IX. Integument
  A. Hydration
  B. Neoplasia (pulmonary metastasis)
  C. Subcutaneous emphysema (fractured ribs)
  D. Parasites (fleas, mites)
    1. Anemia

    E. Burns

      1. Fluid and electrolyte loss

    F. Trauma

X. Musculoskeletal

    A. Weakness

    B. Electrolyte imbalance (hypokalemia)

    C. Ambulatory or nonambulatory

    D. Fractures

PRESURGICAL LABORATORY WORKUP

(See Tables 2-2 and 2-3)

I. Minimum laboratory evaluation

    A. Plasma protein

    B. PCV

    C. Hb

II. Other laboratory tests (see Tables 2-4, 2-5)

    A. CBC

    B. Blood gases

    C. Hemostasis

    D. Temperature

TABLE 2-2

NORMAL HEMATOLOGIC VALUES

	Dog	Cat	Cow	Horse	Sheep	Pig
Plasma protein (g/dl)	5.7-7.8	6.3-8.3	6.7-8.6	6.0-8.5	6.3-7.1	6.0-7.5
PCV (%)	35-54	27-46	23-43	25-45	30-50	30-48
Hb (g/dl)	14-18	9-16	8-13	9-16	10-16	10-15
Total leukocytes ($\times\ 10^9$/L)	6.0-18	6.0-20.0	5-13	5-13	4-12	6.5-20
Neutrophil — segmented ($\times\ 10^9$/L)	3.0-11.5	3.0-13.0	1.4-6.0	2.3-8	1-6	3-15
Neutrophil — band ($\times\ 10^9$/L)	0-0.3	0-0.3	0-0.1	0-0.1	0-0.1	0-0.5
Lymphocytes ($\times\ 10^9$/L)	1.2-5.2	1.2-9.0	1.4-7	1-5	2-8	2-12
Monocytes ($\times\ 10^9$/L)	0.2-1.3	0-0.7	0-0.8	0-0.7	0-0.6	0-0.6
Eosinophil ($\times\ 10^9$/L)	0-1.2	0-1.2	0-2.0	0-0.8	0-1.0	0-0.6
Basophil ($\times\ 10^9$/L)	rare	rare	0-0.2	0-0.3	0-0.1	0-0.1

T A B L E 2 - 3

SERUM CHEMISTRY

	Units	Dog	Cat	Cow	Horse	Yearling	Sheep	Pig
CO_2 combining	mEq/L	16-30	15-25	21-32	25-35	21-33	–	–
Calcium	mg/dl	8.8-11.3	8.3-10.5	8.2-9.9	10-12.6	10.2-14.8	8.1-9.5	–
Phosphorus	mg/dl	2.5-6.1	3.5-7.1	4.3-7.2	2.4-5.2	2.9-6.9	3.5-6.7	5.3-9.6
Glucose	mg/dl	75-125	65-125	55-85	75-105	–	50-80	60-100
Creatinine	mg/dl	0.3-1.3	0.8-1.8	0.6-1.5	1.0-1.8	1.5-2.3	–	1.0-2.7
Bilirubin (T)	mg/dl	0-0.3	0-0.3	0-0.3	0.3-1.0	0.2-5.1	–	–
Bilirubin (D)	mg/dl	0-0.1	0-0.1	0-0.1	0-0.5	–	–	–
Albumin	gm/dl	2.1-3.6	2.3-3.6	2.7-3.7	2.5-3.4	–	2.4-3.0	–
Protein	gm/dl	5.7-7.8	6.3-8.3	6.7-8.6	6.0-8.5	–	6.3-7.1	–
BSP		5% R	5% R	2.5-4 $t_{1/2}$	2.0-3.7 $t_{1/2}$	–	–	3% R
BUN	mg/dl	8-25	15-35	5-23	10-27	15-27	5-20	8-24
Cholesterol	mg/dl	65-240	35-155	75-225	65-115	–	–	–
Alk. Ptase.	IU/L	0-110	1-70	17-80	130-350	141-401	–	–
Amylase	IU/L	330-2300	800-2450	–	–	–	–	–
CPK	IU/L	10-240	0-250	0-225	12-96	26-114	–	–
LDH	IU/L	0-120	0-360	–	108-174	130-282	–	–

R = retention
$t_{1/2}$ = half-life

TABLE 2-3—CONT'D

SERUM CHEMISTRY

	Units	Dog	Cat	Cow	Horse	Yearling	Sheep	Pig
SDH	IU/L	—	—	6-30	4-20	—	—	—
SGOT	IU/L	8-75	11-55	60-140	260-480	147-243	—	—
SGPT	IU/L	7-70	14-70	—	—	—	—	—
Na	mEq/L	140-155	149-162	130-148	131-143	135-147	140-145	139-152
K	mEq/L	3.8-5.3	3.6-5.4	3.6-5.2	3.0-4.4	3.4-4.6	4.9-5.7	4.4-6.7
Cl	mEq/L	105-121	105-135	95-108	92-106	88-104	—	100-105
Mg	mg/dl	1.8-2.4	—	2.2-3.4	2.2-2.8	—	—	—
pH	Units	7.27-7.43	7.25-7.33	7.32-7.45	7.34-7.42	—	—	—
PO$_2$	mm Hg	—	—	—	—	—	—	—
PCO$_2$	mm Hg	28-49	35-49	34-52	39-53	—	—	—
HCO$_3$	mEq/L	18-25	18-22	23-31	23-31	—	—	—
Base excess	mEq/L	-6 to 0.5	-6 to -3	-1 to 6	-1 to 5	—	—	—
Cortisol 0 hr	µg/dl	1-4.8	—	1-2.7	1-4.4	—	—	—
Cortisol 2 hr	µg/dl	5-26	—	2.7-6.0	5.1-14.6	—	—	—
IM ACTH					(8 hr)			
T$_3$ (RIA)	ng/dl	50-200	60-200	—	—	—	—	—
T$_4$ (RIA)	µg/dl	1-4	1.5-5	—	—	—	—	—

TABLE 2-4

ARTERIAL BLOOD GASES

	Normal values	Values routinely observed during anesthesia
pH	7.4 ± 0.2	7.25 to 7.45
$PaCO_2$ mm Hg	40 ± 3	30 to 60*
PaO_2 mm Hg	94 ± 3	250 to 500 (100% O_2)
Room air		Up to 250 (50% O_2)
BE	0 ± 1	−4 to −10

*Note: The development of respiratory acidosis during anesthesia is common, the severity of which is in part dependent upon the drugs used, the depth of anesthesia, the duration of anesthesia, and patient status.

III. Blood chemistry profile
    A. Electrolytes
    B. BUN
    C. Creatinine
    D. SGPT, SGOT
IV. Urinalysis
    A. Specific gravity 1.010-1.030 (normal hydration)
    B. Physiochemical evaluation
        1. pH 7-7.5 (meat diet)
            7-8 (vegetable diet)
        2. Protein: neg.
        3. Acetone: neg.
        4. Bilirubin: neg.
        5. Blood: neg.
    C. Microscopic evaluation of urine sediment
        1. Casts: 0−rare
        2. RBC: neg.
        3. WBC: neg.
        4. Epithelial cells: neg.
        5. Bacteria: neg.
        6. Crystals
            a. oxalate: normal
            b. Triple phosphates: normal
            c. Urates: normal
            d. Calcium carbonate: normal in horse only

FURTHER PRESURGICAL TESTS

I. Electrocardiography
    A. Traumatized patients
    B. Irregular rhythm on physical

T A B L E 2 - 5

HEMOSTASIS AND TEMPERATURE

	Units	Dog	Cat	Cow	Horse	Sheep	Pig
Platelets	1000/μl	150-400	150-400	200-800	100-400	250-800	200-700
OSPT	Seconds	10-12	6.5-9	23-28	15-19	13-17	—
APTT	Seconds	18-24	14-20	55-80	55-110	35-50	—
Normal body temperature							
°F		101.5-102.5 (small breed) 99.5-101.5 (large breed)	100-102.5	101.5-130.5 (calf up to 1 yr) 100-102.5 (ox)	99.5-101.5 (foal) 99-100.5 (adult)	102-104	102-104 (piglet) 100-102 (adult)
°C		38.5-39.2 (small breed) 37.5-38.6 (large breed)	37.8-39.2	38.6-39.8 (calf up to 1 yr) 37.8-39.2 (ox over 1 yr)	37.5-38.6 (foal) 37.2-38 (adult)	38.9-40	38.9-40 (piglet) 37.8-38.9 (adult)

II. Radiology
   A. Thorax
   B. Abdomen

PHYSICAL STATUS

   I. Identify status
      A. Class I: normal patient with no organic disease
      B. Class II: patient with mild systemic disease
      C. Class III: patient with severe systemic disease limiting activity but not incapacitating
      D. Class IV: patient with incapacitating systemic disease that is a constant threat to life
      E. Class V: moribund patient not expected to live 24 hours with or without operation
   II. Emergency operation designated by "E" after appropriate classification

PATIENT PREPARATION

   I. Withhold food 8-12 hours
      A. Chapters 19-21, anesthetic procedures and techniques in horses, ruminants, and small animals, for species specific recommendations
      B. Do not withhold food for excessive periods in neonates, animals under 5 pounds, or birds
   II. Correct or compensate for
      A. Dehydration (hypovolemia)
      B. Anemia or hypoproteinemia
      C. Acidosis
      D. Cardiac dysfunction
      E. Respiratory distress
      F. Renal dysfunction
      G. Hemostatic defects
      H. Temperature
   III. Specific preparation for intended procedure
      A. Thoracic
      B. Abdominal
      C. Orthopedic
      D. Ophthalmologic
   IV. Other considerations
      A. Fluid and caloric needs during and following anesthesia
      B. Special medications (antiarrhythmics)
      C. Duration of surgery
      D. Needs of the surgeon

PLAN FOR ANESTHETIC MANAGEMENT

   I. Formulation of anesthetic care plan
      A. Planned surgical procedure

    B. Positioning
    C. Selection of drugs
    D. Airway management
    E. Fluid management
    F. Body temperature management
    G. Monitoring
    H. Possible untoward effects

II. Assemble emergency drugs and equipment

CHAPTER THREE

Drugs Used for Preanesthetic Medication

"Dying is nothing, but pain is a very serious matter."
HENRY JACOB BIGELOW, 1871

OVERVIEW

The use of drugs classified as preanesthetic medication is an important part of safe animal management. When used appropriately, they can minimize the cardiopulmonary depression and deleterious effects associated with many intravenous and inhalation anesthetics.

Drugs that are routinely used as preanesthetic medication classically fall into one of four categories. *Anticholinergics*, although controversial, have been used to limit excessive salivary secretions and prevent bradycardia. *Phenothiazine and butyrophenone tranquilizers* are used to produce a calming effect to decrease the amount of general anesthetic required to produce anesthesia. *Xylazine and tranquilizer narcotic combinations* are used to produce sedation and sleep without producing general anesthesia. *Narcotics* are used to produce a calming effect and an analgesic effect.

GENERAL CONSIDERATIONS

I. Purpose
  A. Aid in animal restraint
  B. Allay apprehension and/or minimize pain
  C. Decrease the quantity of potentially more dangerous drugs used to produce sedation, analgesia, or general anesthesia

D. Produce safe and uncomplicated induction, maintenance, and recovery from anesthesia
E. Minimize the adverse and potentially toxic effects of concurrently administered drugs used to produce general anesthesia
F. Minimize autonomic reflex activity whether of sympathetic or parasympathetic origin

DRUG CATEGORIES

I. Anticholinergics (atropine, glycopyrrolate, scopolamine)
   A. Competitively antagonize the action of acetylcholine on structures innervated by postganglionic parasympathetic (cholinergic) nerve fibers and on smooth muscles that are influenced by acetylcholine but lack innervation. Referred to as *parasympatholytics, anticholinergics,* or *antispasmodics*
   B. Primarily used to prevent salivary secretions and to inhibit the bradycardic effects of vagal stimulation
   C. Atropine and scopolamine may produce drowsiness and potentiate the effects of CNS depressant drugs. Large doses may stimulate cerebral areas leading to restlessness, disorientation, and delirium. This effect is more common in ruminants
   D. Glycopyrrolate, a quaternary ammonium drug, does not cross the blood brain or placental barriers
   E. Reduce glandular secretions of the respiratory tract, gastrointestinal tract, oral and nasal cavity
      1. The accumulation of excessive secretions in the oral cavity of small animals (cats) may predispose to upper airway obstruction and laryngospasm
      2. A postparasympatholytic rebound phenomenon of increased secretory activity may occur several hours after parasympatholytic drug administration
   F. Gastric pH is increased (less acidic). Reduce gastrointestinal motility and contraction of the bladder and ureter. Intestinal motility may be decreased for several hours in horses. This effect could cause colic
   G. Produce bronchodilation (increased physiological dead space) and mydriasis
   H. Inhibit potentially dangerous bradycardia caused by reflex increases in vagal tone (e.g., laryngeal or ocular stimulation in the dog, vagovagal reflexes)
      1. Parasympatholytics may induce a sinus tachycardia or occasionally precipitate ventricular arrhythmias. Anticholinergics usually cause sinus bradycardia and then progress through various stages of first- and second-degree atrioventricular block prior to the establishment of sinus tachycardia
      2. Atropine sulfate may induce an initial sinus bradycardia due to stimulation of vagal nuclei in the medulla. Glycopyrrolate does not cross the blood-brain or placental barrier and, therefore, is devoid of CNS or fetal effects
      3. Vagovagal reflexes produces by traction on visceral organs are not always successfully treated with parasympatholytic drugs
      4. General anesthetics, narcotics, digitalis, glycosides, hyperkalemia, acidosis, and injection of calcium salts augment vagal effects and may precipitate bradycardia

    a. Halothane, methoxyflurane, enflurane, isoflurane, and barbiturates may enhance parasympathetic influence by suppressing sympathetic tone

    b. Large doses of a phenothiazine tranquilizer may produce a central nervous system–induced cholinergic effect and are adrenolytic

  I. Administered IM or SC (IV for emergencies)

    1. 0.01-0.02 mg/lb of atropine sulfate or 0.005 mg/lb of glycopyrrolate will dry secretions in small animals

      a. Duration of action: atropine sulfate, 60-90 minutes

             glycopyrrolate, 2-4 hours

    2. The routine use of parasympatholytics in large animal species is of questionable value. Therapy should be directed to specific needs. Dosages utilized have not been adequately evaluated

      a. Horse: atropine, 0.02-0.04 mg/lb

           glycopyrrolate, 0.0015-0.003 mg/lb

      b. Ruminants: not recommended. Atropine will temporarily decrease secretions. The secretions become more viscid. Proper positioning is of the utmost importance in order to prevent aspiration

      c. Pig: atropine, 0.02 mg/lb

           glycopyrrolate, 0.0015 mg/lb

  J. Untoward reactions

    1. Atropine may cause an initial bradycardia after intravenous administration

    2. Cardiac arrhythmias, particularly sinus tachycardia and first- and second-degree atrioventricular block, are observed after intravenous administration of atropine or glycopyrrolate. Ventricular arrhythmias may occur after intravenous atropine administration

    3. Atropine may cause depression in dogs and cats; restlessness, delirium, and disorientation in ruminants

    4. Colic in horses due to ileus

II. Tranquilizers, neuroleptics and sedatives (phenothiazines, butyrophenones, benzodiazepines, and xylazine)(see Table 3-1)

  A. Phenothiazines (acepromazine, promazine), butyrophenones (droperidol, lenperone, azaperone)

    1. Mode of action

      a. Calming and neurologic effects appear to be mediated by antidopaminergic actions. Drug actions on the brain stem can cause a loss of vasomotor regulation

      b. Suppression of the sympathetic nervous system (depresses mobilization of catecholamines centrally and peripherally)

      c. Phenothiazine tranquilizers lower seizure threshold in animals with epilepsy. Butyrophenones do not demonstrate this activity

      d. Phenothiazines and butyrophenones produce a marked antiemetic effect by inhibiting dopamine interaction in the chemoreceptor trigger zone (CTZ) in the medulla

    2. Produce *mental calming*, decrease motor activity, and increase threshold to external stimuli. Not noted for analgesic activity, but will increase the analgesic effect of drugs with analgesic activity. Excessive doses

TABLE 3-1

COMMONLY USED ANALGESIC AND TRANQUILIZER COMBINATIONS FOR INTRAVENOUS USE

Animal	Drugs	Recommended IV dosages	Untoward effects
Dog	Acepromazine-meperidine	0.05-0.1 mg/lb 0.1-0.3 mg/lb	Hypotension
	Acepromazine-oxymorphone	0.05-0.1 mg/lb 0.05-0.1 mg/lb	Hypotension
	Diazepam-fentanyl	0.1-0.2 mg/lb 0.005 mg/lb	Bradycardia
	Droperidol-fentanyl (Innovar-Vet)	1 ml/30-60 lb	Bradycardia/apnea
Cat	Acepromazine-oxymorphone	0.1 mg/lb (*Note:* IM) 0.05 mg/lb	Excitement
	Droperidol-fentanyl	1 ml/20 lb (*Note:* IM)	Excitement
Horse	Xylazine-morphine	0.3 mg/lb 0.1-0.3 mg/lb	Hypotension
	Xylazine-meperidine	0.3 mg/lb 0.5 mg/lb	Hypotension
	Xylazine-butorphanol	0.3 mg/lb 0.01 mg/lb	Ataxia
	Xylazine-acepromazine	0.3 mg/lb 0.025 mg/lb	Hypotension
	Meperidine-acepromazine	0.25 mg/lb 0.025 mg/lb	Hypotension
Pig	Droperidol-fentanyl (Innovar-Vet)	1 ml/40 lb (under 200 lb) 1 ml/80 lb (over 200 lb)	Respiratory depression
	Azaperone	0.5-2 mg/lb	
Ruminants			
Cow	Xylazine	0.02-0.05 mg/lb	Respiratory
Sheep	Xylazine	0.05-0.1 mg/lb	depression,
Goat*	Xylazine	0.005-0.05 mg/lb	bradycardia

*Variable response

of phenothiazines and butyrophenones cause apparent involuntary (extrapyramidal) effects and hallucinatory activity in some animals, particularly horses

a. The calming effect can be temporarily reversed with an adequate stimulus. This is most evident in the excitable or apprehensive animals

3. Potentially useful for vicious or nervous animals
4. Cardiopulmonary effects
   a. α-adrenergic blockade (use of epinephrine may cause a paradoxical fall in blood pressure)
      (1) Hypotension: particularly excited or apprehensive patients. Reflex tachycardia may occur in response to hypotension
      (2) Severe reactions include hypotensive crisis and (rarely) bradycardia resulting in death
      (3) Phenylephrine (α-agonists) can be used to increase blood pressure following IV fluid administration
   b. Reflex tachycardia due to hypotension. Centrally induced bradycardia occurs rarely
   c. Antiarrhythmic effects: protect against epinephrine-induced cardiac irregularities by reducing central sympathetic, ganglionic, and peripheral (adrenal) activity
   d. Direct depression of the myocardium and vascular smooth muscle
   e. Ganglionic blocking activity
   f. Reduces respiratory rate first, but may decrease tidal volume when administered in large doses. Alters respiratory center sensitivity to increases in CO_2
5. Potentiates the ventilatory and cardiovascular depressant effects of narcotics and drugs used to produce general anesthesia
6. Useful as antiemetics
7. Most have antihistaminic properties—avoid phenothiazines and butyrophenones when skin testing for allergies
8. Most phenothiazine tranquilizers cross the placental barrier relatively slowly
9. Many phenothiazine tranquilizers, including acepromazine and promazine, can cause erection and temporary or permanent prolapse of the penis in stallions
10. Primary area of detoxification is the liver
11. Clinical effects are present for 4-8 hours, but may last up to 48 hours (especially in geriatric patients)
12. Commonly used phenothiazines include acepromazine and promazine. Butyrophenone tranquilizers presently in use in veterinary practice are droperidol, lenperone, and azaperone (see Table 3-2)
13. Untoward reactions
    a. Akathisia: need for the patient to be in constant motion
    b. Acute dystonic reactions: hysteria, seizures, ataxia
    c. Tachycardia or (rarely) bradycardia
    d. Hypotension
    e. Hypothermia
    f. Inhibited platelet function
    g. Butyrophenone tranquilizers (droperidol, lenperone, azaperone) cause excitement and extrapyramidal effects in horses at relatively low doses

TABLE 3 - 2

INTRAVENOUS DOSAGES OF COMMONLY USED TRANQUILIZERS, SEDATIVES, AND NARCOTICS (mg/lb)

Agent	Dog	Cat	Horse	Cow	Goat	Pig
Major tranquilizers						
Acepromazine	0.05-0.2	0.05-0.3	0.01-0.04	0.02-0.04	0.02-0.04	0.1-0.3
Promazine	0.3-0.5	0.5-1.5	0.1-0.5	0.1-0.5	0.1-0.5	0.5-1.5
Minor tranquilizers						
Diazepam	0.1-0.2	0.1-0.2	0.01-0.04	0.01-0.04	0.01-0.04	0.1-0.2
Midazolam	0.1-0.2	0.1-0.2	0.01-0.02	—	—	—
Sedative						
Xylazine	0.2-0.5	0.2-0.5	0.2-0.5	0.01-0.05	0.01-0.03	Not effective
Chloral hydrate	—	—	10-15	20-30	15-25	20-30
Lenperone	0.1-0.4	—	—	—	—	?
Azaperone	—	—	0.1-0.2	—	—	0.5-1.0

Narcotic agonists and partial agonists*

Morphine	0.2-0.5	0.05-0.1	—	0.02-0.05	—	0.2-0.4
Meperidine	0.2-0.5	0.1-0.2	—	0.2-0.5	—	0.2-0.5
Oxymorphone	0.05-0.1	—	—	0.01-0.05	—	—
Methadone	0.1-0.3	—	—	0.03-0.06	—	—
Fentanyl	0.001-0.003	—	—	—	—	—
Pentazocine	0.1-0.2	0.05-0.01	—	0.2-0.4	—	0.1-0.2
Butorphanol	0.05-0.1	—	—	0.005-0.1	—	—

Neuroleptanalgesics

Fentanyl-droperidol	1 ml/30-60 lb	1 ml/20 lb	—			1 ml/50 lb
(0.4 mg fentanyl + 20 mg droperidol/ml)						

Intramuscular dose is 2-3 times intravenous dose.

*Narcotic antagonists are used whenever narcotic antagonism is desired; remember that analgesia is often reversed also:

Naloxone   15 μg/5 lb
Nalorphine   1 mg/5 lb (small animals)
Levallorphan 0.005 mg/lb

B. Benzodiazepines (diazepam, midazolam) (*Note:* Sometimes referred to as minor tranquilizers)
  1. Mode of action
    a. Benzodiazepine derivatives exert many of their pharmacologic effects by enhancing the activity of central nervous system inhibitory neurotransmitters (γ-aminobutyric acid [GABA], glycine). They may also produce their effects by combining with central nervous system benzodiazepine receptors
    b. Depression of the limbic system, thalamus, and hypothalamus (reduces sympathetic tone), thereby inducing a *mild calming effect*
    c. Reduces polysynaptic reflex activity, resulting in *muscle relaxation*
    d. Causes minimal CNS depression, but does possess *anticonvulsant* effects in most animals. May cause disorientation and agitation after rapid intravenous administration
  2. Physical properties
    a. Diazepam is solubilized by mixing with 40% propylene glycol, ethyl alcohol, sodium benzoate, or benzoic acid
      (1) Propylene glycol is a cardiovascular depressant and may produce hypotension, bradycardia, cardiac arrhythmias, and apnea if administered too rapidly intravenously
    b. Midazolam is water-soluble
  3. Cardiopulmonary effects
    a. Minimal hypotensive effects are observed after intravenous administration
    b. Bradycardia and cardiac arrest have occurred after rapid intravenous administration (a propylene glycol effect)
    c. Respiratory rate and tidal volume are minimally affected
  4. Affords excellent muscle relaxation in animals and is additive with other drugs used to produce general anesthesia
    a. Reduces muscle spasms and spasticity
  5. All benzodiazepines increase seizure threshold
  6. Effects upon gastrointestinal activity are undetermined
  7. Use in pregnancy has not been investigated
  8. Diazepam is eliminated after biodegradation by the liver in the urine and feces
    a. Duration of action is 1-4 hours
  9. Diazepam increases appetite in domestic cats and ruminants, probably in all species
  10. Untoward effects
    a. Ataxia, particularly evident in large animal species
    b. Paradoxical increase in anxiety and fear response in excitable animals
    c. May cause pronounced CNS depression in neonates
    d. Propylene glycol diluent can cause bradycardia, cardiac arrhythmias, hypotension, and respiratory depression
    e. Painful if administered intramuscularly

C. Xylazine hydrochloride
1. Mode of action
   a. Produces central nervous system depression by stimulating α_2 adrenoceptors in the central nervous system. This decreases norepinephrine release centrally and peripherally. *Note*: The central nervous system effects of xylazine can be antagonized by α_2 receptor antagonists (yohimbine)
   b. Detomidine produces similar pharmacologic effects as xylazine but has a longer duration of action
2. General properties
   a. Produces *calming, muscle relaxation*, and *analgesia* lasting approximately 10-30 minutes
   b. Chemical properties
      (1) A derivative of thiazine hydrochloride and close chemical relative of clonidine, an antihypertensive drug
      (2) Demonstrates sedative, analgesic, and muscle relaxing properties
   c. Polysynaptic reflexes are inhibited, but the neuromuscular junction is not influenced. Depresses internuncial neuron transmission
   d. Induces a sleeplike state comparable to phenothiazines, only more pronounced
   e. Additive with other depressants or drugs used to produce general anesthesia
   f. Demonstrates both parasympathetic (bradycardia) and initial sympathetic (α_1 and α_2) receptor stimulatory activity
3. Cardiopulmonary effects
   a. Depresses respiratory centers centrally
   b. Decreases tidal volume and respiratory rate with an overall decrease in minute volume when administered in large dosages intravenously
   c. May induce stridor and dyspnea in horses and brachycephalic dogs with upper airway obstruction
   d. Initially increases blood pressure (α_1 and α_2 adrenoceptor stimulatory effect), then reduces it to below control values
      (1) Increases peripheral vascular resistance initially
   e. Slows heart rate due to increased parasympathetic activity
      (1) May initiate sinus bradycardia, first- or second-degree atrioventricular blockade; this occurs most commonly after intravenous administration
   f. Increases cardiac sensitivity to catecholamine-induced arrhythmias during halothane anesthesia. This effect is caused by α_1 and α_2 adrenoceptor stimulation
   g. Cardiac output may decrease by 30% due to decreases in heart rate and increases in peripheral vascular resistance
4. Gastrointestinal system
   a. Suppresses salivation, gastric secretions, and gastrointestinal mobility

  b. Depresses swallowing reflex

  c. Excellent in obtunding pain produced by colic

  d. Causes vomiting in the dog and cat

 5. Absorption, fate, and excretion

  a. Relatively rapidly metabolized by the liver and excreted in the urine

  b. Metabolites may retain activity

   (1) 20 metabolites identified, with sulfate and carbon dioxide being end products

  c. 70% excreted via the kidneys and 30% via the liver and bile

 6. Other

  a. Of questionable clinical value in pigs due to relatively rapid metabolism

  b. Highly excited or nervous animals may react adversely to the drug or demonstrate little response

  c. May produce profound sleep in dogs, cats, foals, and small ruminants. This is partially reversible with doxapram hydrochloride in the appropriate dosage. Yohimbine (0.25 mg/lb IV) and another α_2 adrenoceptor antagonist, tolazoline (1-2 mg/lb IV), are more specific antagonists

  d. Xylazine crosses the placenta, but an abortificient effect has *not* been noted in pregnant mares; neither were there observable effects upon gestation or parturition. Xylazine may induce premature delivery in cattle

  e. Demonstrates an oxytocin-like effect in ruminants. This activity has not been reported in mares or small animals

  f. Blood and urine glucose levels increase significantly after xylazine administration. This effect is transient and of questionable clinical significance

 7. Untoward effects

  a. Severe respiratory depression (respiratory acidosis)

  b. Profound bradycardia

  c. Hypotension

  d. Ataxia in large animals

  e. Occasional severe inflammatory response if administered subcutaneously in horses or cattle

III. Narcotics

 A. Mode of action

  1. Act by reversible combination with one or more specific (opiate) and nonopiate receptors in the brain and spinal cord to produce a variety of physiological effects, including *sedation, euphoria, excitement, dysphoria,* and *analgesia*

  2. Referred to as narcotic agonists; several possess agonist-antagonist activity

   a. This group of drugs consists of a wide variety of naturally occurring (opiate) derivatives and synthetically manufactured drugs

   b. Classified according to analgesic activity or addiction potential

      c. Commonly used narcotics include morphine, meperidine, oxymor-
         phone, methadone, and fentanyl. Pentazocine and butorphanol are
         narcotic-like substances with narcotic agonist-antagonist effects
      d. Analgesic potency

(1) Morphine	1
(2) Meperidine	0.5
(3) Oxymorphone	5-10
(4) Fentanyl	100
(5) Pentazocine	0.1
(6) Butorphanol	2-5
(7) Etorphine	10,000

   3. Narcotic agonists or partial agonists do not interfere with:
     a. Touch
     b. Vibration
     c. Vision
     d. Hearing

B. Are used prior to, during, or after surgery for analgesia
   1. Fentanyl, sufentanyl, alfentanyl and oxymorphone are generally used dur-
     ing surgery as a part of a balanced anesthetic technique

C. Analgesic action is produced at doses lower than are needed for sedation
   (dosage tailored to individual animal)

D. The sedative actions are generally accompanied by:
   1. Miosis in the dog and pig, mydriasis in the cat and horse
   2. Decrease of tidal volume and respiratory rate. Dogs may pant due to
     resetting of the thermoregulatory center
   3. Bradycardia
   4. Hypothermia
   5. Reduction in response to external stimuli (animal may not recognize
     owner)
   6. Sweating, particularly in horses
   7. Behavioral changes (euphoria or dysphoria)

E. Effects are additive when used with other depressants (tranquilizers, barbiturates, inhalation anesthesia)

F. Cardiopulmonary effects
   1. Positive inotropic action when used in low dosages (morphine only)—
     due to release of epinephrine and norepinephrine from the adrenal
     medulla
   2. Bradycardia—stimulation of medullary vagal nuclei
   3. Hypotension may occur due to the release of histamine
   4. Respiratory depression is dose-dependent (rate and tidal volume)
   5. Reduces respiratory reserve capabilities
   6. Raises the threshold of the respiratory center to CO_2

G. Gastrointestinal effects
   1. Salivation
   2. Nausea

    3. Vomiting in those species that can

    4. Nonpropulsive gastrointestinal hypermotility, increases in sphincter tone

    5. Defecation

H. Alter thermoregulatory control

    1. Dogs decrease their body temperatures by panting

I. Produce excellent sedation in dogs, but may cause excitement when given rapidly IV. Cats and horses are particularly susceptible to the excitatory effect of narcotics. This is typified by increased motor activity and pacing in horses

J. May be a problem from a drug control standpoint

K. Narcotics cross the placental barrier relatively slowly, but because their depressant effects can be antagonized, they are useful for cesarean section

L. May be used in combination with tranquilizers for analgesia and sedation— neuroleptanalgesia (see Table 3-1)

M. Narcotics are extensively metabolized by the liver, and metabolites are eliminated in the urine. Although the narcotic agonists vary in biological half-life, their clinical duration of action ranges from 30 minutes to 3 hours in most species. Morphine may produce effects lasting 6-8 hours in horses

N. Agonist-antagonists

    1. Pentazocine, butorphanol, and nalbuphine antagonize the effects of other narcotic agonists (morphine, meperidine, oxymorphone, fentanyl), but can produce mild central nervous system depression, euphoria and analgesia when administered in therapeutic doses

    2. Butorphanol is an excellent cough suppressant

O. Narcotic antagonists

    1. Classification

        a. Pure antagonist (naloxone)

        b. Partial antagonists (nalorphine, levallorphan, diprenorphine)

        c. Narcotic antagonists may possess many of the same properties as narcotics but decrease depressant characteristics by competitive antagonism. Naloxone possesses the least narcotic agonistic effects

    2. Mechanism of action

        a. Opioid antagonists compete with morphine-like drugs for their specific receptor sites

            (1) Naloxone is almost entirely devoid of agonistic effects

        b. Partial antagonists act in a fashion similar to opioid antagonists

            (1) Nalorphine and levallorphan can also produce autonomic, endocrine, analgesic, and respiratory depressant effects

            (2) Nalorphine is about two thirds as potent as morphine as an analgetic

            (3) Nalorphine may add to existing respiratory depression produced by CNS depressants

    3. Metabolism

        a. Rapidly metabolized in the liver

    4. Dosage
       a. Naloxone   1-15 μg/lb IV
       b. Nalorphine   1mg/5 lb IV
       c. Levallorphan   0.1 mg/lb IV
  P. Untoward reactions
    1. Excitement, dysphoria
    2. Apnea
    3. Bradycardia
    4. Ataxia and incoordination
    5. Excessive vomiting
    6. Excessive sweating in horses

IV. Neuroleptanalgesia
  A. A state of central nervous system depression and analgesia produced by the combination of a tranquilizer and analgesic drug (see Glossary, Chapter 1)
  B. The animal may or may not retain consciousness and is responsive to auditory stimuli. Many animals will defecate.
  C. The only commercial combination is that of fentanyl (narcotic) and droperidol (tranquilizer)
    1. Fentanyl
       a. Actions are similar to morphine, but 100 times more potent as an analgesic on a milligram-to-milligram basis
       b. Respiratory and cardiovascular depressant
         (1) Decreases the minute volume response to CO_2 increase by shifting the normal threshold
         (2) Does not cause vomiting in most instances
         (3) May produce a dramatic decrease in heart rate
    2. Droperidol
       a. A butyrophenone derivative tranquilizer
       b. Can be compared in its action to the phenothiazine derivatives. A potent antiemetic
       c. Prevents arrhythmias produced by exogenous epinephrine (adrenergic blocking action)
       d. Enhances the actions of barbiturates
    3. This drug combination may cause dramatic behavior modification and aggressiveness in aged dogs
    4. The veterinary product contains 0.4 mg/ml of fentanyl and 20 mg/ml of droperidol (Innovar-Vet)
  D. The combination of these agents results in
    1. Depression of ventilation (apnea may occur)
    2. Bradycardia
    3. Defecation and flatulence
    4. Analgesia for periods up to 40 minutes
  E. Overdosages usually result in profound hypotension and respiratory depression

    1. Respiratory depression can generally be reversed by a narcotic antagonist (nalorphine, levallorphan, naloxone)

F. Most animals are premedicated with a parasympatholytic (glycopyrrolate) to prevent bradycardia and excessive salivation

G. Neuroleptanalgesics are used in combination with barbiturates in dogs to eliminate stimulatory effect of loud noises and produce better muscle relaxation
    1. Thiamylal (1 mg/lb) after Innovar-Vet (1 ml/30 lb) IV
    2. Sodium pentobarbital (3 mg/lb) after Innovar-Vet (1 ml/20 lb) IV

H. Other combinations of narcotics and tranquilizers have been used to produce sedation and analgesia similar to that of Innovar-Vet
    1. Acepromazine (0.1-0.2 mg/lb) in combination with morphine (0.2-0.4 mg/lb IV or SC), meperidine (0.5-1.0 mg/lb IV), or oxymorphone (0.05-0.1 mg/lb IV) is used to produce neuroleptanalgesia in dogs
    2. The combination of xylazine (0.3 mg/lb IV) and morphine (0.1-0.3 mg/lb IV) or xylazine (0.3 mg/lb IV) and butorphanol (0.01-0.02 mg/lb IV) is very popular for horses

I. Useful for short operative procedures and, because of analgesia and reversibility, for cesarean section in small animals

J. Untoward effects
    1. Respiratory depression
    2. Bradycardia
    3. Ataxia

CHAPTER FOUR

Local Anesthesia Drugs and Techniques

"Pleasure is nothing else but the intermission of pain."

JOHN SELDEN

OVERVIEW

Local anesthetics are used to produce desensitization and analgesia of skin surfaces (topical anesthesia), local tissues (infiltration and field blocks), and regional structures (conduction anesthesia, intravenous regional). Local anesthetic techniques are used as an alternative or adjunct to intravenous and inhalation anesthesia in high-risk patients. A number of local or regional analgesic drugs are available; they vary as to potency, toxicity, and cost. The most commonly used local analgesic drugs in veterinary medicine are lidocaine hydrochloride and mepivacaine hydrochloride, representing drugs of intermediate analgesic duration lasting 90-180 minutes, having a rapid onset of action, and providing anesthesia over a wide field. Vasoconstrictors (epinephrine) are occasionally incorporated or can be added to a local analgesic drug to increase intensity and prolong analgesic activity. If hyaluronidase is added, tissue penetration in the region of infiltration is increased, and the time of onset is hastened.

GENERAL CONSIDERATIONS

I. Use sterile solutions and injection equipment
II. Do not inject into inflamed areas
III. Use undamaged needles
IV. Use as small a gauge of needle as possible
V. Aspirate before injecting
VI. Use smallest possible concentration of local anesthetic agent

VII. Use smallest possible amount of local anesthetic (consider the use of a vaso-constrictor)

LOCAL ANESTHETICS

I. Mechanism of membrane and impulse conduction
   A. All clinically used local anesthetics are membrane-stabilizing agents
   B. Enter and occupy the membrane channels (by polar association) through which ions normally move
   C. Most immediate and apparent effect is to prevent the inflow of Na^+ and, therefore, block all subsequent ionic flow
   D. Prevent depolarization and, therefore, stop or retard conduction or impulses

II. Uptake
   A. The salt of the anesthetic base is an ionizable quaternary amine with little or no anesthetic properties of its own because it is not lipid-soluble and is not absorbed in the nerve membrane
   B. After deposition in tissue, which is slightly alkaline and has considerable buffering capacity, the anesthetic base is liberated:

$$RNH^+ Cl^- \rightleftharpoons Cl^- + RNH^+ \rightleftharpoons RN + H^+$$
$$\text{salt} \qquad\qquad \text{cation} \quad \text{base}$$

   The free anesthetic base is absorbed at the outer lipid nerve membrane, where anesthetic action appears to take place

III. Effect of tissue pH
   A. If sufficient local buffering capacity exists to remove the dissociated H^+, this reaction proceeds to the right to liberate active base and thus exert an anesthetic effect
   B. The pH is considerably below normal (more acid) in inflamed or infected tissues
   C. Local anesthetics have poor buffering capacity. When in the presence of acid conditions, little free base dissociates from the anesthetic salt, resulting in a poor anesthetic result

IV. Absorption
   A. Poor absorption through intact skin
   B. Absorption from
      1. Injured skin
      2. Mucous membranes
      3. Respiratory epithelium
      4. Intramuscular depot
      5. Subcutaneous depot
      6. Intravenous administration

V. Classification and function of nerve fibers
   A. Myelinated A-fibers
      1. α: motor, proprioception
      2. β: motor, touch

3. γ: muscle spindles

4. δ: pain, temperature

B. Myelinated B-fibers

1. Preganglionic sympathetic

C. Nonmyelinated C-fibers

1. Pain, temperature

VI. Priority of blockade

A. B, C ≫ A$_δ$ > A$_α$-fibers

B. Sensation disappears in the following order: pain, cold, warmth, touch, joint, and deep pressure

VII. Blocking quality

A. Potency: binding affinity to receptor protein: tetracaine > lidocaine > procaine

B. Latency: time between injection and maximum effect

C. Duration of action: related to the logarithm of the concentration (e.g., doubling the concentration increases the duration by only approximately 30%)

D. Recovery time

1. Time to return of normal sensation

2. Dependent not only on outflow diffusion, but also on gradual release of bound local anesthetic from the nerve membrane

3. May be 2-200 times longer than induction time

VIII. Autoclaving of local analgetic drugs

A. Ampules of hydrochloride salts can be autoclaved at 120° C for 20-30 minutes

DRUGS USED FOR VASOCONSTRICTION

I. Epinephrine (adrenaline) or L-norepinephrine (levarterenol) 1:50,000 (1 mg in 50 ml of saline) or 1:200,000 (1 mg in 200 ml saline). Effects of vasoconstriction:

A. Maximal vasoconstriction is probably produced by the lower of these concentrations, but because of the instability of epinephrine, the higher concentration is used especially in commercially prepared solutions

B. Vasoconstrictors delay absorption of the local anesthetic agent, reducing the toxicity and increasing the margin of safety

C. Increases the intensity and prolongs analgetic activity

D. Increases the risk of cardiac arrhythmia and ventricular fibrillation

II. Hyaluronidase

A. Increases the area of diffusion, resulting in a larger total area being desensitized

B. Effective anesthesia often develops more rapidly

C. Anesthesia time is usually shortened because of increased absorption, unless a vasoconstrictor is used

D. Cannot be used as a substitute for precise, accurate technique; fascial planes act as a barrier

E. Units: one turbidity unit per milliliter of local anesthetic solution

TABLE 4-1

LOCAL ANESTHETICS

Agent (generic name)	Trade name (registered by)	Chemical name	Potency (procaine = 1)
Procaine	Novocaine (Winthrop Stearns Inc.)	Para-aminobenzoic acid ester of diethylamino-ethanol	1:1
Chloroprocaine	Nesacaine (Wallace & Tiernan, Inc.)	Para-amino-2-chlorobenzoic acid ester of B-diethylamino-ethanol	2.4:1
Lidocaine	Xylocaine (Astra Pharmaceutical Products, Inc.)	Diethylaminoacet -2,6-xylidide	2:1
Mepivacaine	Carbocaine (Winthrop Laboratories)	1-methyl-2', 6'-pipecoloxylidide monohydrochloride	2.5:1
Tetracaine	Pontocaine (Winthrop Laboratories)	Parabutylamino benzoyl-dimethylamino-ethanol-HCl	12:1
Hexylcaine	Cyclaine (Merck, Sharpe and Dohme)	1-cyclo-hexamino 2-propylbenzoate	1-2:1
Dibucaine	Nupercaine (CIBA Pharmaceutical Products)	a-butyl-oxycin-choninic acid of diethylethylene-diamide	20:1
Bupivacaine	Marcaine (Breon Laboratories Inc.)	1-butyl-2', 6'-pipecoloxylidide-HCl	8:1

III. Combinations

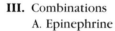

A. Epinephrine ⎫
                ⎬ + procaine
Hyaluronidase ⎭

→ Doubles the area anesthetized

→ Increases duration of local anesthesia almost five times

Toxicity (procaine = 1)	Dosage	Stability	Comments
1:1	1-2% for infiltration and nerve block	Aqueous solutions are heat-resistant, decomposed by bacteria	Hydrolyzed by liver and plasma esterase
0.5:1	1-2% for infiltration and nerve block	Multiple autoclaving accelerates hydrolysis and impairs potency	Immediate onset of action; 2 hr duration with epinephrine
0.5% 1:1 1% 1.4:1 2% 1.5:1	0.5-2% for infiltration and nerve block; topically 2-4%	Aqueous solutions are thermostable; multiple autoclaving possible	Excellent penetrability; rate of onset twice as fast as procaine; 2 hr duration with epinephrine
Less toxic than lidocaine	1-2% for infiltration and nerve block	Resistant to acid and alkaline hydrolysis; multiple autoclaving possible	Absence of vasodilator effect makes addition of a vasoconstrictor unnecessary
10:1	0.1% for infiltration and nerve block; topically 0.2%	Crystals and solutions should not be autoclaved	Slow onset of anesthesia (5-10 min); 2 hr duration; for eye installation
2-4:1	0.5-1% for infiltration; 2% for nerve block; 5% topically	Crystals and solutions are thermostable	Recommended for epidural and topical anesthesia
15:1	Topically 0.1%	Thermostable but precipitation by alkalies	Slowly detoxified
Greater margin of safety than lidocaine	0.25% for infiltration; 0.5% for nerve block; 0.75% for epidural block	Stable compound	Intermediate onset, lasting 4-6 hr

IV. Ester-linked drugs (see Table 4-1)
- A. Cocaine (alkaloid of the leaf of *Erythroxylon coca*)
- B. Procaine hydrochloride (Novocaine)
  - 1. Prototype of all other local anesthetics
  - 2. Standard drug for comparison of anesthetic effects

      3. Hydrolyzed in plasma by pseudocholinesterase
- C. Chloroprocaine hydrochloride (Nesacaine)
  1. Minimal toxicity
  2. Good penetrance
- D. Tetracaine hydrochloride (Pontocaine)
  1. 10-15 times more potent than procaine
  2. Relatively toxic
  3. Prolonged anesthetic effect

V. Amide-linked drugs
- A. Lidocaine hydrochloride (Xylocaine, Lignocaine)
  1. Most stable; not decomposed by boiling, acids, or alkali
  2. Superior penetrance, compared to procaine: Effects are evident in 1/3 the time; effects persist $1\frac{1}{2}$ times longer; spreads over a wider field
  3. No tissue damage or irritation
  4. No allergy or hypersensitivity
  5. Sedative effects
  6. Antiarrhythmic
- B. Mepivacaine hydrochloride (Carbocaine)
  1. Similar to lidocaine
  2. No irritation or tissue damage
- C. Dibucaine hydrochloride (Nupercaine)
  1. 20 times more potent than procaine
  2. Three to five times longer anesthetic effect

TOPICAL ANESTHETICS

I. Commonly used topicals
- A. Butacaine (Butya sulphate)
- B. Tetracaine (Pontocaine)
- C. Piperocaine (Metycaine)
- D. Proparacaine (Ophthaine)
- E. Cetacaine (Benzocaine)

II. Vascular effect
- A. Local anesthetic drugs are vasodilators
  1. Exceptions
     a. Cocaine (a vasoconstrictor)
     b. Lidocaine (minimal effect)

III. Toxicity dependent upon
- A. Rate of absorption
- B. Rate of detoxification

METHODS OF LOCAL ANESTHETIC APPLICATION

I. Surface anesthesia
- A. Spray or brush on mucous membranes (mouth, nose)
- B. Drop into the eye
- C. Infuse into the urethra

    D. Inject subsynovially (synovial membranes)

II. Infiltration anesthesia

    A. Diffuse infiltration of operation area

        1. Sensitive: skin, nerve trunks, blood vessels, periosteum, synovial membranes, mucous membranes near the orifices (mouth, nose, rectum, anus)

        2. Insensitive: subcutaneous, fat, muscles, tendons, fascia, bone, cartilage, visceral peritoneum

    B. Techniques

        1. Bleb (very localized deposition of a small quantity of local anesthetic)

        2. Layer by layer

    C. Uses

        1. Treatment of wounds

        2. Skin incision

            a. Surgical removal of superficial tumors

            b. Repositioning of fractured bones

III. Regional (perineural) anesthesia

    A. Linear block

    B. Field block

        1. Contraindications

            a. Fissures of bones

            b. Fractures of bones

            c. Epidural block

            d. Paravertebral block

IV. Intra-articular anesthesia

V. Subsynovial anesthesia

VI. Intravenous regional anesthesia (IVRA)

VII. Refrigeration or hypothermic anesthesia

CHAPTER FIVE

Local Anesthesia in Cattle, Sheep, Goats, and Pigs

OVERVIEW

Injection of local anesthetic agents into the surgical site (local or infiltration anesthesia) and perineural injection of local anesthetics around major nerves (regional anesthesia, are commonly used in food animals (for example, cattle, sheep, goats, and pigs). The most popular techniques in ruminants are surface (topical) anesthesia, infiltration anesthesia, nerve block (conduction) anesthesia, epidural anesthesia, and intravenous regional anesthesia. The standing position is optimal for surgical procedures of ruminants, as it reduces the problems associated with: bloat, salivation, recumbency-related regurgitation, and nerve or muscle damage.

The most popular local anesthetic techniques in properly tranquilized pigs are infiltration anesthesia, lumbosacral epidural anesthesia, and intratesticular injection.

CATTLE: LOCAL ANESTHESIA FOR STANDING LAPAROTOMY

I. At least five techniques for inducing anesthesia of the paralumbar fossa in ruminants have been described
   A. Infiltration anesthesia
   B. Proximal paravertebral anesthesia
   C. Distal paravertebral anesthesia
   D. Segmental dorsolumbar epidural anesthesia
   E. Thoracolumbar subarachnoid anesthesia

II. These anesthetic techniques may be used for abdominal surgeries such as:
  A. Rumenotomy
  B. Cecotomy
  C. Correction of gastrointestinal displacement
  D. Intestinal obstruction
  E. Volvulus
  F. Cesarean section
  G. Ovariectomy
  H. Liver or kidney biopsy
III. Infiltration anesthesia
  A. Line block
   1. Area blocked: skin, muscle layers, and parietal peritoneum along the line of incision
   2. Needle used: 18 gauge, $1\frac{1}{2}$–3-inch
   3. Anesthetic: 50 ml of 2% lidocaine
   4. Method: multiple subcutaneous injections of 0.5-1.0 ml of anesthetic, 1.0-2.0 cm apart, followed by infiltration of the muscle layers and parietal peritoneum through the desensitized skin
   5. Advantages
     a. Easiest of all techniques
     b. Can be done with routinely available sizes of needles
   6. Disadvantages
     a. Relatively large volume of local anesthetic
     b. Lack of muscle relaxation
     c. Possibility of incompletely blocking the deeper layers of the abdominal wall
     d. Formation of hematomas along the incision line
     e. Increased cost due to larger doses of anesthetic and time required
   7. Complications
     a. Toxicity after injection of significant amounts of anesthetic solution into the peritoneal cavity
     b. Interference with the healing process
  B. Inverted L block (Fig. 5-1)
   1. Area blocked: along the caudal border of the last rib, along a line ventral to the lumbar transverse processes from the last rib to the fourth lumbar vertebra
   2. Needle used: 18 gauge, 3-inch
   3. Anesthetic: up to 100 ml of 2% lidocaine
   4. Method: injection of the anesthetic into the tissues bordering the dorsocaudal aspect of the last rib and ventrolateral aspect of the lumbar transverse processes, creating a wall of anesthetic enclosing the incision site
   5. Advantages
     a. Similar to line block
     b. Absence of anesthetic agent from the incision line

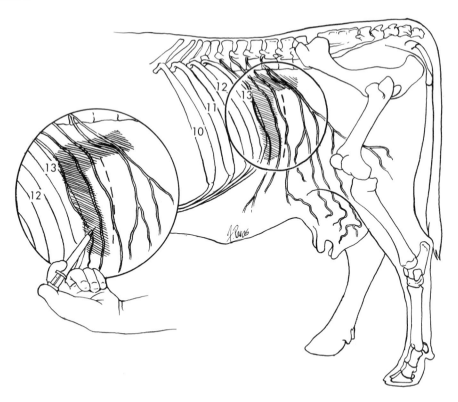

FIG. 5-1 Regional anesthesia of the cow's flank using inverted L infiltration pattern.

      6. Disadvantages
         a. Large volume of anesthetic required
         b. Time required to infiltrate such a long line
      7. Complications: similar to line block
IV. Specific nerve anesthesia
    A. Proximal paravertebral anesthesia (Farquharson technique)
      1. Area blocked: flank on the same side where the nerve block is performed
      2. Nerves blocked: T13, L1, and L2 (and occasionally L3—the animal may become ataxic)
      3. Site: Position 5 cm from midline (see Fig. 5-2). T13 just in front of transverse process of L1; L1 just in front of transverse process of L2; L2 just in front of transverse process of L3
      4. Needle used: 14 gauge, 1/2-inch needle, creating passage for a 16 or 18 gauge needle, 4 1/2-inch (up to 6 inches for bull)
      5. Anesthetic: 20 ml of 2% lidocaine at each site
      6. Method: Palpate the lumbar transverse processes, starting from L5 and moving forward. L1 may be difficult to feel. Measure 5 cm (2 1/2 inches) from midline. Palpate the lumbar dorsal processes; site for injection is at 90° angle to the spaces between the dorsal processes. Pass the needle

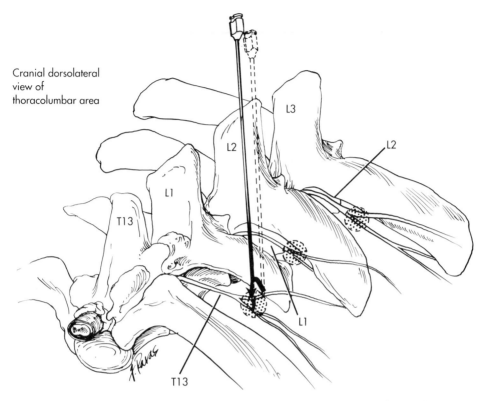

Cranial dorsolateral
view of
thoracolumbar area

FIG. 5-2 Needle placement for proximal paravertebral anesthesia in cattle. A left dorso-lateral aspect of thoracolumbar vertebrae T13 to L3 with needle tip placed at spinal nerve T13.

vertically down until you hit the cranial edge of the transverse process, and proceed down through the intertransverse ligament. Inject 15 ml of 2% lidocaine below the ligament to block the ventral branch of the nerve (minimal resistance). Withdraw the needle, and inject 5 ml of 2% lidocaine above ligament, level with dorsal surface of transverse process to block the dorsal branch (resistance to injection). If the first lumbar transverse process cannot be palpated, anesthetize the other nerves first, and then measure the distance between injection sites to find the site for blocking nerve T13

7. Advantages of paravertebral nerve block over field block
   a. Anesthesia of skin, musculature, and peritoneum
   b. No additional restraint required
   c. Infiltration to produce nerve block does not require large quantities of local anesthetic
   d. Short postsurgical convalescent period
8. Disadvantages of paravertebral nerve block
   a. Difficult to perform

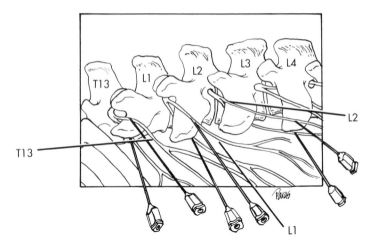

FIG.5-3 Needle placement for distal paravertebral anesthesia in cattle. A left lateral aspect of thoracolumbar vertebrae T13 to L4 with needle tip placed at spinal nerves T13, L1, and L2.

      b. Paralysis of back muscles
      c. Anesthesia of abdominal viscera
    9. Complications
      a. Potential for penetration of the aorta
      b. Potential for penetration of the thoracic longitudinal vein (posterior) or vena cava
  B. Distal paravertebral anesthesia (Magda, Cakala technique)
    1. Area blocked: flank on the same side where the nerve block is performed
    2. Nerves blocked: T13, L1, and L2
    3. Site: distal ends of lumbar transverse processes of L1, L2, and L4 (see Fig. 5-3)
    4. Needle used: 18 gauge, 3-inch
    5. Anesthetic: 10-20 ml of 2% lidocaine at each site
    6. Method: The needle is inserted ventral to the tips of the respective transverse process. Anesthetic (up to 20 ml) is injected in a fan-shaped infiltration pattern. The needle is completely withdrawn and reinserted dorsal to the transverse process, in a slightly caudal direction, where approximately 5 ml of the anesthetic is injected
    7. Advantages of distal paravertebral nerve block over proximal paravertebral block
      a. Use of more routinely sized needles
      b. Lack of risk of penetrating a major blood vessel
      c. Lack of scoliosis
      d. Minimal weakness in the pelvic limb or ataxia
    8. Disadvantages
      a. Large doses of anesthetic

b. Variations in efficiency, particularly if the nerves vary in their anatomic pathway
9. Complications: none
C. Segmental dorsolumbar epidural block
1. Area blocked: flank
2. Nerves blocked: T13 and anterior lumbar nerves depending upon the total dose administered
3. Site: epidural space between L1 and L2 vertebrae
4. Needle used: spinal, preferably 18 gauge, 4^{1}/2-inch
5. Anesthetic: 8 ml of 2% lidocaine
6. Method: To reach the epidural space, the spinal needle is inserted for a distance of 8-12 cm while being directed ventrally and medially at an angle of 10-15° from vertical. Piercing of the interarcuate ligament is felt as slight resistance during the insertion process. No blood or cerebrospinal fluid upon needle aspiration, and also no resistance to the injection of the anesthetic result after correct needle placement
7. Advantages of segmental dorsolumbar epidural anesthesia as compared with proximal or distal paravertebral anesthesia
a. Use of only one injection
b. Use of small quantity of anesthetic
c. Uniform anesthesia and relaxation of the skin, musculature, and peritoneum
8. Disadvantages
a. Difficulty in performing the technique
9. Complications
a. Loss of motor control of the pelvic limbs due to overdose or subarachnoid injection
b. Physiologic disturbance due to overdose or subarachnoid injection
c. Potential for trauma to the spinal cord or venous sinuses

ANESTHESIA FOR OBSTETRIC PROCEDURES AND RELIEF OF RECTAL TENESMUS

I. Caudal epidural anesthesia and desensitization of the internal pudendal nerve are commonly used techniques in ruminants for obstetric manipulations, caudal surgical procedures, and as an adjunct treatment for control of rectal tenesmus. The techniques are not effective in pigs
II. Cattle
A. Low posterior, or caudal, epidural anesthesia (see Fig. 5-4)
1. Area blocked: anus, perineum, vulva, vagina
2. Nerves blocked: coccygeal and posterior sacral nerves
3. Site: First intercoccygeal space
4. Needle used: 18 gauge, 1^{1}/2-inch (average dairy cow)
5. Anesthetic: 5-6 ml of 2% lidocaine
6. Method: Locate the sacrococcygeal joint by moving the tail up and down; this joint moves very little and is located just anterior to the anal folds. The first intercoccygeal joint is easily located by its movement;

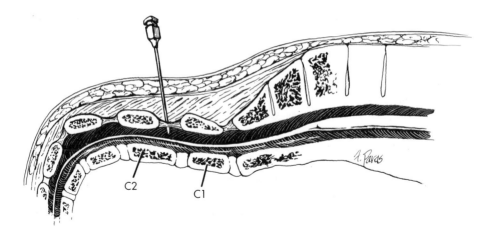

FIG. 5-4 Needle placement for caudal epidural anesthesia in cattle. C1: first coccygeal vertebra. C2: second coccygeal vertebra.

it is much wider and is posterior to the anal folds. Insert the needle exactly at the midline of the space at right angles to the skin surface. Push the needle ventrally through the interarcuate ligament to the floor of the neural canal, which is at about 2 to 4 cm (3/4-1 1/2 inches). Withdraw the needle slightly into epidural space and test with air if there is no resistance

7. Advantages
   a. Minimal effect on cardiovascular and respiratory systems
   b. Little effect on organ systems
   c. Little problem with toxicity
   d. Good muscle relaxation
   e. Good postoperative analgesia
   f. Rapid recovery
   g. Relatively simple
   h. Inexpensive

8. Disadvantages
   a. Technically difficult if C1-C2 interspace is not identified
   b. Technically difficult if the sacrococcygeal interspace is ossified in older cow

9. Complications
   a. Rare
   b. Infection resulting in draining tracts or permanently paralyzed tail
   c. The animal becomes ataxic and collapses in the rear quarters due to overdosage
   d. Hemorrhage due to puncture of a venous sinus

B. Internal pudendal nerve block
   1. Indications
      a. Anesthesia and relaxation of the penis for examination

      b. Relief of tenesmus associated with vaginal and uterine prolapse

   2. Nerves blocked: internal pudendal, caudal rectal (middle hemorrhoidal), and pelvic splanchnic nerves

   3. Site: identified by rectal palpation

   4. Needle used: spinal, preferably 18 gauge, $3^1/2$-inch

   5. Anesthetic: 30 ml of 2% lidocaine per side

   6. Method: Rectal palpation is used to locate the lesser sciatic foramen, a soft, circumscribed depression in the sacrosciatic ligament. The nerve is found a finger's width dorsal to the pulsating pudendal artery present in the fossa. The needle is passed through the disinfected skin in the ischiorectal fossa. About 20 ml of 2% lidocaine is deposited around the nerve. The needle is withdrawn 2-3 cm caudodorsally, and another 10 ml is injected in the area of the pelvic splanchnic nerve. The procedure is repeated on the opposite side

   7. Advantages

      a. No loss of tail tone

      b. No sciatic nerve involvement

   8. Disadvantages

      a. Technically difficult

      b. Anesthesia lasts 3-6 hours

   9. Complications: The bull's penis must be protected from injury by replacing it into the prepuce and taping the external preputial orifice

III. Sheep and Goats

   A. The technique for low posterior, or caudal, epidural anesthesia in sheep and goats is similar to the technique used in cattle. Similarly, 0.5-1.0 ml of 2% lidocaine per 50 kg of bodyweight is injected at the first coccygeal interspace

ANTERIOR EPIDURAL ANESTHESIA

  I. Anterior epidural anesthesia is indicated for all procedures caudal to the diaphragm. The lumbosacral space is commonly used in calves, sheep, and goats because the injection sites are usually palpable. This space is the only practical injection site for producing anterior anesthesia in pigs. Proper techniques should provide anesthesia of:

   A. Perianal region

   B. Inguinal region

   C. Flank

   D. Abdominal wall up to the umbilicus

 II. Increasing the dose of the anesthetic increases the area of blockade

III. Rapid epidural injections have to be avoided in order to:

   A. Minimize discomfort to the patient

   B. Avoid increased rate of vascular absorption, which can result in less drug for neural uptake and subsequent:

      1. 15% decrease of duration of action

      2. Higher incidence of incomplete analgesia

      3. Only a slight increase in segmental spread

IV. The technique is contraindicated in animals with known:
  A. Cardiovascular disease
  B. Bleeding disorders
  C. Low blood pressure
V. Complications that may arise from faulty techniques (overdose, subarachnoid injection) include:
  A. Loss of consciousness
  B. Flexor spasm
  C. Rapid muscular contractions
  D. Respiratory paralysis
  E. Hypotension
  F. Hypothermia
VI. Small ruminants (sheep and goats)
  A. Landmarks and techniques for injection at the lumbosacral space are similar to those used in dogs (see Figs. 7-3 and 7-4)
  B. Dose: 1 ml of 2% lidocaine per 10 lb of body weight
  C. Effect
    1. Onset of posterior paralysis occurs in 2-15 minutes
    2. Extent of anesthesia generally reaches three quarters of distance from pubis to umbilicus
    3. Duration of anesthesia is generally 1-2 hours
    4. Similar extent and duration of anesthesia can be achieved if only half the dose (0.5 ml/10 lb) is injected subarachnoidally
    5. True spinal anesthesia will result with onset of posterior paralysis within 1-3 minutes
VII. Pigs
  A. Landmarks and techniques for injection at the lumbosacral space are similar to those used in dogs (see Figs. 7-3 and 7-4)
  B. Dose when using 2% lidocaine:

For standing castration	For cesarean section
4 ml/200 lb	10 ml/200 lb
6 ml/400 lb	15 ml/400 lb
8 ml/600 lb	20 ml/600 lb

  C. Effect
    1. Onset of anesthetic action is generally in 5 minutes
    2. Maximum effect is within 15-20 minutes
    3. Duration: 60 minutes

LOCAL ANESTHESIA FOR DEHORNING

I. Cattle
  A. Area blocked: horn and base of the horn
  B. Nerve blocked: cornual branch of zygomaticotemporal nerve
  C. Site: temporal ridge, 2 cm from the base of horn (see Fig. 5-5)
  D. Needle used: 18 gauge, 1- or 1$\frac{1}{2}$-inch
  E. Anesthetic: 5-10 ml of 2% lidocaine

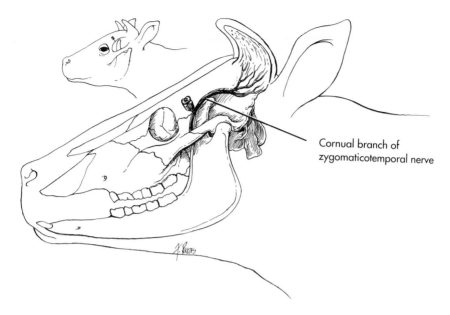

FIG.5-5 Needle placement for desensitizing the cornual branch of the zygomaticotemporal nerve in the cow.

F. Method: Palpate the lateral temporal ridge of the frontal bone. The nerve is relatively superficial, 7-10 mm deep ($1/4$-$1/2$ inch) on the upper third of the ridge, lying between the thin frontalis muscle and the temporal muscle. It can usually be palpated. Inject only 2-3 cm in front of the horn if the horns are well developed, to block the posterior branch of the nerve

G. Advantages
    1. Minimal systemic effects on the cardiopulmonary system
    2. Relatively simple

H. Disadvantages
    1. Cornual anesthesia does not result if the anesthetic is injected too deeply in the aponeurosis of the temporal muscle
    2. A second injection posterior to the horn may be required in adult cattle with well-developed horns
    3. Anesthesia of a fracture horn involving the frontal bone or sinuses requires the Peterson eye block

I. Complications: none

II. Goats
    A. Area blocked: horn and base of the horn
    B. Nerves blocked: cornual branch of the zygomaticotemporal (lacrimal) nerve and cornual branch of the infratrochlear nerve
    C. Site: halfway between lateral canthus of the eye and lateral base of the horn (lacrimal nerve) (see Fig. 5-6, A) and halfway between medial canthus of the eye and medial base of the horn (cornual branch of infratrochlear nerve) (see Fig. 5-6, B)

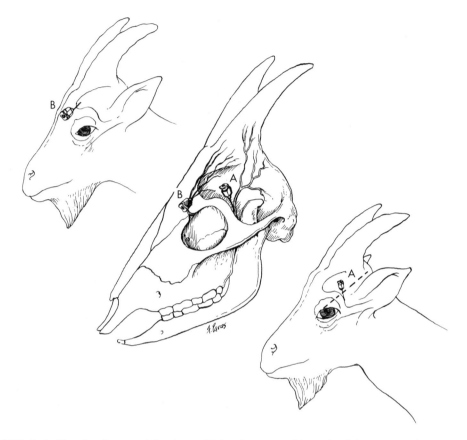

FIG. 5-6 Needle placement for desensitizing the cornual branch of the zygomaticotemporal (lacrimal) nerve (*A*) and cornual branch of the infratrochlear nerve (*B*) in the goat.

    D. Needle used: 22 gauge, 1-inch
    E. Anesthetic: 2-3 ml 2% lidocaine at each site in the adult goat. No more than 0.5 ml 2% lidocaine for ring block at the horn base in young kids 7-14 days of age
    F. Method: To reach the cornual branch of the zygomaticotemporal nerve, the needle is inserted as close as possible to the caudal ridge of the supraorbital process and 1.0-1.5 cm deep (see Fig. 5-6, *A*). To reach the cornual branch of the infratrochlear nerve, the needle is inserted dorsal and parallel to the dorsomedial margin of the orbit. The anesthetic is injected in a line, as this nerve is frequently branched (see Fig. 5-6, *B*)
    G. Advantages
        1. Alleviation of pain during dehorning
        2. Alleviation of pain during disbudding
    H. Disadvantages
        1. Sedation of the animal is required if the frontal sinus will be entered during horn removal

    2. A total dose of 10 mg/kg (0.5 ml of 2% lidocaine) must not be exceeded to minimize adverse reactions

I. Complications

    1. Toxicity due to overdose of lidocaine includes any of the following clinical signs

      a. Excitation

      b. Lateral recumbency

      c. Generalized tonoclonic convulsions

      d. Opisthotonus

      e. Respiratory depression

      f. Cardiac arrest

LOCAL ANESTHESIA FOR THE EYE

I. At present, topical and regional anesthetic techniques are used to facilitate surgery of the eye and its associated structures. Paralysis of the eyelids (without analgesia) is accomplished by selectively desensitizing the auriculopalpebral branch of the facial nerve (akinesia). Anesthesia of the eye and orbit and immobilization of the globe are commonly achieved by:

    A. Peterson technique

    B. Modification of Peterson technique

    C. Retrobulbar injection of local anesthetic

II. Peterson eye block (Fig. 5-7)

    A. Area blocked: eye and orbit, orbicularis oculi muscle, eyelids

    B. Nerves blocked: oculomotor, trochlear, and abducens nerves and the three branches of the trigeminal nerve (ophthalmic, maxillary, and mandibular)

    C. Sites: at the emergence of these nerves from the foramen rotundum

    D. Needle: 14 gauge, 1-inch to serve as a cannula
                18 gauge, 4$1/2$-inch

    E. Anesthetic: 7-15 ml of 2% lidocaine at the foramen
                 orbitorotundum
              5-10 ml of 2% lidocaine for desensitizing
                 the auriculopalpebral nerve

    F. Method

      1. Cow's head is fully extended with frontal and nasal bones parallel to the ground

      2. Prepare area posterior and ventral to the eye

      3. Inject several milliliters of anesthetic with a small gauge needle into the skin and subcutaneously into the notch formed by the zygomatic and temporal process of the malar bone (where the supraorbital process of the frontal bone meets the zygomatic arch)(see Fig. 5-7)

      4. Place a 14 gauge $1/2$- or 1-inch needle (to serve as a cannula) through the skin as far anterior and ventral as possible in the notch

      5. Direct a straight 18 gauge 4$1/2$-inch needle with no syringe attached (to feel the bony landmarks) through the cannula in a horizontal and

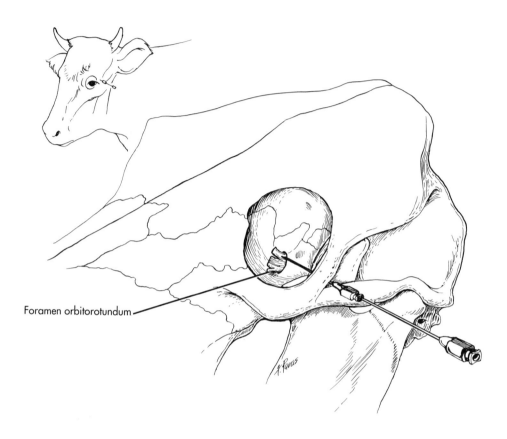

FIG.5-7 Needle placement for Peterson eye block, with needle tip at the foramen orbito-rotundum.

slightly posterior direction, until it strikes the coronoid process of the mandible

6. The needle's point is positioned anteriorly until it passes medially around this bone

7. Advance needle slightly posteriorly and somewhat ventrally until it strikes a solid bony plate, which is at a depth of about 3-4½ inches

8. Inject 15 ml of 2% lidocaine anterior to the foramen rotundum

9. To block the auriculopalpebral branch of the facial nerve (see Fig. 5-8), a 10 ml syringe filled with local anesthetic is attached to the needle, and the cannula is partially withdrawn

10. The needle is withdrawn until it almost leaves the skin, and it is directed posteriorly for 2-3 inches lateral to the zygomatic arch as lidocaine is injected

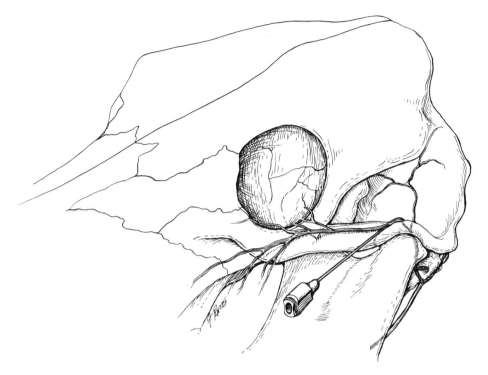

FIG.5-8 Needle placement for akinesia of the eyelids in the cow.

11. If the upper lid is involved in the surgical procedure, a line of infiltration with local anesthetic should be made subcutaneously about 1 inch from the margin of the lid

G. Advantages
   1. Useful for enucleation of the eyeball and removal of tumors from eye and eyelids
   2. The technique is quick, easy, safe, and effective if done properly
   3. Less edema and inflammation result than when eyelids and orbit are infiltrated
   4. Surgery of cornea (removal of tumors and dermoids) can be done easily without retraction or fixation forceps if the eyeball is proptosed
   5. Peterson eye block is safer than retrobulbar injections of local anesthetic, which often lead to orbital hemorrhage, direct pressure on the globe, penetration of the globe, damage to the optic nerve, or injection into the optic nerve meninges

H. Disadvantages
   1. The cow's head is difficult to keep horizontal when the animal is in a chute or stanchion with the head tied to one side; this makes the landmarks difficult to locate
   2. If the needle point strikes the pterygoid crest, no anesthesia will result following injection of the local anesthetic

3. In 50% of the cases, incomplete anesthesia of the upper eyelid results because of sensory innervation from other nerves
4. Blinking is prevented for several hours
5. Sterile saline solution should be applied to the eye frequently during surgery to keep the cornea moist
6. Antibiotic eye ointments should be applied to the cornea after orbital replacement of the globe
7. Sunlight, dust, and wind in the eye must be avoided to prevent keratoconjunctivitis
8. The lids may be sutured together until motor activity of the lids returns

I. Complications
1. In procedures other than enucleation, keratitis may result from postoperative drying of the cornea because effective block will prevent blinking for several hours
2. Penetration of the turbinates and injection with local anesthetic into the nasopharynx and optic nerve meninges can cause severe CNS toxicity including the following clinical signs
   a. Hyperexcitability
   b. Lateral recumbency
   c. Tonoclonic convulsions
   d. Opisthotonus
   e. Respiratory arrest
   f. Cardiac arrest

LOCAL ANESTHESIA OF THE FOOT

I. Local anesthesia of the foot may be induced by:
  A. Infiltrating the tissues around the limb with local anesthetic solution (ring block)
  B. Injecting local anesthetic solution into an accessible superficial vein in an extremity isolated from circulation by placing a tourniquet on the animal's leg (intravenous regional anesthesia)
  C. Desensitizing specific nerves (regional anesthesia)

INTRAVENOUS REGIONAL ANESTHESIA (IVRA)

I. Regional anesthesia technique
  A. Area blocked: extremity distal to tourniquet
  B. Site: lateral digital vein (see Fig. 5-9)
  C. Needle used: 18 gauge, 1 1/2-inch
  D. Anesthetic: 10-30 ml 2% lidocaine
  E. Method: A rubber tourniquet is placed proximal to the metatarsal or metacarpal region for foot surgery, or at a more proximal position for surgery of the carpal or tarsal region. Local anesthetic is rapidly injected into the prominent lateral/dorsal metatarsal or metacarpal vein, with the needle directed either proximally or distally
  F. Advantages

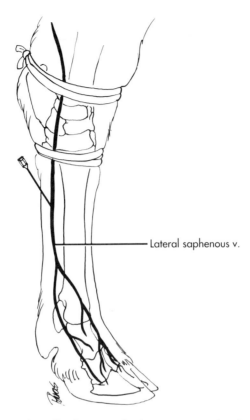

Lateral saphenous v.

FIG. 5-9 Tourniquet and needle placement for intravenous regional anesthesia of the cow's right pelvic limb, with needle tip placed at the cranial branch of the lateral saphenous vein.

    1. No special skill or knowledge of anatomy of the limb is needed
    2. Only one injection is required, with little risk of introducing bacteria
    3. Rapid onset of anesthesia distal to the tourniquet (5-10 minutes)
    4. Rapid recovery after removal of tourniquet (5-10 minutes)
  G. Disadvantages
    1. 7% inexplicable failure rate
    2. Occasional hematoma at the injection site
    3. Failure due to tourniquet slipping or extravascular injection
  H. Complications
    1. Lameness and edema if tourniquet is left in place for longer than 2 hours

TEAT AND UDDER ANESTHESIA OF CATTLE

  I. Surgical procedures on the foreudder and foreteats may be performed using:
    A. Paravertebral anesthesia of L1, L2, and L3
    B. Segmental epidural anesthesia
  II. Both techniques have been described as difficult, and they often result in the cow's lying down

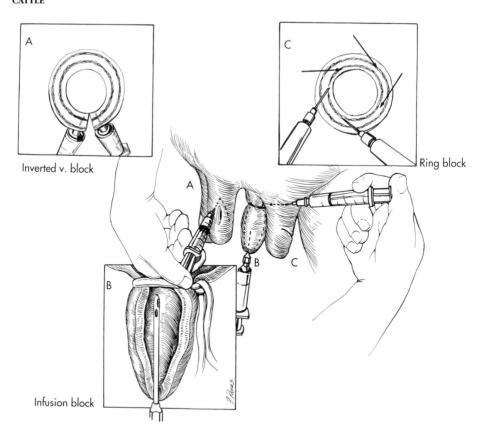

FIG.5-10 Needle placement for the cow's teat inverted V block (*A*); tourniquet and cannula placement for teat cistern infusion (*B*); teat ring block (*C*).

III. Surgical procedures of the caudalmost teats and escutcheon areas of the udder may be performed after:
   A. Desensitizing the perineal nerve in the standing cow
   B. High caudal epidural anesthesia in recumbent ruminants
   C. Lumbosacral epidural anesthesia in recumbent ruminants
IV. Most surgical procedures on the teat (repair of a stenotic teat sphincter, repairs of teat fistulae and lacerations) are generally performed under local anesthesia
   A. Needle used: 20-22 gauge, 1/2-inch or teat cannula
   B. Anesthetic: 6-10 ml of 2% lidocaine
   C. Method
      1. Ring block: Local anesthetic is infused into the skin and muscular tissue of base of the teat, after thorough cleaning of the external surface of the teat and quarter (see Fig. 5-10)
      2. Inverted V block: Line infusion of the anesthetic using an inverted V pattern, which encloses the teat skin defect (see Fig. 5-10)

3. Teat infusion block
   a. Teat opening is cleaned
   b. Tourniquet is placed at the base of the teat
   c. 10 ml of 2% lidocaine is infused into teat cistern (see Fig. 5-10)
   d. The mucous membrane of the teat cistern is anesthetized within 5 minutes; the muscular and skin layers remain sensitive

CHAPTER SIX

Local Anesthesia in Horses

OVERVIEW

Many diagnostic and surgical procedures are performed safely and humanely in the horse using physical restraint, sedation, and surface (topical) anesthesia, infiltration anesthesia, nerve block (regional) anesthesia, and epidural anesthesia. The techniques vary with each procedure and personal preference. Peripheral nerve blocks, intra-articular and intrabursal injections, and local infiltrations (ring block) are used to aid diagnosis of equine lameness and as a means of providing analgesia to a potential surgery site. Desensitization of the auriculopalpebral nerve is most frequently used for examination and treatment of the eye, since voluntary closure of the eyelids (akinesia) is prevented. Although regional anesthesia of the head can be induced by various techniques, the most frequently desensitized nerves of the head are the supraorbital, infraorbital, and mandibular alveolar.

Caudal epidural anesthesia is used to facilitate surgery involving the tail, perineum, anus, rectum, vulva, vagina, urethra, and symptomatic relief of painful conditions during obstetrical manipulations. Improper injection technique contributes to inadequate anesthesia. Overdosing leads to more serious complications including ataxia of hindlimbs, hindlimb motor blockade, and recumbency.

REGIONAL ANESTHESIA OF THE HEAD

I. The most frequently desensitized nerves of the head are the:
    A. Supraorbital (frontal)
    B. Auriculopalpebral
    C. Infraorbital
    D. Mandibular alveolar

ANESTHESIA OF UPPER EYELID AND FOREHEAD

I. Area blocked: upper eyelid except medial and lateral canthi
II. Nerve blocked: supraorbital (or frontal) nerve

III. Site: supraorbital foramen (Fig. 6-1, *A*)
IV. Needle used: 22-25 gauge, 1-inch
V. Anesthetic: 5 ml of 2% lidocaine
VI. Method: The needle is inserted into the supraorbital foramen to a depth of 1.5-2 cm. The foramen is palpated about 5-7 cm above the medial canthus where it perforates the bone of the supraorbital process of the frontal bone. Injections: 2 ml of anesthetic into the foramen, 1 ml as the needle is withdrawn, and 2 ml subcutaneously over the foramen
VII. Use
   A.   Desensitization of the upper eyelid
   B.   Blockade of the palpebral motor supply derived from the auriculopalpebral nerve

AKINESIA OF THE EYELIDS

I. Area blocked: paralysis of orbicularis occuli muscles
II. Nerve blocked: auriculopalpebral nerve (Fig. 6-1, *B*)
III. Site: highest point of zygomatic arch (or caudal to posterior ramus of the mandible)
IV. Needle used: 22-25 gauge, 1-inch
V. Anesthetic: 5 ml of 2% lidocaine
VI. Method: The needle is inserted 3 cm ventral to the highest point of the dorsal border of the zygomatic arch, directed dorsally, and pushed along the bone until the tip almost reaches the dorsal border of the zygomatic arch. Local anesthetic is injected subfascially as the needle is withdrawn
VII. Use
   A.   For examination of the eye
   B.   Successful blockade of the motor nerve supply prevents the horse from closing the eyelids

ANESTHESIA OF THE UPPER LIP AND NOSE

I. Area blocked: lip and nostril, roof of nasal cavity, and related skin up to the infraorbital foramen
II. Nerve blocked: infraorbital nerve
III. Site: at its point of emergence from infraorbital canal (Fig. 6-1, *C*)
IV. Needle used: 22-25 gauge, 1-inch
V. Anesthetic: 5 ml of 2% lidocaine
VI. Method: The perineural injection is performed at the site where the bony lip of the foramen can be felt, which is about halfway along and 2.5 cm dorsal to a line connecting the nasomaxillary notch and the anterior end of the facial crest. The flat levator labii superioris muscle, which runs over the foramen, can be pushed upward by the fingertips
VII. Use: for simple laceration in quiet or sedated horses

ANESTHESIA OF THE LOWER LIP

I. Area blocked: lower lip, all parts of mandible back to the third premolar tooth (PM3)

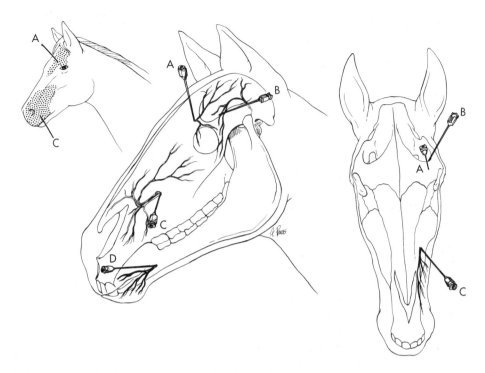

FIG. 6-1 Needle placement for nerve blocks on the head: *A*, supraorbital (or frontal); *B*, auriculopalpebral; *C*, infraorbital; *D*, mandibular alveolar nerves.

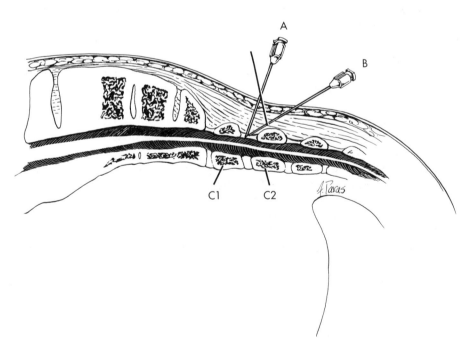

FIG. 6-2 Needle placement into caudal epidural space (*A* or *B*) at the first intercoccygeal space (C1-C2).

II. Nerve blocked: mandibular alveolar nerve

III. Site: in mandibular canal (Fig. 6-1, *D*)

IV. Needle used: 20 gauge, 3-inch

V. Anesthetic: 10 ml of 2% lidocaine

VI. Method: The needle is inserted into the mandibular canal as far as possible in a ventromedial direction. The lateral border of the foramen is palpated as a ridge along the lateral aspect of the ramus in the middle of the interdental space. Injection of local anesthetic requires pressure, and fluid might partially drain back from the canal under the skin, which is responsible for unreliable results

VII. Use: for simple laceration in quiet or sedated horses

CAUDAL EPIDURAL ANESTHESIA

I. Area blocked: tail, perineum, anus, rectum, vulva, vagina

II. Nerves blocked: caudal nerves and last three pairs of sacral nerves

III. Site: epidural space between first intercoccygeal space (C1-C2) (Fig. 6-2)

IV. Needles used: spinal with stylet: 18 gauge, 2-3–inch; 2 gauge, 2-inch

V. Anesthetic: 6-10 ml of 2% lidocaine

VI. Method

    A. Proper restraint should be used depending on the horse's temperament. The injection site is clipped, surgically scrubbed, and disinfected. There is no relationship between origin of first tail hairs, caudal folds of the tail, and palpable depression between the first and second coccygeal vertebrae. Make a skin wheal, and infiltrate the tissues down to the interarcuate ligament to minimize movement during insertion of the spinal needle

    B. Method A (see Fig. 6-2, *A*): Insert the spinal needle into the epidural space in the center of the first intercoccygeal space at a right angle to the general contour of the croup, and press the needle ventrally in a median plane until it strikes the floor of the vertebral canal. The needle is withdrawn for about 0.5 cm

    C. Method B (see Fig. 6-2, *B*): Insert the spinal needle about 1 inch posterior to the first intercoccygeal space and slide its point ventrocranially at an angle of about 30° to the horizontal plane to its full length into the vertebral canal

    D. Test with a syringe of air for resistance to the injection. Inject local anesthetic and leave needle in place with stylet reinserted. Maximum blockade may require 10-30 minutes, and it is not advisable to redose during this time if surgery is to be done with the horse standing

VII. Use

    A. For anesthesia of pelvic viscera without loss of hindleg motor control during obstetric manipulations

    B. For anesthesia of genitalia without loss of hindleg motor control during obstetric manipulations

    C. For surgical procedures of viscera and genitalia to be done standing

        1. Caslick operation

        2. Rectovaginal fistula repair

        3. Prolapsed rectum repair

        4. Tail amputation

VIII. Common causes for inadequate anesthesia or incomplete block
  A. Improper injection technique
    1. Use of solutions of diminished potency
    2. Inadequate dispersal of anesthetic
  B. Inappropriate angulation of the spinal needle
    1. Needle point strikes the dorsal aspect of the vertebral arch
    2. Deviation of the needle from the midline
  C. Horses that have had previous epidural injections
    1. Anatomic peculiarities
    2. Presence of septa within the epidural space
    3. Presence of patent intervertebral foramina
IX. Complications
  A. Trauma to coccygeal nerve(s)
  B. Infection of the neural canal
  C. Extensive cranial migration of local anesthetic solution causing:
    1. Ataxia
    2. Staggering
    3. Excitement
    4. Recumbency

REGIONAL ANESTHESIA OF THE LIMB

  I. Peripheral nerve blocks should be performed on the most distal branches of the nerve trunks in order to gain as much information as possible in diagnosis of equine lameness; then the examination should proceed proximally
  II. The palmar (volar) digital nerves of the forelimb or the plantar digital nerves of the hindlimb branch dorsal to the fetlock at the level of the sesamoids, forming three digital nerves
  A. The dorsal or anterior digital nerve, supplying sensory fibers to the anterior two thirds of the hoof
  B. The middle digital nerve (relatively unimportant)
  C. The palmar digital nerve (PDN) (most important clinically), supplying sensory fibers to the posterior third of the hoof, including portions, if not all, of the navicular area

PALMAR (VOLAR) OR PLANTAR DIGITAL NERVE BLOCK

See Figs. 6-3, *A* and 6-4, *A*
  I. Area blocked: posterior third of the foot, including the navicular bursa
  II. Nerves blocked: digital nerves
  III. Site: in the palmar (volar)/plantar region of the pastern joint
  IV. Needle used: 20-25 gauge, 1-inch
  V. Anesthetic: 2 ml of 2% lidocaine at each site
  VI. Method: The palmar (volar) or plantar nerve is palpated just palmar/plantar to the vein and artery, dorsal to the flexor tendon. The needle is inserted in the palmar/plantar region of the pastern joint, medially and/or laterally with the leg elevated or bearing weight
  VII. Use: diagnosis of equine lameness

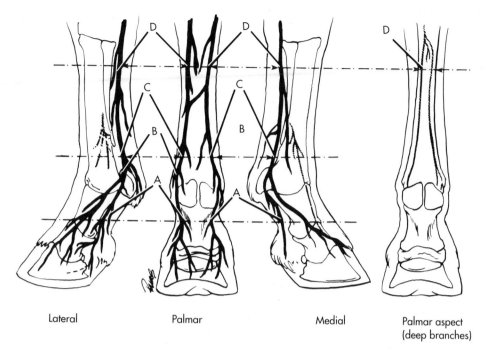

Lateral   Palmar   Medial   Palmar aspect
(deep branches)

FIG. 6-3 Injection sites for nerve blocks on the left forelimb in the horse: *A*, palmar (volar); *B*, abaxial sesamoidean; *C*, low palmar; *D*, high palmar nerve.

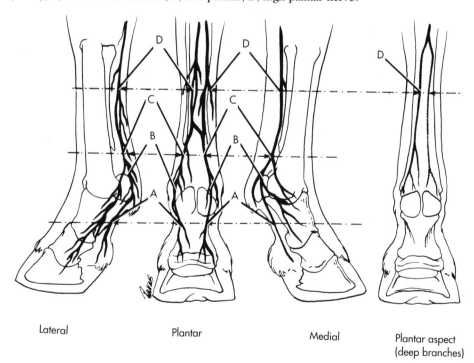

Lateral   Plantar   Medial   Plantar aspect
(deep branches)

FIG. 6-4 Injection sites for nerve blocks on the left hindlimb in the horse: *A*, plantar digital; *B*, abaxial sesamoidean; *C*, low plantar; *D*, high plantar nerve.

ABAXIAL (BASILAR) SESAMOIDEAN NERVE BLOCK

See Figs. 6-3, *B*, and 6-4, *B*

 I. Area blocked: entire foot
 II. Nerves blocked: digital nerves
 III. Site: in palmar region of the fetlock joint over abaxial surface of proximal sesamoids
 IV. Needle used: 20-25 gauge, 1-inch
 V. Anesthetic: 3 ml of 2% lidocaine at each site
 VI. Method: The digital nerve is palpated in the palmar region of the fetlock joint over the abaxial surface of proximal sesamoids, just palmar/plantar to the digital artery and vein. The needle is inserted subcutaneously at this site
 VII. Use: diagnosis of equine lameness

PALMAR (VOLAR) OR PLANTAR NERVE BLOCK

 I. The palmar (volar) or plantar nerves can be desensitized at either a low site (low palmar/volar [LVNB] or low plantar nerve block [LPNB]) or a high site (high palmar/volar [HVNB] or higher plantar nerve block [HPNB])
 II. Midregion blocks (midmetacarpal or midmetatarsal) should be avoided due to the anastomotic branch, which transverses in a downward direction from medial to lateral

LOW PALMAR (VOLAR) OR PLANTAR NERVE BLOCK

See Figs. 6-3, *C* and 6-4, *C*

 I. Area blocked: almost all structures distal to the fetlock and fetlock joint except for the dorsal fetlock joint
 II. Nerves blocked: palmar or plantar nerves (medial/lateral)
 III. Site: medially and laterally at the level of the distal enlargements of the metacarpal II and IV and metatarsal II and IV (splints)
 IV. Needle used: 20-25 gauge, 1-inch
 V. Anesthetic: 2-3 ml of 2% lidocaine at each site
 VI. Method
   A. The palmar nerves (medial/lateral) are desensitized by injecting the anesthetic between the flexor tendon and suspensory ligament
   B. The palmar metacarpal and metatarsal nerves (medial/lateral) are desensitized by injecting the anesthetic between the suspensory ligament and the splint bone
 VII. Use: diagnosis of equine lameness

HIGH PALMAR (VOLAR) OR PLANTAR NERVE BLOCK

See Figs. 6-3, *D* and 6-4, *D*

 I. Area blocked: palmar (volar) metacarpal or plantar metatarsal region and all of the digit distal to the fetlock
 II. Nerves blocked: palmar or plantar nerves (medial/lateral)
 III. Site: proximal quarter of the metacarpus or metatarsus proximal to the communicating branch of the medial and lateral palmar (volar) or plantar nerves
 IV. Needle used: 22 gauge, 1 1/2-inch

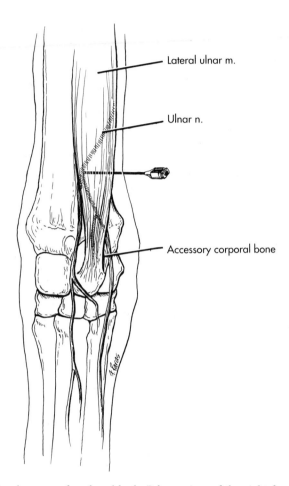

Lateral ulnar m.

Ulnar n.

Accessory corporal bone

FIG. 6-5 Needle placement for ulnar block. Palmar view of the right forelimb: ulnaris lateralis muscle, ulnaris nerve, accessory carpal bone.

   V. Anesthetic: 5 ml of 2% lidocaine at each site
  VI. Method: The medial and lateral palmar (volar) and plantar nerves are desensitized by injecting the anesthetic subfascially into the groove between the suspensory ligament and the deep flexor tendon on both the medial and lateral sides
 VII. Use
     A. Diagnosis of equine lameness
     B. To complete anesthesia of the forelimb from the carpus distally, the ulnar, median, and musculocutaneous nerves must be desensitized

ULNAR NERVE BLOCK

See Fig. 6-5
    I. Area blocked: lateral, or dorsal and palmar skin area (as illustrated with stippled area in Fig. 6-6)

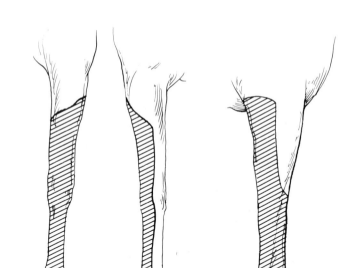

Palmar   Dorsal   Lateral

FIG. 6-6 Desensitized area after ulnar nerve block.

II. Nerve blocked: ulnar nerve

III. Site: 10 cm proximal to the accessory carpal bone

IV. Needle used: 22 gauge, 1-inch

V. Anesthetic: 5-10 ml of 2% lidocaine

VI. Method: The nerve is desensitized 1.5 cm deep beneath the fascia between the flexor carpi ulnaris and ulnaris lateralis muscle

VII. Use: anesthesia of part of the forelimb

MEDIAN NERVE BLOCK

See Figs. 6-7 and 6-8

I. Area blocked: lateral, medial, palmar, and dorsal skin areas (as illustrated with stippled area in Fig. 6-8)

II. Nerve blocked: median nerve

III. Site: medial aspect of the forelimb 5 cm ventral to the elbow joint

IV. Needle used: 20-22 gauge, 1½-inch

V. Anesthetic: 10 ml of 2% lidocaine

VI. Method: The median nerve is desensitized between the posterior border of the radius and the muscular belly of the internal flexor carpi radialis

VII. Use: anesthesia of part of the distal limb

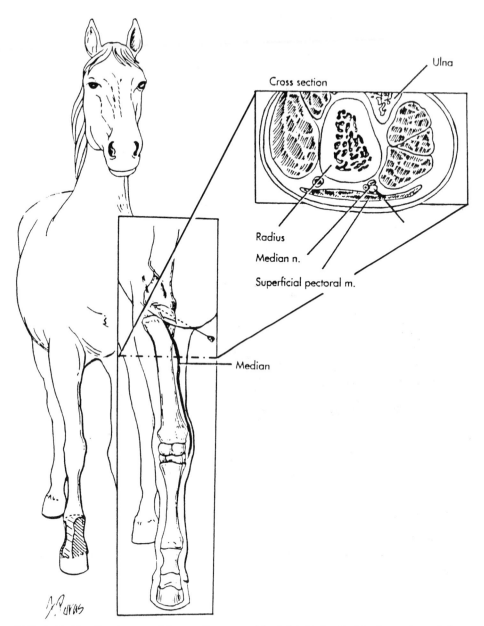

Cross section

Ulna

Radius

Median n.

Superficial pectoral m.

Median

FIG. 6-7 Needle placement for median nerve block (right forelimb). *A*, craniomedial aspect; *B*, cross section; *C*, desensitized cutaneous area.

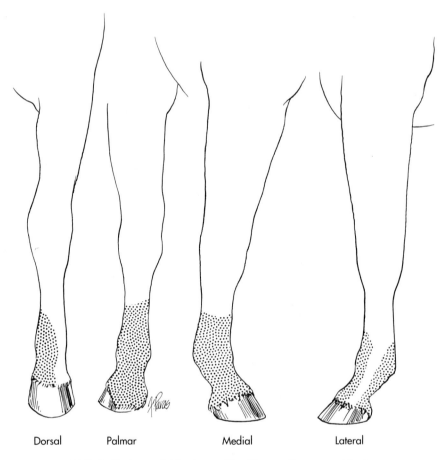

Dorsal   Palmar   Medial   Lateral

FIG. 6-8 Area of skin desensitized by median nerve block.

MUSCULOCUTANEOUS NERVE BLOCK

See Fig. 6-9, *A*

   I. Area blocked: medial, palmar, and dorsal skin area (as illustrated with striped area in Fig. 6-9, *B*)

  II. Nerve blocked: cutaneous branch of musculocutaneous nerve

 III. Site: anteromedial aspect of the forelimb halfway between the elbow and carpus

  IV. Needle used: 22 gauge, 1-inch

   V. Anesthetic: 10 ml of 2% lidocaine

  VI. Method: The musculocutaneous nerve is desensitized subcutaneously where it is easily palpated just cranial to the cephalic vein

 VII. Use

    A. Anesthesia of part of the forelimb

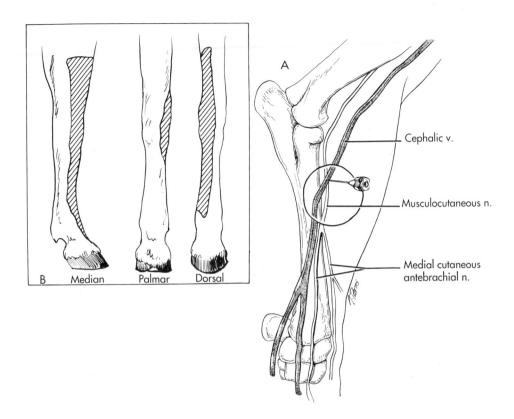

F I G. 6-9 Needle placement for musculocutaneous nerve block (left forelimb). *A*, medial aspect; *B*, desensitized cutaneous area of left forelimb.

B. For further discussion of other anesthetic techniques, see Practical regional anesthesia, in Mansmann RA, McAllister ES, Pratt PW (eds): *Equine Medicine and Surgery*, ed. 3. Santa Barbara, Calif, American Veterinary Publications, 1982, vol 1, pp 229-238; and Local and regional analgesia, in Short CE (ed): *Principles and Practice of Veterinary Anesthesia*. Baltimore, Williams and Wilkins, 1987, pp 91-133

CHAPTER SEVEN

Local Anesthesia
in Dogs and Cats

OVERVIEW

Local anesthetic techniques are taught but rarely practiced in the dog and cat because of the preference for using general anesthesia. On the other hand, dogs or cats that are considered high risks to the depressent effects of general anesthesia may benefit from lumbosacral epidural anesthesia, continuous epidural anesthesia, brachial plexus block, and selected nerve blocks in the head.

Epidural anesthesia is the injection of local anesthetic into the epidural space. Spinal anesthesia is the injection of local anesthetic into the subarachnoid space; this is potentially dangerous in the dog and cat since this space is small in these species.

REGIONAL ANESTHESIA OF THE HEAD

I. When combined with effective sedation, the desensitization of the following nerves of the head can be routinely considered
   A. Infraorbital
   B. Maxillary
   C. Ophthalmic
   D. Mental
   E. Alveolar mandibular

ANESTHESIA OF THE EYE

I. Area blocked: eye, orbit, conjunctiva, eyelids, and forehead skin
II. Nerves blocked: lacrimal, zygomatic, and ophthalmic (ophthalmic division of the trigeminal nerve)
III. Site: at the orbital fissure (Fig. 7-1, C)
IV. Needle used: 22-25 gauge, 1-inch
V. Anesthetic used: 2 ml of 1% lidocaine
VI. Method: The needle is inserted ventral to the border of the zygomatic process at the lateral canthus of the eye. The needle is directed in a mediodorsal and somewhat caudal direction until it reaches the orbital fissure

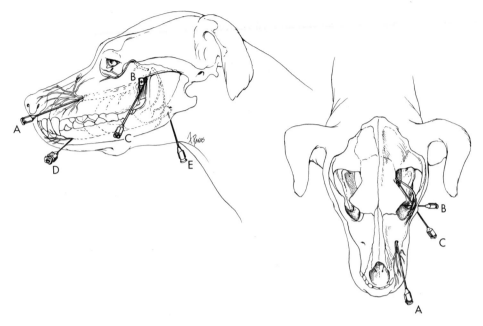

F I G . 7 - 1   Needle placement for nerve blocks on the head: *A*, infraorbital; *B*, maxillary; *C*, ophthalmic; *D*, mental; *E*, mandibular alveolar.

ANESTHESIA OF MAXILLA, UPPER TEETH, NOSE, AND UPPER LIP

I. Area blocked: maxilla, upper teeth, nose, and upper lip
II. Nerve blocked: maxillary
III. Site: at the perpendicular portion of the palatine bone between the maxillary foramen and foramen rotundum (Fig. 7-1, *B*)
IV. Needle used: 22-25 gauge, 1-inch
V. Anesthetic: 2 ml of 1% lidocaine
VI. Method: The needle is inserted through the skin at an angle of 90°, in a medial direction, ventral to the border of the zygomatic process and approximately 0.5 cm caudal to the lateral canthus of the eye. The needle is advanced to close proximity of the pterygopalatine fossa

ANESTHESIA OF UPPER LIP AND NOSE

I. Area blocked: upper lip and nose, roof of nasal cavity, and related skin up to the infraorbital foramen
II. Nerve blocked: infraorbital
III. Site: at its point of emergence from the infraorbital canal (Fig. 7-1, *A*)
IV. Needle used: 22-25 gauge, 1-inch
V. Anesthetic: 2 ml of 1% lidocaine
VI. Method: The needle is inserted either intra- or extraorally approximately 1 cm cranial to the bony lip of the infraorbital foramen. The needle is advanced

to the infraorbital foramen, which is felt between the dorsal border of the zygomatic process and the gum of the canine tooth.

ANESTHESIA OF THE LOWER LIP

I. Area blocked: lower lip
II. Nerve blocked: mental
III. Site: rostral to the mental foramen (Fig. 7-1, *D*)
IV. Needle used: 22-25 gauge, 1-inch
V. Anesthetic: 2 ml of 1% lidocaine
VI. Method: The needle is inserted over the mental nerve, rostral to the middle mental foramen at the level of the second premolar tooth

ANESTHESIA OF THE MANDIBLE

I. Area blocked: cheek teeth, canine, incisors, skin and mucosa of the chin and lower lip
II. Nerve blocked: inferior alveolar branch of the mandibular nerve
III. Site: at its entry into the mandibular canal at the mandibular foramen (Fig. 7-1, *E*)
IV. Needle used: 22-25 gauge, 1-inch
V. Method: The needle is inserted at the lower angle of the jaw approximately 1.5 cm rostrad to the angular process. The needle is then advanced 1.5 cm dorsally against the medial surface of the ramus of the mandible to the palpable lip of the mandibular foramen

ANESTHESIA OF THE FOOT

I. Anesthesia of the foot may be induced by:
   A. Infiltrating the tissues around the limb with local anesthetic solution (ring block)
   B. Infiltration of the brachial plexus by local anesthetic (brachial plexus block)
   C. Intravenous injection of anesthetic into an accessible superficial vein in a distal extremity isolated from circulation by placing a tourniquet on the animal's leg (intravenous regional anesthesia)
   D. Injection of local anesthetic into the lumbosacral epidural space (anesthesia of the hindlegs)

BRACHIAL PLEXUS BLOCK

I. Area blocked: distal foot, up to the elbow region
II. Nerves blocked: radial, median, ulnar, musculocutaneous, and axillary nerves
III. Site: medial to the shoulder joint (see Fig. 7-2)
IV. Needle used: 22 gauge, 3-inch
V. Anesthetic: 10-15 ml of 2% lidocaine
VI. Method: The needle is inserted medial to the shoulder joint toward the costochondral junction and parallel to the vertebral column. The anesthetic is injected slowly as the needle is withdrawn. Anesthesia can be obtained within 20 minutes and for 2 hours

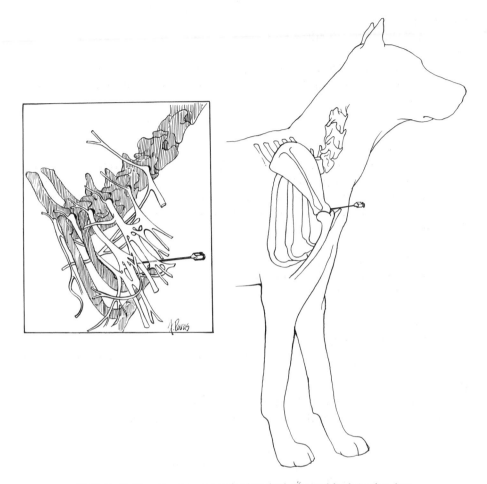

FIG. 7-2 Needle placement for brachial plexus block in the dog.

INTRAVENOUS REGIONAL ANESTHESIA (IVRA)

  I. Area blocked: extremity distal to tourniquet
 II. Nerves blocked: nerve endings in peripheral tissues
III. Site: any superficial vein distal to tourniquet
 IV. Needle used: 22 gauge, 1 1/2-inch
  V. Anesthetic: 2-3 ml of 1% lidocaine (without epinephrine)
 VI. Method: A rubber tourniquet is placed around the forearm just proximal to the elbow for thoracic limb surgery or proximal to the hock for pelvic limb surgery. Local anesthetic is injected with light pressure
VII. Advantages
    A. Safe and simple technique
    B. Lack of toxicity to organs if the occlusion of blood supply is limited to 2 hours
    C. Blood-free surgery site

VIII. Disadvantages

    A. Anesthesia time limited to 2 hours

  IX. Complications

    A. Shock occurs if tourniquet is removed after 4 hours (reversible)

    B. Death occurs if tourniquet is removed after 8-10 hours, due to sepsis and endotoxemia

EPIDURAL ANESTHESIA

  I. Indications

    A. Animals that are severely depressed, are in shock, or require immediate surgery of the rear quarters

    B. Animals that are at high risk, that are aged, or in which the use of other analgesic or anesthetic agents is contraindicated

  II. Specific procedures

    A. Tail amputations

    B. Anal sac therapy or perianal surgery

    C. Rear limb lacerations or fractures

    D. Urolithiasis therapy

    E. Abdominal surgery

    F. Cesarean sections

    G. Obstetrical manipulations

    H. Surgical procedures of the tail, perineum, vulva, vagina, rectum, and bladder

 III. Landmarks and anatomy (Figs. 7-3 and 7-4)

    A. Right and left cranial dorsal iliac wings of the ilium

    B. Spinous process of the seventh lumbar vertebra and the medium sacral crest

    C. Important anatomical features

      1. Shape of lumbar and sacral spinous processes

      2. Interspinous ligament

      3. Ligamentum flavum

      4. Terminal portion of the dural sac

      5. Filum terminale

      6. Intervertebral disc

    D. The spinal cord usually ends at vertebral body L6 in the dog and S1 in the cat; therefore, the procedure is more hazardous when performed in the cat

  IV. Equipment

    A. 2- or 4-inch, 18 or 20 gauge short beveled spinal needle with stylet (disposable needle preferred)

    B. One 2.5 cc and one 5 cc syringe

    C. Thin-walled, 18 gauge, 3-inch needle if a polyethylene catheter is to be placed for continuous epidural anesthesia

  V. Procedure

    A. This is a sterile procedure and it should be performed after proper surgical preparation

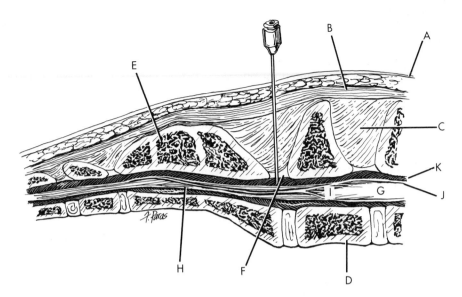

FIG. 7-3 Needle placement into lumbosacral epidural space in the dog. *A*, skin; *B*, supraspinous ligament; *C*, interspinous ligament; *D*, L7; *E*, sacrum; *F*, ligamentum interarcu-atum (flavum); *G*, spinal cord; *H*, cauda equina; *I*, cerbrospinal fluid; *J*, arachnoid membrane; *K*, dura mater.

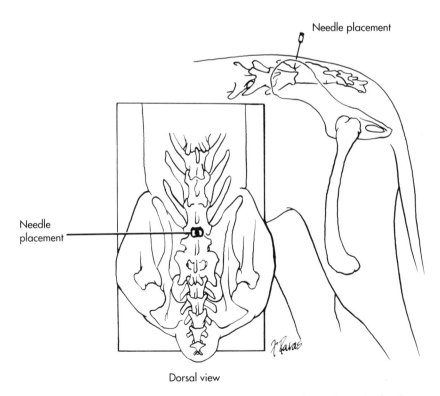

Needle placement

Needle placement

Dorsal view

FIG. 7-4 Needle placement for lumbosacral epidural anesthesia in the dog.

B. The spinal needle should be placed perpendicular to the skin surface at the midline of the lumbosacral space. This space can be palpated halfway between the dorso-iliac wings and just caudal to the dorsal spinous process of the seventh lumbar vertebra (Fig. 7-3)
   1. This may be facilitated by prior infusion of the area with 2% lidocaine
   2. The spinal needle is pushed ventrally in a slight cranial or caudal angle as needed
C. Upon reaching the ligamentum flavum, resistance is usually encountered
   1. A distinct "pop" is usually felt when the needle is advanced through this ligament
D. Upon penetrating the ligamentum flavum, you are in the epidural space
   1. Needle depth may vary from $1/2$ to $1\,1/2$ inches depending on animal size
   2. Remove the stylet and examine the needle for blood or CSF
      a. If no blood or CSF is observed, the needle should be aspirated
   3. 1-2 ml of air is injected to check for proper needle placement
      a. If subcutaneous crepitus is felt, the needle is incorrectly placed and should be repositioned
      b. No resistance should be felt to the injection of air or local anesthetic agent
VI. Dosages
   A. The dosage varies depending upon the desired effect
   B. 2% lidocaine or 0.75% bupivacaine is the agent of choice; 1 ml of local anesthetic is injected for each 10 pounds of body weight and will produce anesthesia as far cranial as L2. If anesthesia is required up to T5, the dose may be increased to 1 ml of local anesthetic per 7.5 pounds of body weight
      1. Small amounts of 1:200,000 epinephrine have been added to lidocaine in order to delay the rate of absorption and thus prolong anesthetic action
   C. Bupivacaine with epinephrine (Marcaine) produces 4-6–hour periods of anesthesia
VII. Continuous epidural anesthesia in dogs
   A. Procedure
      1. The procedure is similar to that previously described, only a larger needle is used through which a catheter is passed
      2. The needle is withdrawn, but the catheter is left in place
      3. Only $1/2$ inch of catheter should be advanced into the epidural space
VIII. Factors influencing cranial level of blockade
   A. Size of patient
   B. Conformation of patient
   C. Volume of drug injected
   D. Drug mass
   E. Rate of injection
   F. Direction of needle bevel
   G. Age of patient

TABLE 7-1

PROPOSED SITE OF ACTION AFTER EPIDURAL INJECTION

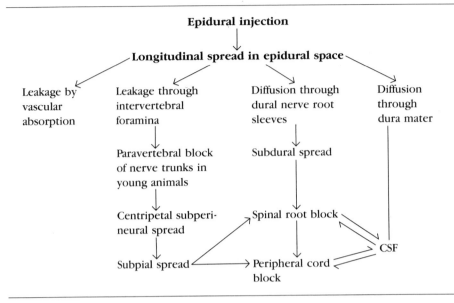

H. Obesity of patient
I. Presence and size of abdominal mass
J. Position of patient
IX. Proposed site of action after epidural injection (see Table 7-1)
X. Possible complications
   A. Injection of local anesthetic in the vertebral sinuses
      1. Vomiting, tremors
      2. Decreased blood pressure due to peripheral vasodilation
      3. Convulsions
      4. Paralysis
   B. Respiratory paralysis due to drug overdose in dogs and cats
      1. The drug must advance to approximately C5 or C7 to produce complete respiratory paralysis due to blockade of the phrenic nerves
      2. Keep the head elevated
   C. Temperature may fall in small animals due to a loss of shivering
      1. The patient's rear quarters should be kept warm by wrapping them in a towel or a water blanket
   D. Concurrent drugs that have been used
      1. Phenothiazine tranquilizers (0.05-0.2 mg/lb acepromazine IM) can be used if the animal is apprehensive
      2. Cyclohexamines (2-5 ml/lb ketamine IM) may be used successfully in cats)
      3. Xylazine (0.2-0.5 mg/lb IM) for mild sedation

CHAPTER EIGHT

Specific Intravenous
Anesthetic Drugs

"To sleep: perchance to dream"
WILLIAM SHAKESPEARE

OVERVIEW

A variety of injectable anesthetic drugs can be used to induce chemical restraint and general anesthesia. Proper use of pre-anesthetic medication (tranquilizers, sedatives, analgesics) is imperative for anesthetic drugs to produce the desired effect and to avoid detrimental side effects. Injectable anesthetic drugs are often more convenient and economical to use than inhalational anesthetic drugs. Their principal disadvantage is that once administered, they are not rapidly eliminated, although several injectable drugs (thiobarbiturates, methohexital, etomidate) have a very short duration of action. This section outlines the properties of injectable anesthetic drugs useful for chemical restraint and general anesthesia.

GENERAL CONSIDERATIONS

I. All degrees of central nervous system depression can be produced, from drowsiness and mild sedation to anesthesia and coma
II. The rate of onset and degree of depression depends upon:
   A. The anesthetic drug used
   B. Dose
   C. Route of administration (IM, IP, IV)
   D. The animal's level of consciousness (excited vs. depressed) at the time of drug administration

    E. Drug tolerance

    F. Drug interactions with other anesthetics

    G. Acid-base and electrolyte balance. Acidosis enhances barbiturate depression

III. Most injectable anesthetic drugs depress the cerebral cortex and probably the thalamus

    A. Used in the control of convulsions

    B. Barbiturates increase the threshold of spinal reflexes

        1. Can be used clinically in treatment of strychnine poisoning

IV. Routes of administration

    A. Most injectable drugs are routinely administered intravenously

    B. Sodium salts of barbiturates can be injected in up to 10% solutions, guaifenesin in up to 15% solutions, and chloral hydrate in up to 7% solutions

    C. Due to the extreme alkalinity of barbiturate solutions, subcutaneous injections may result in necrosis and sloughing

        1. Thiobarbiturates are *not* injected intramuscularly or subcutaneously

V. Dose is calculated based on lean body mass (body weight minus fat)

BARBITURATE ANESTHESIA

I. Classification of barbiturates according to duration of action

    A. Long: many hours (8-12)

    B. Intermediate: several hours (2-6)

    C. Short: 45 minutes to 1.5 hours

    D. Ultrashort: 5-15 minutes

II. Official Names

	Approximate duration of action
Phenobarbital sodium	Long
Barbital sodium	Long
Amobarbital sodium	Intermediate
Pentobarbitol sodium	Short (see Table 8-1)
Secobarbital sodium	Short
Thiopental sodium	Ultrashort
Thiamylal sodium	Ultrashort
Thialbarbitone sodium	Ultrashort
Methohexital	Ultrashort

III. General anesthetic actions of barbiturates

    A. Effects on the central nervous system

        1. All degrees of central nervous system depression can be produced, from drowsiness and mild sedation to coma

        2. Response to barbiturate anesthesia

            a. Pentobarbital sodium and the ultrashort-acting barbiturates decrease cerebral blood flow (CBF), metabolic rate ($CMRO_2$), and neuronal activity of the brain (e.g., dog). The $CBF/CMRO_2$ ratio is unchanged or increased. There are minimal changes in CSF pressure

T A B L E   8 - 1

INTRAVENOUS (mg/lb) DRUGS COMMONLY USED TO PRODUCE ANESTHESIA OF SHORT DURATION

Agent	Horse	Dog	Cat	Pig	Cow	Goat
1. Thiamylal	3-5	4-6	4-6	4-6	2-5	2-5
2. Thiopental	3-5	4-6	4-6	4-6	2-5	2-5
3. Etomidate	—	0.5-2.0	0.5-2.0	0.5-2.0	—	—
4. Guaifenesin	30-60	20-40	—	20-40	30-60	30-60
5. Chloral hydrate	—	—	—	6-9 g/100 lb	6-10 g/100 lb	6-10 g/100 lb
6. Ketamine	—	—	1-3	1-3	—	1-3
7. Telazol	—	2.0-5.0	1.0-5.0	2.0-5.0	2.0-5.0	1.0-5.0
8. Guaifenesin	20-40	15-40	—	15-40	20-40	20-40
Thiamylal	1-3	1-3	—	1-3	1-3	—
9. Guaifenesin	20-40	15-40	—	—	20-40	—
Ketamine	0.5-0.7	0.5	—	—	0.3-0.5	0.3-0.5
10. Chloral hydrate (7% soln.)	10 ml/100 lb*	—	—	20-30 ml/100 lb	20-30 ml/100 lb	20-30 ml/100 lb
11. Chloropent	10ml/100 lb	—	—	—	10 ml/100 lb	10 ml/100 lb
Thiamylal	1-3	—	—	—	1-3	1-3
12. Acepromazine	—	0.1	0.2	0.2	—	—
Ketamine	—	5.0	1-3	1-3	—	—
13. Xylazine	0.5	0.3	0.3	0.3	0.04	0.02
Ketamine	0.5-1.0	3	1-3	1-3	1-3	1-3
14. Xylazine	0.5	0.2	0.3	—	0.05	0.04
Telazol	0.5-1.0	3	1-3	—	1-3	1-3
15. Diazepam	—	0.15	0.2	0.1	0.1	—
Ketamine	—	2-3	2-3	2-3	2-3	—
16. Innovar-Vet	—	1 ml/30 lb	—	1 ml/40 lb	—	—
Pentobarbital	—	1-3	—	1-3	—	—
17. Xylazine, Guaifenesin, Ketamine	(See Chapter 20)					

*Sedative dose

   b. Barbiturates minimally depress arterial blood pressure and intracranial pressure; cerebral perfusion pressure is increased
   c. Usually used to produce a general anesthesia (short) or to induce (ultrashort) a patient to surgical anesthesia
   d. Barbiturates are universally poor analgesics at subhypnotic dosages
B. Organ system effects and responses
   1. Action on the respiratory system
      a. Barbiturates are major respiratory depressants
         (1) They depress respiratory centers in the medulla and the mechanisms responsible for the characteristic rhythmic pattern of respiratory movement (apneustic and pneumotaxic centers)
         (2) The degree of respiratory depression is related to dose and rate of administration
      b. Coughing, sneezing, hiccoughing, and laryngospasm occur frequently. These effects are caused by excessive salivary secretion and may be minimized with proper preanesthetic medication (atropine, glycopyrrolate)
         (1) Laryngospasm is one of the chief respiratory complications of barbiturate anesthesia in dogs and cats
         (2) Short periods of apnea frequently occur after intravenous bolus administration
      c. When respiratory arrest occurs, attention should be directed toward establishing an airway and ventilating the patient
         (1) Respiratory stimulants may be necessary if the animal does not begin to ventilate spontaneously
   2. Effects on the cardiovascular system
      a. Barbiturates produce significant cardiovascular effects when given as a bolus or in extremely large dosages
      b. Cardiac arrhythmias may occur
         (1) Thiobarbiturates sensitize the heart to epinephrine and induce autonomic imbalance. Arrhythmias, particularly ventricular extrasystoles and bigeminy, are seen with ultrashort-acting barbiturates much more frequently than with short-acting barbiturates
         (2) During induction to anesthesia, thiobarbiturates increase both parasympathetic and sympathetic tone. This may lead to atrial or ventricular arrhythmias; sinus bradycardia; or first-, second-, or third-degree heart block and cardiac arrest
         (3) Thiobarbiturates may produce transient episodes of ventricular extrasystoles and ventricular bigeminy
      c. Barbiturates may cause a transient fall in blood pressure. If the patient is already in a state of surgical anesthesia, small doses of a barbiturate may cause dramatic decreases in cardiac contractility and arterial blood pressure

(1) Barbiturates should be administered slowly to shock patients
(2) Concentrations greater than 4% are toxic to tissues and may injure the capillary musculature, causing capillary dilation and vascular shock
(3) Thiobarbiturates may cause an initial increase in blood pressure due to tachycardia and an increase in peripheral vascular resistance caused by increases in sympathetic tone
3. Actions on the gastrointestinal tract
   a. Depress intestinal motility
      (1) Thiobarbiturates may depress GI tract motility initially, then increase both tonus and motility
   b. Diarrhea or intestinal stasis is generally not observed at recommended dosages
4. Kidney and liver
   a. No direct effect on the kidney has been observed unless large dosages are given, which may decrease renal blood flow
      (1) Systemic hypotension may cause a cessation in urine production
   b. Single administrations at therapeutic doses have no effect on liver function
      (1) In patients with liver damage, large doses may cause injury
5. Effects on the uterus and fetus
   a. Barbiturates readily diffuse across the placenta into the fetal circulation
      (1) Thiopental reaches mixed fetal cord blood within 45 seconds
   b. Doses of barbiturates that do not produce anesthesia in the mother can completely inhibit fetal respiratory movements
IV. Absorption, fate, and excretion
  A. Absorption
    1. Barbiturates are absorbed readily from the GI tract after oral administration
    2. Intravenous administration
      a. IV administration should be attempted with adequate provisions available to support respiration and circulation
      b. Short-acting barbiturates require approximately 5-10 minutes to produce maximal CNS effect after their intravenous administration
      c. Ultrashort-acting barbiturates attain maximum concentration in the brain within 30 seconds of administration
  B. Fate
    1. Barbiturates are eliminated by renal excretion and/or destroyed by oxidative activity of hepatic tissues
    2. The amount of active (non-ionized, non-protein-bound) drug present is increased by acidosis
    3. Redistribution: Ultrashort-acting barbiturates are greatly dependent on redistribution of drug to lean body tissues (muscle) for their duration of action

      a. Emergence from sleep depends on shift from brain to other tissues

      b. Muscle and skin become saturated about 15-30 minutes after thiobarbiturate injection

      c. Saturation of fat may take several hours

      d. Repeated doses have a cumulative effect

      e. Extremely thin, heavily muscled animals (e.g., greyhounds, whippets) demonstrate prolonged recoveries (3-5 hours) from thiobarbiturate anesthesia

      f. Obesity retards drug elimination because of high solubility of barbiturates in fat

      g. "Acute tolerance" is rarely observed with the administration of thiobarbiturates in people, horses, and dogs. The mechanism is unknown. Alternative anesthetic techniques should be used if this occurs

C. Excretion

   1. Long-acting barbiturates are excreted in the urine over a period of several days

      a. Severe toxicity depression and coma may occur when used in patients with renal disease

   2. Hepatic metabolism

      a. The barbiturates are metabolized by both hepatic and extrahepatic mechanisms

      b. Oxybarbiturates are transformed primarily by the liver

      c. Liver disease may prolong drug's duration of action. Avoid using short-acting barbiturates in presence of liver disease

      d. Hypothermia and depressed cardiovascular function may prolong hepatic metabolism of barbiturates

V. Dosage and administration of specific barbiturate drugs

A. Pentobarbital sodium (Nembutal)

   1. Oral administration: neither safe nor practical for dog or cat

   2. Intravenous anesthetic dose varies from 3 to 13 mg/lb of body weight depending upon the type and amount of preanesthetic medication

      a. When administered as the only source of anesthesia, approximately half the anticipated dose should be injected, the rest to effect

   3. Morphine or other preanesthetic drugs prior to barbiturates make the animal easier to handle and decrease the dose of barbiturates

   4. Provides good surgical anesthesia. May be used in combination with other anesthetics to produce surgical anesthesia

   5. Complete recovery occurs in 8-24 hours

   6. Atropine sulfate or glycopyrrolate decrease salivary secretions, the potential for laryngospasms, and vagal activity

   7. The minimum lethal dose (MLD) in dogs is 23 mg/lb IV

   8. The anesthetic duration can be prolonged by administration of 50% glucose IV. This is termed the *glucose effect*

   9. Overdose is treated by cardiopulmonary support, respiratory stimulants, alkalinizing the patient, and diuresis

B. Thiopental sodium (Pentothal) and thiamylal sodium (Surital, Biotal)
  1. Used as a 2-10% solution
     a. Solution should be destroyed after being stored for 3 days at room temperature. Precipitated solutions should not be used
     b. More concentrated solutions cause severe tissue damage if accidentally administered subcutaneously
  2. Thiamylal is similar to thiopental, but slightly more potent (1.5 times). Therefore, it is potentially more toxic than thiopental on a mg/mg basis
  3. Subcutaneous injection causes necrosis of tissue
     a. Tissue necrosis may be minimized by infiltrating the area with saline. Pain can be minimized by injecting 2% lidocaine
  4. Given to effect intravenously to produce anesthesia (3-8 mg/lb) for induction to anesthesia
  5. Calculate dose on lean body weight
  6. Dose for induction and intubation: 4-6 mg/lb of body weight. Solutions up to 10% are used in the horse
     a. Repeated doses have a cumulative effect, resulting in prolonged recovery from anesthesia
  7. Anesthesia usually occurs in 20-60 seconds
  8. Ventricular arrhythmias are occasionally observed following induction to anesthesia
  9. Apnea is commonly associated with rapid IV injections. Ventilation should be supported early in anesthesia
  10. Recovery occurs in 10-30 minutes, but the animal may remain depressed for many hours depending on dose. Cumulative effect with repeated doses
  11. Overdose is best treated with continuous O_2 controlled ventilation and alkalinization of the plasma and urine
C. Methohexital (Brevane)
  1. Similar to other ultrashort-acting drugs, only not as cumulative (rapidly metabolized)
  2. Preferred in slight hounds (greyhounds, whippets, borzois, etc.) due to the prolonged effect produced by thiobarbiturates in these breeds
  3. 3-7 mg/lb provides light anesthesia in small animals
  4. Duration: 5-10 minutes
  5. Respiratory depression and apnea are common
  6. Recovery may be accompanied by pronounced involuntary excitement and convulsions (emergence delirium). CNS effects are prevented by diazepam (0.1 mg/lb)
  7. Not routinely used in large animals. Occasionally used in cattle

NONBARBITURATE ANESTHESIA

I. Specific nonbarbiturate drugs
  A. Etomidate (Amidate)
     1. An ultrashort-acting, nonbarbiturate intravenous anesthetic

2. General anesthetic actions
   a. Produces hypnosis (sleep), minimal analgesia at subhypnotic doses
   b. Produces depression of the brainstem reticular formation
   c. Enhancement of monosynaptic reflex activity may result in myoclonal activity
   d. Decreases CBF and $CMRO_2$; $CBF/CMRO_2$ increases
3. System effects and responses
   a. Respiratory system
      (1) Tidal volume and respiratory rate are minimally affected during anesthetic maintenance. Respiration may increase
      (2) Brief periods of apnea may occur immediately after intravenous injections
   b. Cardiovascular system
      (1) Produces little change in heart rate, arterial blood pressure, and cardiac output when administered at induction dosages
      (2) Cardiac contractility is mildly depressed
      (3) Etomidate does not sensitize the myocardium to catecholamine-induced cardiac arrhythmias
      (4) Etomidate does not produce histamine release
   c. Gastrointestinal system
      (1) Nausea and vomiting are occasionally observed during induction and following anesthesia
      (2) Minimal effects on GI motility
   d. Endocrine system
      (1) Produces an antiglucocorticoid and mineralocorticoid effect. ACTH stimulation tests and glucose tolerance tests may be invalid.
      (2) Adrenocorticoid function is suppressed for 2-3 hrs in dogs after a single intravenous administration of etomidate
4. Fate and excretion
   a. Rapidly distributed to the brain, heart, spleen, lung, liver, and intestine
   b. Anesthetic duration of action is dependent on drug redistribution and capacity—limited ester hydrolysis by the liver
   c. No cumulative effect; acquired tolerance has not been demonstrated after repeated administrations
5. Other
   a. Produces good muscle relaxation during anesthesia. Involuntary muscle movements and myoclonic reactions occur during induction and recovery
   b. Does not trigger malignant hyperthermia in susceptible pigs, but predisposes susceptible pigs to a more rapid onset of malignant hyperthermia if triggered by other drugs
   c. Pain may occur during intravenous injection
   d. Decreases intraocular pressure

    6. Clinical uses

       a. Short-term (5-10 minutes) anesthesia in the dog and cat. Etomidate produces excessive muscle ridigity and seizures in horses and cattle

       b. As an induction agent for general anesthesia

    7. Dosages

       a. 0.25-1.5 mg/lb IV in dogs and cats

       b. The best results are obtained after sedating the animal with diazepam, xylazine, or acepromazine

B. Chloral hydrate

    1. Chemistry

       a. Physical properties

          (1) Colorless, translucent crystals that volatilize on exposure to air

       b. Chemical properties

          (1) Readily soluble in both water and oil

          (2) Largely reduced to trichloroethanol in the body

          (3) Bitter, caustic taste; quite irritating to the skin and mucous membranes

    2. General anesthetic actions

       a. Sedative-hypnotic, depressing the cerebral cortex, resulting in hyporeflexia

       b. Central nervous system depression believed to be due to trichloroethanol. CBF is decreased or unchanged; $CMRO_2$ is decreased

       c. Subanesthetic doses depress motor and sensory nerves and produce mild sedation

       d. Anesthetic doses produce deep sleep lasting for several hours; recovery is prolonged (6-24 hours)

       e. A poor analgesic at subhypnotic doses. Excitement or delirium occur upon painful stimulation

    3. System effects and responses

       a. Respiratory system

          (1) Hypnotic doses depress both respiratory rate and tidal volume

          (2) Anesthetic doses markedly depress ventilation through depression of the respiratory centers. Death is usually caused by progressive respiratory center depression

       b. Cardiovascular system

          (1) Anesthetic doses produce depression of the myocardium (decreased contractility)

          (2) Potentiates vagal (parasympathetic) activity, causing bradycardia, P-R interval prolongation, and sinus arrest or A-V block

          (3) Supraventricular arrhythmias and transient period of atrial fibrillation have been observed after chloral hydrate anesthesia in horses

       c. Gastrointestinal system

          (1) Increases gastrointestinal secretions and motility due to parasympathomimetic effect; diarrhea may occur following anesthesia

        (2) Induces nausea and vomiting, salivation, and defecation when given orally

    d. Liver and kidney

        (1) Effects on these systems appear to be secondary to parasympathetic and cardiovascular effects

    e. Uterus and fetus

        (1) Will readily cross the placenta

  4. Absorption, fate, and excretion

    a. May be administered orally, rectally, intravenously, or intraperitoneally; very irritating if given perivascularly, intramuscularly, or intraperitoneally

    b. A small amount is excreted unchanged in the urine. The majority is reduced to trichloroethanol, a less potent hypnotic, and then conjugated with glycluronic acid, after which it is excreted in the urine

  5. Clinical uses

    a. Chloral hydrate is frequently used as a sedative and adjunct to surgical anesthesia in horses and cattle. The dosage for anesthesia is variable (100-300 mg/lb)

    b. Casting harnesses or hobbles are generally necessary

    c. Generally used in combination with pentobarbital and magnesium sulfate

    d. Pharmaceutical companies no longer supply chloral hydrate for veterinary use, but it can be obtained from chemical companies (Sigma, Aldrich).

  6. Dosage

    a. Sedation: 1-3 g/100 lb

    b. Anesthesia: 6-10 g/100 lb

C. Guaifenesin (glyceryl guaiacolate)

  1. Chemistry

    a. Physical properties

        (1) A white, finely granular powder that is soluble in water

    b. Chemical properties

        (1) A common decongestant and antitussive also noted for its muscle relaxant properties

        (2) Very similar to mephenesin chemically. Mephenesin is an aromatic glycerol ether

  2. General anesthetic actions

    a. Guaifenesin blocks impulse transmission at the internuncial neurons of the spinal cord and brainstem

    b. Produces *relaxation of skeletal muscles*, but does not affect function of the diaphragm

    c. Relaxes both laryngeal and pharyngeal muscles, thus potentiating intubation of the trachea

    d. Potentiates other preanesthetic and anesthetic agents and is compatible with them

e. Produces excitement-free induction and recovery from anesthesia

f. Excessive doses produce a paradoxical increase in muscle rigidity

3. System effects and responses

a. Respiratory system

(1) Little, if any, effect on overall respiration

(2) Ventilatory rate may be increased initially, with decreases in tidal volume

(3) Excessive doses produce an apneustic pattern of breathing

b. Cardiovascular system

(1) Initial mild decrease in blood pressure, which returns to normal

(2) Myocardial contractile force and cardiac rate are relatively unchanged

c. Gastrointestinal system

(1) Increases gastrointestinal motility, but does not appear to abnormally affect the function of this organ system or that of the liver or kidney

d. Uterus and fetus

(1) Guaifenesin will cross the placental barrier, but appears to have minimal effects on the fetus

4. Absorption, fate, and excretion

a. Excreted in the urine after conjugation in the liver to a glucuronide

5. Clinical uses

a. Used for restraint and muscle relaxation in large and small animal species

b. Used for short anesthetic procedures of up to 30-60 minute duration

c. Used as a 5, 10, or 15% solution. High concentrations (> 10%) may cause hemolysis and hemoglobinuria in cattle. Solutions greater than 15% cause hives, hemolysis, and apneustic breathing in horses

d. Often made by mixing 50 g of guaifenesin with 50 g of dextrose and 1 L warm sterile water

e. Guaifenesin is compatible with other intravenous and inhalation anesthetic drugs

6. Dosage

a. The dose varies from 30 to 70 mg/lb

b. Guaifenesin may be administered to effect in 1 L solutions with the following agents

(1) 5% or 10% guaifenesin, 2 g thiamylal or thiopental

(2) 5% or 10% guaifenesin, 2.5 g pentobarbital

c. The margin of safety is three times the therapeutic dose

d. Excessive dosages cause muscle ridigity and an apneustic pattern of breathing

DISSOCIOGENIC AGENTS

I. This group includes the cyclohexamines, of which *ketamine*, *phencyclidine*, and *tiletamine* are members

A. Anesthesia is characterized by profound *amnesia, superficial analgesia* and *catalepsy*
   1. Oral, ocular, and swallowing reflexes remain intact and muscle tone generally increases
      a. Large doses of these agents produce convulsions. This can be controlled with small doses of Na^+ pentobarbital, thiobarbiturates, or diazepam
B. Psychosomatic effects such as hallucinations, confusion, agitation, and fear have occurred in humans and seem to occur in animals
C. Muscle rigidity can be minimized by the addition of small doses of tranquilizers, barbiturates, or benzodiazepines (diazepam)
D. Effects are partially reversed by adrenergic and cholinergic blockade
E. Specific agents
   1. The most commonly used cyclohexamine is ketamine HCl (Vetalar, Ketaset). Telazol (tiletamine-zolazepam drug combination) is gaining popularity (see Table 8-1)
   2. Ketamine increases CBF and causes no change or an increase in $CMRO_2$; the $CBF/CMRO_2$ ratio increases. Arterial blood pressure and intracranial pressure increase; cerebral perfusion pressure decreases
      a. Used for restraint and minor surgical procedures
      b. Palpebral, conjunctival, corneal, and swallowing reflexes persist. Nystagmus is common
   3. Telazol, a 1:1 drug combination of zolazepam and tiletamine, is being investigated as a dissociogenic drug combination for use in all species of animals. It may be very useful in exotic animals
   4. Tiletamine produces the most profound central nervous system side effects. Although it possesses anticonvulsant activity, tremors, oculogyria, tonic spasticity, and convulsions occur when excessive dosages are administered
F. Salivation and lacrimation may become copious
G. Analgesia is selective, with the best results obtained in superficial pain models. Visceral pain is not abolished
H. Muscle relaxation is poor. Ketamine and other cyclohexamines should be used with muscle relaxants to produce the best effects
I. Animals are hyper-responsive and ataxic during recovery (emergence delirium has occurred)
J. System effects and responses
   1. Respiratory system
      a. Apneustic pattern of breathing; respiratory rate may be increased; arterial PO_2 generally falls after intravenous administration
      b. Possible increases in PCO_2 and decreases in arterial pH due to the irregular pattern of breathing
   2. Cardiovascular system
      a. Increased heart rate
      b. Increased blood pressure
      c. Decreased cardiac contractility

       d. Ketamine and other cyclohexamines minimally sensitize the heart to catecholamine-induced arrhythmias

   3. Kidney and liver

      a. Ketamine HCl is metabolized by the liver and excreted unchanged by the kidneys.

         (1) Ketamine should be used with caution in animals with hepatic or renal disease. Ketamine can be used in cats with urethral obstruction, provided renal disease is absent or not severe and the obstruction is eliminated

K. Dose range of ketamine

   1. Cat: 2-15 mg/lb IM or s.c.; 0.5-1.0 mg/lb IV. Doses as small as 1.0-3.0 mg *total* are administered IV to sick animals and cats with urethral obstruction

   2. Dog: xylazine 0.3 mg/lb IV and ketamine 3-5 mg/lb IV; diazepam 0.15 mg/lb IV and ketamine 2.5 mg/lb IV

   3. Pigs: 2-10 mg/lb IM of ketamine may be used with thiamylal following Innovar-Vet 1 ml/80 lb IM or azaperone 1 mg/lb IM

CHAPTER NINE

Inhalation Anesthesia

"O sleep! O gentle sleep!
Nature's soft nurse, how have I frightened thee,
That thou no more wilt weigh my eyelids down
and steep my senses in forgetfulness?"

WILLIAM SHAKESPEARE

OVERVIEW

Inhalational anesthetic drugs are used to produce general anesthesia. They are suitable for use in all species, including reptiles, birds, and both domestic and zoo animals. Their safe use requires knowledge, not only of their pharmacologic effects, but of their physical chemical properties. Ideally, these drugs should produce unconsciousness (hypnosis), hyporeflexia, and analgesia. The ideal inhalation anesthetic should be easy to control, should permit rapid induction and recovery from anesthesia, and should contain no adverse side effects. This section outlines the basic principles of inhalational anesthetic uptake and distribution.

GENERAL CONSIDERATIONS

I. Inhalation agents are vapors or gases administered directly into the respiratory system
II. They must be absorbed from the alveoli into the bloodstream and pass to the brain in order to produce a cortical tension (partial pressure) in the brain
III. Inhalation anesthetics are not primarily dependent on body detoxification mechanisms for the duration of clinical effect but are relatively rapidly eliminated by the lungs

IV. Because of the relative rapidity of uptake and elimination, there is good control of the depth of anesthesia, but constant patient monitoring is required

PROPERTIES OF A DESIRABLE GENERAL ANESTHETIC

See Table 9-1
I. Nonirritant and free from disagreeable odors
II. Potent: produces pleasant, rapid induction and rapid recovery
III. Produces adequate muscular relaxation and analgesia for surgical procedures
IV. Should not promote capillary bleeding
V. Wide margin of safety—potentially reversible or easily controlled
VI. Easily and inexpensively produced
VII. Not explosive; stable during storage
VIII. Nontoxic to the patient and to human personnel

FACTORS CONTROLLING THE BRAIN TENSION OF VOLATILE ANESTHETIC

I. Factors governing production and delivery of a suitable concentration of anesthetic for inhalation
  A. Physical and chemical properties of the agent
    1. Vapor pressure of the agent governs the volatility of the agent
    2. Boiling points for inhalation agents (other than nitrous oxide) are higher than room temperature (70° F or 27° C)
  B. Anesthetic system
    1. The concentrations delivered to the patient depend on the type of anesthetic system, fresh gas flow rate, type of vaporizer, and other equipment
    2. Frequent inspection and maintenance is necessary to prevent malfunctions due to leaks, sticky valves, etc.
II. Factors responsible for delivery of inhalation anesthetic to lungs and alveoli
  A. The partial pressure of inhalation anesthetic in the brain is directly controlled by the alveolar partial pressure of anesthetic. The alveolar level of anesthetic is the result of: (1) delivery of anesthetic to the lungs, and (2) uptake from the lungs. Delivery to the lungs is dependent on: (1) inspired concentration, and (2) level of alveolar ventilation
  B. Inspired concentration
    1. Concentration effect: the higher the inspired concentration administered, the more rapid the rate of rise in alveolar concentration
    2. *Second gas effect:* Passive increase in inspired ventilation due to rapid uptake of *either* large volumes of a less blood-soluble agent (e.g., nitrous oxide) *or* smaller volumes of a highly blood-soluble agent (e.g., ether or, potentially, methoxyflurane) may have secondary consequence when a second gas is given concomitantly (e.g., halothane). This increase in alveolar ventilation accelerates the *rate of rise* of the second gas regardless of its concentration
    3. The net result of a 50-80% flow of nitrous oxide is to augment the inflow and accelerate the uptake of a low concentration of a second gas (e.g., halothane) in the inspired mixture

TABLE 9-1

BOILING POINTS, VAPOR PRESSURES, AND VAPORIZATION OF INHALATION AGENTS

Drug	Boiling point (°C)	Vapor pressure at 20°C (torr/mm Hg)	Maximum concentration of vapor delivered by saturation vaporizer at 20°C (%)	Useful ranges of concentration (agent used alone) (%)	
				Induction (%)	Maintenance (%)
Volatile anesthetics:					
Ether	36	443	58	10-40	3-12
Isoflurane	48	252	33	2-6	1-3
Halothane	50	243	32	1-4*	0.5-2
Enflurane	57	180	24	3-7	1-3
Methoxyflurane	105	24	3	Up to 3	0.25-1
Anesthetic gases:					
Nitrous oxide	−89	39,500 (50 atm)			
Cyclopropane	−33	4,800 (6 atm)			

*Up to 5% may be used in induction of large animals.

C. Alveolar ventilation
1. Generally, the greater the ventilation, the more rapid the approach of the alveolar gas level to the inspired gas level (see Eger EI (ed): *Anesthetic Uptake and Action*, Baltimore, Williams and Wilkins, 1974.
2. Limited by lung volume; the larger the functional residual capacity (FRC), the longer it takes to wash in a new gas
3. Large increases in alveolar ventilation may decrease cerebral blood flow, thus slowing induction
4. Factors affecting ventilation
   a. Decreased tidal volume as a result of drug-induced respiratory depression
   b. Increased dead space (anatomical and physiologic) during anesthesia will decrease effective alveolar ventilation
   c. Effective alveolar ventilation is dependent upon a patent airway

III. Factors responsible for uptake of anesthetic from the lungs
A. Solubility: This term describes how an anesthetic is distributed between two phases (e.g., between blood and gas, between tissue and blood). Solubility is usually expressed as a partition coefficient. Ostwald's partition coefficient between blood and gas is commonly used to describe anesthetic uptake in terms of solubility:

Agent	Blood/gas partition coefficient (Ostwald's coefficient)
Diethyl ether	15.2
Methoxyflurane	13.0
Halothane	2.36
Enflurane	1.91
Isoflurane	1.41
Nitrous oxide	0.49
Cyclopropane	0.42

[handwritten: 15.2 blood / 1 alveoli]

A gas with a blood-gas partition coefficient of 2 will have *one* volume in the alveoli per *two* volumes in the blood at equilibrium
1. Anesthetic solubility and anesthetic uptake are not the same as potency, but they are primary determinants of the rapidity of onset of anesthetic effect
2. The greater the blood/gas partition coefficient, the greater the uptake of anesthetic by blood. Tension of anesthetic in arterial blood, therefore, rises slowly for drugs with high blood/gas coefficients. Onset of clinical effect is dependent on a tension of anesthetic developing in the blood sufficient for transfer of anesthetic to the brain. Very soluble agents, such as methoxyflurane, have long induction and recovery periods because large amounts of anesthetic must be taken into the blood before the tension or partial pressure of the anesthetic rises. Clinically, slow induction may be overcome by raising the inspired concentrations to levels in excess of those necessary to maintain anesthesia

[handwritten margin note: Rapid uptake by blood ≠ rapid rise of tension in blood. If its very soluble in blood, it won't be transferred well to brain.]

3. The lower the blood/gas partition coefficient, the less soluble the agent (only small quantities are carried in the blood; thus both alveolar concentration and tension will rise rapidly). Less soluble agents, such as nitrous oxide and isoflurane have relatively short induction and short recovery periods

4. Drugs with high blood/gas partition coefficients exhibit long induction and recovery times, whereas drugs with low blood/gas partition coefficients exhibit short induction and recovery times

B. Cardiac output: Blood carries anesthetic from the lungs; thus the greater the cardiac output, the greater the uptake of anesthetic and the slower the rate of rise of alveolar concentration and tension. Thus the greater the cardiac output, the slower the rate of induction. Animals with depressed cardiac output may be induced very rapidly. Changes in cardiac output will have the greatest effect on the most soluble agents (e.g., methoxyflurane)

C. Alveolar-venous anesthetic tension difference: During induction, tissues remove nearly all the anesthetic brought to them. Venous blood returning to the lungs contains little anesthetic; thus there is maximal anesthetic uptake. As time passes, increasing tissue saturation raises the venous blood concentration, and less anesthetic is taken up in the lungs. However, anesthetic uptake is continuous

D. Shunts
   1. Right-to-left intracardiac or intrapulmonary shunts (e.g., Fallot's tetralogy) delay induction; important for poorly soluble agents (nitrous oxide)
   2. Body shunts (left to right) may speed the rate of induction if cardiac output is low; endotoxic shock mimics a body shunt

E. Pathological changes in alveoli: If the alveolar membranes are affected by changes resulting in exudate, transudate, emphysema, or pulmonary fibrosis, diffusion may be impaired. Uptake of anesthetic will thus be reduced

IV. Factors governing brain and tissue uptake of anesthetic
   A. Same as those determining uptake from the lungs
      1. Tissue blood flow
      2. Solubility (tissue/blood)
      3. Arterial blood–tissue anesthetic tension difference
   B. The uptake by tissue is primarily dependent on blood flow to that tissue and its capillary density. Tissues can be divided into four groups according to blood supply
      1. Vessel rich group (VRG): 75% cardiac output (e.g., brain, heart, intestine, liver, kidney, spleen)
      2. Vessel moderate group, or muscle group (MG): 15-20% cardiac output (e.g., muscle, skin)
      3. Neutral fat group (FG): 5% cardiac output (e.g., adipose tissue)
      4. Vessel poor group (VPG): 1-2% cardiac output (e.g., bone, tendons, cartilage)
   C. Tissue/blood partition coefficients vary far less than blood/gas coefficients (except for fat)

1. Lowest is about 1 (nitrous oxide in lung tissue)
2. Highest is about 4 (halothane in muscle tissue)

D. Important considerations
1. Equilibration of an anesthetic agent in the VRG is complete in 5-20 minutes
2. Equilibration in the MG may take $1^1/2$-4 hours
3. Arterial-tissue partial pressure difference, and thus uptake, decreases far more rapidly in VRG than in MG
4. Solubility of an inhalation agent in VRG and MG may affect recovery time
5. The fat group occupies 10-30% of body mass and receives about 5% of the cardiac output. The FG has a higher tissue solubility for inhalation anesthetics than most other tissues, and thus has a greater and more prolonged capacity to absorb anesthetic. Due to its low blood flow, the fat group has little effect on induction of anesthesia. The FG may affect recovery time after prolonged anesthetic periods (over 4 hours)

Fat/blood partition coefficient

Diethyl ether	4.2
Methoxyflurane	61.0
Halothane	65.0
Enflurane	37.0
Isoflurane	48.0
Nitrous oxide	2.3
Cyclopropane	15.0

6. VPG tissues have very little effect on anesthesia
7. Rubber solubility: Agents such as halothane and methoxyflurane are freely absorbed into rubber components of the anesthetic system. During recovery, they will be excreted back into the anesthetic circuitry

ELIMINATION OF INHALATION ANESTHETICS

I. By lung
A. Inhalation anesthetics are excreted largely unchanged by the lungs
B. The same factors that affect the rate of anesthetic uptake are important in anesthetic elimination
1. Pulmonary ventilation
2. Blood flow
3. Solubility in blood and tissue
C. As anesthetic gas washes out of the lungs, the arterial blood tension falls first, followed by that in tissues. Because of the high blood flow to the brain, its tension of anesthetic gas falls rapidly and accounts for the rapid awakening from anesthesia with insoluble agents such as N_2O. Release from other tissues is progressively slower and dependent on blood flow
II. Other routes through which small quantities of inhalation anesthetic agent may be excreted: skin, milk, mucous membrane, urine

TABLE 9-2

MINIMAL ALVEOLAR CONCENTRATION OF INHALATION ANESTHETICS IN VARIOUS SPECIES

	Human	Dog	Cat	Horse
Diethyl ether	1.92	3.04	2.10	—
Methoxyflurane	0.16	0.29	0.23	0.22
Halothane	0.76	0.87	1.19	0.88
Enflurane	1.68	2.06	2.40	2.12
Isoflurane	1.2	1.30	1.63	1.31
Nitrous oxide	101.0	188-200	150.0	190.0

Modified from Eger EI (ed): *Anesthetic Uptake and Action.* Baltimore, Williams and Wilkins, 1974, p 5.

III. Biotransformation
   A. Anesthetic gases are metabolized in the body to variable degrees.
   B. Metabolism is generally by hepatic microsomal enzyme systems. Various intermediate metabolites are formed. These may be responsible for certain toxic effects or after effects
      1. Approximately 10-20% of inspired halothane is metabolized, compared to up to 50% of methoxyflurane. Approximately 2.5% of enflurane and 0.25% of isoflurane are metabolized.
      2. Toxic metabolites are primarily inorganic fluoride and bromide ions
IV. Diffusion hypoxia
   A. This effect may occur at the end of anesthesia and will be described in the discussion of nitrous oxide (see Chapter 10: Pharmacology of Inhalation Anesthetic Drugs). Briefly, the rapid elimination of N_2O from the blood into the alveoli results in the dilution of alveolar oxygen and hypoxemia if ventilation is not maintained

POTENCY OF INHALATION ANESTHETICS

   I. Anesthetic potency can be expressed in several ways. One commonly accepted method is to measure the minimum alveolar concentration (MAC) of the inhalation anesthetic (Table 9-2). MAC is the minimum alveolar concentration of an anesthetic, at 1 atmosphere, that produces no response in 50% of patients exposed to a painful stimulus
   A. MAC is generally measured as the end-tidal concentration of anesthetic
   B. MAC values are not vaporizer settings
   C. MAC values are used to compare the potency of anesthetics
   II. MAC values vary with species and with:
   A. Age—aged patients require less inhalation anesthetic
   B. Temperature—hypothermia reduces MAC
   C. Administration of other CNS depressants
   D. Disease
      1. Hyper- or hypothyroidism
      2. Hypovolemia, anemia

       3. Septicemia

       4. Extreme acid-base imbalances

    E. Pregnancy

III. Studies using dogs suggest that:

    A. 1.0 × MAC: produces light anesthesia

    B. 1.5 × MAC: produces moderate surgical anesthesia

    C. 2.0 × MAC: produces deep anesthesia

CHAPTER TEN

Pharmacology of Inhalation Anesthetic Drugs

"Reality is for people who cannot handle drugs."
ANONYMOUS

OVERVIEW

Inhalation anesthetic drugs are pharmacologically active chemicals that cause unconsciousness and changes in organ system function. Their administration requires familiarity with a variety of equipment (vaporizers, flow meters, pressure valves, etc.) needed to vaporize the anesthetic liquid and deliver the anesthetic to the patient. Theoretically, the depth of anesthesia is easily controlled. It is the intent of this chapter to outline the pharmacologic properties and the interactions of inhalation anesthetic drugs.

GENERAL CONSIDERATIONS

I. The ability of an inhalation anesthetic to produce general anesthesia is dependent on its direct membrane effects and physicochemical properties (see Table 10-1)
   A. Factors that influence anesthetic uptake and delivery to the brain include:
      1. Alveolar ventilation
      2. Blood/gas partition coefficient
      3. Cardiac output
      4. Alveolar–to–mixed venous anesthetic partial pressure difference
II. Ventilation/perfusion abnormalities and hypoventilation may hinder the rate of anesthetic induction
III. Left-to-right intracardiac shunts may hinder the rate of anesthetic induction

TABLE 10 - 1

SUMMARY OF PHYSICOCHEMICAL PROPERTIES OF INHALATION AGENTS

Properties	Ether	Nitrous oxide	Halothane	Methoxyflurane	Enflurane	Isoflurane
Chemical formula	$(C_2H_5)_2O$	N_2O	Br F H-C-C-F Cl F	Cl F H H-C-C-O-C-H Cl F H	Cl F F H-C-C-O-C-H F F	F Cl H F-C-C-O-C-H F H F
Molecular weight	74.0	44.0	197.4	165.0	184.5	184.5
Boiling point (at 760 mm of Hg)	36.5° C	−89° C	50.2° C	104.7° C	56.5° C	48.5° C
Specific gravity (g/ml)	0.72	1.53	1.87	1.41	1.52	1.52
Vapor pressure (torr) (at 20° C)	443	39,500	243	24	180	252
Odor	Pungent; unpleasant	Sweet; pleasant	Sweet; pleasant	Fruity; pleasant	Ethereal; pleasant	Pleasant
Preservative	Necessary	Unnecessary	Necessary (thymol)	Necessary (butylated hydroxytoluene)	Unnecessary	Unnecessary
Stability:						
To metal	May react	Nonreactive	May react	May react	Nonreactive	Nonreactive
To alkali	Stable (traces aldehydes)	Stable	Slight decomposition	Stable	Stable	Stable
To UV light	Decomposes	Stable	Decomposes	Decomposes	Stable	Stable
Explosiveness	Explosive (in air or oxygen)	None	None	None	None	None
Partition coefficients	See Chapter 9					
MAC values	See Table 9-2					
Presentation at room temperature	Colorless liquid	Colorless gas (liquid under pressure)	Colorless liquid	Colorless liquid	Colorless liquid	Colorless liquid

IV. Hypothermia decreases the need for anesthesia
V. The anesthetic system used (in-circle vs. out-of-circle) influences anesthetic depth
VI. Inhalation anesthetics produce more than unconsciousness and may markedly change organ system physiology
VII. The metabolites of inhalation anesthetics can be toxic

DIETHYL ETHER (ETHER)

I. Ether was once a frequently used inhalation anesthetic. Its use is now limited to occasional applications in laboratory animals and to make tape sticky
II. Ether is an ideal anesthetic in some respects because it maintains respiration at light levels of anesthesia and minimally depresses cardiac output
III. Ether may cause nausea and vomiting during induction and recovery
IV. Ether is highly flammable and explosive
V. The signs and stages of anesthesia, developed for ether anesthesia, can be loosely applied to other anesthetics (see Table 10-2)
   A. Stage I: the stage of *analgesia* (that period from the beginning of induction to the loss of consciousness)
      1. Disorientation with normal or hyperreflexia are the most common features displayed
      2. Fear and subsequent release of epinephrine with increased heart rate and rapid respirations may occur
      3. Excessive salivation
      4. Urine and feces may be voided
   B. Stage II: a stage of *delirium* or *excitement*, which represents the period of early loss of consciousness
      1. The hazards of stage II are struggling, physical injury, and increased sympathetic tone
      2. Voluntary center controls are abolished
      3. The patient reacts to any sort of external stimuli with exaggerated reflex struggling
      4. Respirations are generally irregular in depth and rate, and breath holding may occur
      5. The eyelids are widely open, and the iris is dilated because of sympathetic stimulation
      6. Reflex vomiting is common unless food has been withheld for 6 or more hours before anesthesia. Defecation and urination may occur
      7. The duration of stage II should be decreased if possible, but there is a maximum limit to the rate of administration of an anesthetic in order not to depress the respiratory center
   C. Stage III
      1. Plane I: marked by the appearance of full rhythmic and mechanical respiration
         a. CO_2 retention during the preceding stages may double tidal volume for the first minute

T A B L E 10 - 2

STAGES OF ETHER ANESTHESIA*

Stage of anesthesia	Respiration	Pupil	Eye movement	Abolition of reflexes	Somatic muscles	Pulse rate and blood pressure (BP)
I. Analgesia	Regular	Normal	Voluntary	All present	Normal tone	Rapid pulse; elevated BP
II. Delirium	Irregular	Dilated	Involuntary	All present	Excited movement	Rapid pulse; elevated BP
III. Surgical Plane I	Increased depth, rate	Constricted	Involuntary fixed	Conjunctival; pharyngeal; cutaneous	Slight relaxation	Normal pulse; normal BP
Plane II	Regular rate, depth	Normal		Laryngeal; corneal; peritoneal	Moderate relaxation	Normal pulse; normal BP
Plane III	Decreased rate, depth	Slightly dilated			Marked relaxation	Rapid, normal, or slow fall in BP
Plane IV	Abdominal breathing	Moderately dilated				Slow, weak pulse; then no pulse; fall in BP to zero

*The classical stages described by A.E. Guedel

b. Preanesthetic medication has a direct bearing on the rate and volume of respiration throughout anesthesia

c. Responses to pain are still present, and minute volume is directly proportional to the amount of stimulation from the operative field

d. Cardiovascular function is only minimally affected

2. Plane II: Tidal volume is usually somewhat decreased; respiratory rate may be increased or decreased. Cardiovascular function is mildly depressed

3. Plane III: Entrance into this plane is marked by the beginning of paralysis of the intercostal muscles

a. Potentially a dangerous level of anesthesia

b. Respiratory depression is marked

c. Cardiovascular function is noticeably depressed, dependent on the specific characteristics of the anesthetic drug used

4. Plane IV: complete paralysis of intercostal muscles

a. Passage into plane IV is marked by cessation of all respiratory effort and dilation of the pupil

b. Cardiovascular function is generally impaired, producing hypotension and decreased cardiac contractility

D. Stage IV

1. Respiratory arrest followed by circulatory collapse

a. Death ensues within 1-5 minutes

NITROUS OXIDE

I. General anesthetic properties (see Table 10-1)

A. A gas at room temperature but readily compressible at 30-50 atm to a colorless liquid. Returns to gaseous state when released from the cylinder to atmospheric pressure

B. Nonflammable but supports combustion by decomposing into nitrogen and oxygen

II. Effect on systems

A. Nervous system

1. Mild analgesic and anesthetic action produced by cerebrocortical depression

2. Dangerous in excessive concentrations due to hypoxia (>70% of total gas flow)

B. Respiratory system

1. Nonirritating to the respiratory tract

2. Cough reflex retained

3. Minimal respiratory depression in the presence of hypoxia; respiratory rate may increase

C. Cardiovascular system

1. Few side effects except in the presence of hypoxia

2. Heart rate, cardiac output, and arterial blood pressure remain relatively unchanged

      3. Tachycardia may develop

      4. Does not sensitize the myocardium to catecholamines

   D. Gastrointestinal system

      1. Ileus may occur secondary to gas accumulation within the gastrointestinal tract

      2. No significant effect on the kidney or liver

   E. Muscular system

      1. Produces no muscle relaxation

      2. Does not potentiate muscle relaxants

   F. Uterus and fetus

      1. Passes placental barrier

      2. Fetal hypoxemia may develop

III. Absorption, fate, and excretion

   A. N_2O rapidly crosses alveolar membranes because of its administration in relatively large inspired concentrations (40-75%)

   B. Nitrous oxide speeds the uptake of inhalation anesthetics (second gas) into the blood (second-gas effect). The enhanced uptake of the second gas is caused by a nitrous oxide–dependent increase in alveolar ventilation

   C. Diffusion into closed air cavities: Nitrous oxide is 30 times more soluble in blood than nitrogen. When nitrous oxide is given in high concentrations (over 50%), it will diffuse into an air-containing cavity faster than nitrogen will diffuse out. If the cavity is closed (e.g., pneumothorax, obstructed bowel, air embolism, blocked paranasal sinuses) and N_2O administered, then either the volume or pressure inside the cavity increases. Volume or pressure increases until the alveolar nitrous oxide ratio is in equilibrium with the closed cavity. The relative volume increase can be calculated using the formula: $M = 100/FiN_2O$. M = magnitude of volume change; FiN_2O = fraction of inspired N_2O. Example: If a patient is exposed to 50% N_2O, $FiN_2O = 50\%$. $M = 100/50 = 2$. Volume will increase by a factor of 2

   D. Does not combine with hemoglobin; and has no value as an O_2 source nor does it form any chemical combinations in body. It is carried in simple solution

   E. Elimination through the lungs is rapid and complete in two minutes

   F. *Diffusion hypoxia*: a result of the low blood/gas partition coefficient. Rapid diffusion of nitrous oxide into the alveoli at the end of anesthesia produces an "alveolar dilution effect"; alveolar oxygen tension may be drastically reduced, especially if the patient is breathing room air. Hypoxia is prevented by giving high flow rates of oxygen for at least 5-10 minutes at end of nitrous oxide administration

   G. Recovery is fast and devoid of unpleasant sequelae

   H. Circumstantial evidence suggests that there is some biotransformation; bone marrow depression may occur after prolonged exposure. Nitrous oxide may be teratogenic especially after prolonged exposure of females in the first trimester of pregnancy

IV. Clinical use
  A. Used as an analgesic in veterinary species
  B. Nitrous oxide adds to the effect of other inhalation anesthetics, so less of these more potent agents is needed to produce general anesthesia
  C. Often used to supplement narcotic or inhalation anesthetic techniques
  D. Hypoxia must be prevented; a minimum of 30% O_2 must be present
  E. The patient should be denitrogenated by administering O_2 at the beginning of the anesthetic period
  F. Closed-circuit administration of N_2O is potentially dangerous because of the low flow rates of nitrous oxide and oxygen used. High flow rates and efficient expiratory valves are essential for safe anesthesia without hypoxia
  G. The ratio of N_2O to O_2 delivered by the anesthetic machine must be continually monitored

V. Dosages
  A. Up to 70% N_2O is used
  B. Maintenance concentrations are usually 66% (N_2O:O_2 = 2:1)
  C. If the patient's cardiopulmonary status deteriorates while receiving nitrous oxide, it should be discontinued
  D. Nitrous oxide is not potent enough in many species to make administration of less than 40% in oxygen worthwhile

HALOTHANE (FLUOTHANE)

I. General anesthetic properties (see Table 10-1)
  A. Nervous system
    1. Central nervous system depression
    2. Depression of body temperature–regulating centers. Hyperpyrexia has been associated with the production of the malignant hyperthermia-stress syndrome in man, pigs, horses, dogs, and cats
    3. Stages of anesthesia are not the same as classical signs described for ether: Pupils may be constricted at all stages, respiration may be shallow but rapid, and the abdominal muscles are relaxed only at deeper planes of anesthesia. The arterial blood pressure may provide the best information about the depth of halothane anesthesia
    4. Cerebral blood flow is increased

II. Effect on systems
  A. Respiratory system
    1. Depressed at all levels of halothane anesthesia
    2. There is less ventilation for any level of $Paco_2$ than in the conscious state, but ventilation is usually adequate
    3. The response to hypercarbia is lost in deeper anesthesia, and ventilation becomes inadequate
    4. Tachypnea may occur; the mechanism is uncertain
    5. Tidal volume is decreased
    6. Respiratory depression is pronounced in ruminants

B. Cardiovascular system
   1. Hypotension occurs, related to the depth of anesthesia
   2. Direct depression of vascular smooth muscle causing vasodilatation (e.g., in cerebral, skeletal muscle, and peripheral tissue) and decreases in total peripheral resistance
   3. Directly depresses myocardium. Cardiac output, stroke volume, and cardiac contractility are all decreased
   4. Decreases efferent sympathetic nervous system activity
   5. Cardiac rate is less consistently affected, but is usually decreased at deeper planes of anesthesia
   6. Sinus node depression and ventricular arrhythmias may be seen, especially if acidosis, hypoxia, or other causes of sympathetic stimulation are present
   7. Halothane sensitizes the heart to catecholamines, occasionally producing cardiac arrhythmias
C. Gastrointestinal system
   1. Motility, tone, and peristalic activity of the intestinal tract are decreased
   2. Liver: A number of reports in man have related halothane with jaundice and postanesthetic fatal liver necrosis. Biotransformation of halothane to hepatotoxic metabolites may produce a hypersensitivity response in a small number of individuals. The effect has not been verified clinically in veterinary species. The effect is believed to be related to halothane administration in conjunction with tissue hypoxia
D. Renal system
   1. No reported nephrotoxic effects other than those resulting from hypotension
E. Muscular system
   1. Relaxation is only moderate in light anesthetic planes
   2. Muscle relaxing agents may be needed if pronounced muscle relaxation is required
   3. Halothane potentiates the action of nondepolarizing muscle relaxants
F. Uterus and fetus
   1. Decreases uterine tone; may decrease uterine involution postpartum
   2. Readily passes placental barrier
III. Absorption, fate, and excretion
   A. Absorption takes place rapidly through the lungs
   B. Up to 12% of inspired halothane is metabolized by liver microsomes. Trifluoroacetic acid and bromide and chloride radicals are produced and excreted in the urine for many hours to days
   C. Metabolites may persist for many days in the liver
   D. The major portion of halothane administered is excreted unchanged via the lungs
IV. Clinical uses
   A. Halothane is one of the most useful anesthetics because it is nonflammable, potent, nonirritating, controllable, and relatively nontoxic

    B. Can be used in all species

    C. Accurate concentrations of halothane can be delivered from precision thermostable or thermocompensated, calibrated vaporizers

    D. Decomposes slowly when exposed to light. It is stored in dark bottles with thymol added as a preservative. Thymol is potentially tissue-toxic

    E. Rebreathing and nonrebreathing techniques can be used

V. Dosage

    A. 2-4% used at induction; up to 5% in large animals. Careful observation must be made to avoid overdosage

    B. Induction time is decreased if nitrous oxide is given concomitantly, due to the second-gas effect

    C. Concurrent use of nitrous oxide reduces the amount of halothane required

    D. Maintenance: 0.5-1.5% in small animals; 1-2% in large animals

METHOXYFLURANE (METOFANE, PENTHRANE)

I. General anesthetic properties (see Table 10-1)

    A. The vapor pressure of methoxyflurane is low. The highest concentrations that can be produced at room temperature are between 2.5% and 3.0%

    B. Nervous system

        1. Potent depressor of the central nervous system

        2. Reticular activating system is depressed

        3. Excitement (delirium) may occur during mask induction of anesthesia

        4. Good muscle relaxation and analgesia

II. Effect on systems

    A. Nervous system

        1. Dose-dependent central nervous system depression

        2. Similar to halothane

    B. Respiratory system

        1. More respiratory depression than halothane

        2. Ventilation may need to be assisted in order to prevent hypercarbia

        3. The rate and depth of spontaneous respiration can be used to monitor the depth of anesthesia

        4. Nonirritating to the respiratory tract

    C. Cardiovascular system

        1. Cardiac depression is similar to halothane, but less intense during spontaneous ventilation

        2. Mild to moderate hypotension in light planes of anesthesia

        3. Cardiac contractility and cardiac output decrease with increasing depth of anesthesia

        4. There may be changes in heart rate (bradycardia) and rhythm similar to effects of halothane

        5. Methoxyflurane sensitizes the heart to catecholamines, but less so than halothane

    D. Gastrointestinal system

        1. Smooth muscle tone and motility are decreased

E. Renal system
   1. Methoxyflurane is incriminated in the production of a high-output renal failure in humans. Polyuria, weight loss, and dehydration may last for days after the anesthetic period. Inorganic fluoride, a metabolite, is thought to be responsible
   2. Acute renal failure has been reported in humans after methoxyflurane anesthesia and is frequently associated with obese patients, those with renal disease, those given concurrent nephrotoxic drugs (tetracyclines, aminoglycosides), or those undergoing extensive surgical procedures
   3. Acute methoxyflurane administration has not produced renal failure in animals except when administered with other nephrotoxic drugs (aminoglycosides, tetracycline, etc.)
F. Muscular system
   1. Excellent muscle relaxation and analgesia at relatively low inspired concentrations
   2. Muscle relaxation is due to drug effects on the central nervous system (spinal cord) rather than the neuromuscular junction
G. Uterus and fetus
   1. Rapidly crosses the placental barrier
   2. Motility and tone are relatively unaffected
III. Absorption, fate, and excretion
   A. Absorption is via the lung
   B. Primarily excreted unchanged by the lung
   C. Up to 50% of absorbed methoxyflurane may be metabolized by the liver. Metabolites include inorganic fluoride
   D. Metabolites are excreted by the kidney
IV. Clinical use
   A. Good muscle relaxation is produced. Potent relaxation is produced; therefore, low concentrations of methoxyflurane can be used clinically for many minor surgical procedures
   B. Methoxyflurane is the most potent anesthetic, but the rate of onset of anesthesia action is prolonged, as is recovery
   C. Analgesia may continue into the recovery period
   D. Accurate concentrations can be delivered by precision heat-compensated, calibrated vaporizer; however, simple draw-over wick vaporizers can be used
   E. If nitrous oxide is used, the amount of methoxyflurane required is reduced
V. Dosages
   A. Methoxyflurane is rarely used by mask induction because of the slow onset of anesthesia and the possibility of excitement or delirium
   B. After barbiturate induction, 2-3% is used to induce surgical anesthesia
   C. Maintenance: 0.2-1.0%

ENFLURANE (ETHRANE)

I. General anesthetic properties (see Table 10-1)
   A. Similar to methoxyflurane in general anesthetic properties

B. Relatively rapid induction and recovery from anesthesia
C. Comparatively marked cardiorespiratory depression

II. Effects on body systems
   A. Nervous system
      1. Potent depressor of the central nervous system
      2. Involuntary muscle twitching has been reported (jerks)
      3. EEG pattern changes occur with increasing depth of anesthesia—high-voltage, high-frequency spike complexes (*burst suppression*) may alternate with electrical silence. Seizure activity with associated motor activity occasionally occurs
   B. Respiratory system
      1. Nonirritating to the respiratory tract
      2. Profound respiratory depressant. Assisted or controlled ventilation is usually required
      3. Provokes a sigh response similar to ether
   C. Cardiovascular system
      1. Cardiac depression is related to the depth of anesthesia; cardiac contractility is decreased to a greater degree than with any other inhalation anesthetic
      2. Blood pressure decreases
      3. Heart rate remains relatively constant without significant bradycardia
      4. Cardiac output, stroke volume, and cardiac contractility decrease with increasing depth of anesthesia
      5. Enflurane minimally sensitizes the heart to catecholamines
   D. Gastrointestinal system
      1. Smooth muscle tone and motility are decreased
      2. No hepatic toxicity recorded, although BSP clearance may be prolonged
   E. Renal system
      1. No changes in renal function observed
   F. Muscular system
      1. Muscle relaxation and analgesia are excellent
      2. Nondepolarizing muscle relaxants are markedly potentiated
   G. Uterus and fetus
      1. Crosses the placenta rapidly
      2. Safety in pregnancy has not been established

III. Absorption, fate, and excretion
   A. Absorption and elimination are primarily by the alveoli
   B. Primarily eliminated unchanged via the lung
   C. No toxic effects have been produced by enflurane or its metabolites. Biotransformation of low concentrations (up to 2.5%) result in low levels of serum fluoride ion, much lower than levels known to cause renal damage

IV. Clinical use
   A. Alternative to halothane or methoxyflurane because of good analgesia and muscle relaxation
   B. Rapid induction and recovery and low biodegradation

    C. Patient must be adequately tranquilized for smooth induction and to avoid "emergence delirium" on recovery

    D. Calibrated vaporizers should be used

    E. Enflurane is compatible with nitrous oxide

    F. Contraindicated in patients with a history of cerebrocortical abnormalities

    G. Relatively expensive

V. Dosages

    A. Uptake of enflurane is faster than with halothane, but enflurane is less potent; thus induction times may be similar

    B. Induction with barbiturates is preferred

    C. Surgical anesthesia is induced with 4-6% enflurane

    D. Maintenance: 1.0-3.0%; ventilation may have to be supported

ISOFLURANE (FORANE, AARANE)

  I. General anesthetic properties (see Table 10-1)

    A. Isoflurane is an isomer of enflurane and is exceptionally stable

II. Effect on systems

    A. Nervous system

      1. Generalized central nervous system depression

      2. No involuntary jerking or seizure activity is observed as with enflurane

      3. Burst suppression is observed in moderate to deep surgical anesthesia

    B. Respiratory system

      1. Respiratory depression similar to halothane. Respiratory patterns may be different

      2. Tidal volume increases initially with depth of anesthesia; respiratory rate decreases; unrelated to anesthetic depth

      3. $PaCO_2$ concentration increases with time, although surgical stimulation partly compensates for the respiratory depression and thus prevents a large rise in $PaCO_2$

    C. Cardiovascular system

      1. Cardiac depression is less than with halothane or enflurane

      2. Cardiac contractility is depressed, but cardiac output is maintained

      3. Progressive vasodilation occurs with increasing depth of anesthesia; this may be due to increased muscle and skin blood flow

      4. Mean arterial blood pressure and peripheral vascular resistance decrease with depth of anesthesia similarly to halothane and enflurane

      5. Isoflurane does not sensitize the heart to catecholamines

    D. Gastrointestinal system

      1. Smooth muscle tone and motility are decreased

      2. No hepatotoxicity reported (metabolism is very low)

    E. Renal system

      1. No changes in renal function reported; very little metabolism to tri-fluoroacetic acid

    F. Muscular system

      1. Produces excellent muscle relaxation

      2. Markedly potentiates nondepolarizing muscle relaxants

    G. Uterus and fetus
       1. Crosses the placenta rapidly
       2. Safety in pregnancy has not been evaluated
III. Absorption, fate, and excretion
    A. Absorption and elimination is by the alveoli
    B. Primarily excreted unchanged via the lung
    C. There is very little biodegradation; approximately 0.25% may be metabolized to inorganic fluoride (trifluoroacetic acid); thus isoflurane can be considered the most stable and inert inhalation agent
IV. Clinical use
    A. Although a respiratory depressant, isoflurane is inert and nontoxic and produces minimal cardiovascular effects at surgical planes of anesthesia. It is a useful anesthetic agent but is expensive
    B. Isoflurane produces fast, smooth induction and recovery periods in all species tested
    C. Calibrated vaporizer should be used
    D. Isoflurane can be used with nitrous oxide
    E. Expensive
V. Dosages
    A. Induction: 2.5-4.5% is usually necessary
    B. Induction is facilitated by the use of a barbiturate or nitrous oxide
    C. Maintenance: 1.0-3.0%

CHAPTER ELEVEN

Neuromuscular Blocking Drugs

"Don't fight forces; use them."

R. BUCKMINSTER FULLER

OVERVIEW

Neuromuscular blocking drugs, commonly referred to as "muscle relaxants," interfere with or block neuromuscular transmission. They are useful adjuncts to general anesthesia. They provide no analgesia, sedation, amnesia, or hypnosis and stop ventilation, necessitating controlled ventilation and constant patient monitoring.

GENERAL CONSIDERATIONS

I. Neuromuscular blocking agents (NMBAs) produce skeletal muscle (SM) relaxation as a primary pharmacological effect

II. Other clinically useful drugs and some toxins evoke SM weakness or paralysis as an adverse effect

III. Potential mechanisms of SM relaxation

    A. Interfere with cholinergic neuromuscular transmission in the peripheral somatic nervous system

    B. Enhance activity of endogenous inhibitory mechanisms in the CNS, which normally modulate SM tone

IV. NMBAs are occasionally used adjunctively during anesthesia, specifically to produce controlled transient SM weakness

V. *No analgesia* or *hypnotic* effect is produced; only muscle relaxation

VI. Any clinical dose of a neuromuscular blocking agent may cause complete respiratory paralysis. Mechanical or manual support of ventilation is necessary during respiratory paralysis

VII. Hypothermia is an important secondary effect of prolonged SM relaxation in small animals

VIII. These drugs are positively charged and therefore do not pass blood-brain barrier or placenta in significant amounts

IX. Potentiated by many intravenous and inhalation anesthetic drugs

X. Various electrical stimulators and stimulation protocols should be used to determine the degree of neuromuscular blockade

NORMAL NEUROMUSCULAR TRANSMISSION

I. Release of acetylcholine (ACh) in the resting state
   A. Random, infrequent fusion of intraneuronal synaptic vesicles containing ACh with membranes of the unmyelinated nerve terminal
   B. Random, infrequent release of ACh packets
   C. Random ACh release causes mini-endplate potentials (MEPPS) at postsynaptic muscle membrane, which are insufficient to evoke muscle contraction

II. Action potential (AP)–dependent ACh release
   A. AP causes large depolarization in nerve terminals of α-motor neurons
   B. Depolarization and extracellular Ca^{++} causes nearly simultaneous fusion of many ACh-containing vesicles with the terminal nerve membrane
   C. Release of many ACh packets evokes a large endplate potential (EPP), leading to muscle contraction

III. Combination of ACh with postjunctional receptors
   A. Receptors on the muscle endplates are nicotinic type IV cholinergic receptors
   B. Strength of muscle contraction is proportional to the number of receptors activated by ACh

IV. Hydrolysis of ACh, reuptake of choline, synthesis and packing of ACh
   A. The duration of ACh activity at *any* cholinergic synapse is limited by the action of acetylcholinesterase. ACh $\rightarrow$ acetic acid + choline at synaptic cleft (ACh esterase)
   B. Choline produced by hydrolysis of ACh is taken up by the nerve terminals and resynthesized into ACh. Choline + acetyl CoA $\rightleftharpoons$ ACh (choline acetyl transferase at nerve terminal membrane)
   C. ACh is packaged into vesicles or stored freely in the cytoplasm of the nerve terminals

MECHANISMS OF SM RELAXATION EVOKED BY INTERFERENCE WITH NORMAL PERIPHERAL NEUROMUSCULAR TRANSMISSION

I. At presynaptic site
   A. Inhibition of ACh synthesis; e.g., hemicholinium blocks choline uptake
   B. Inhibition of ACh release
      1. Calcium deficiency: Mg^{++} release

2. Procaine
3. Tetracyclines and aminoglycoside antibiotics
4. Some β-blockers
5. Botulinum toxin

II. At postsynaptic site
  A. Persistent depolarization with an agonist that has longer duration of action than ACh, e.g., succinylcholine chloride
  B. Competitive block of ACh receptors causing nondepolarizing blockade, e.g., curare, pancuronium

TYPES OF NEUROMUSCULAR BLOCKS

I. Phase I block: depolarizing block (succinylcholine)
II. Phase II block: nondepolarizing block (pancuronium)
III. Mixed block: any combination of I and II
IV. Dual block: excessive amounts of depolarizing agents producing phase II block
V. Nonacetylcholine block (procaine, botulinum, decreased Ca^{++}, increased Mg^{++}, increased K^+, decreased K^+)

SEQUENCE OF MUSCLE RELAXATION

I. Oculomotor m. >palpebral m. >facial m. >tongue and pharynx >jaw and tail >limbs >pelvis m. >caudal abdominal m. >cranial abdominal m. >intercostal m. >larynx >diaphragm
II. Intercostal and diaphragmatic muscles are thought to be affected last
III. Recovery is in the reverse order of paralysis
IV. It is possible but difficult to titrate the specific neuromuscular blocking agent in order to paralyze the muscles of the eye yet maintain diaphragmatic function

SPECIFIC NEUROMUSCULAR BLOCKING AGENTS

See Table 11-1
I. Depolarizing agents act like ACh
  A. Succinylcholine chloride (Sucostrin, Anectin, Quillicine, Suxamethonium)
  B. Decamethonium bromide (C-10, Syncurine)
II. Nondepolarizing agents; competitive blocking agents
  A. d-Tubocurarine chloride (curare, Metubine)
  B. Gallamine triethiodide (Flaxedil)
  C. Pancuronium bromide (Pavulon)
  D. Vecuronium bromide (Norcuron)
  E. Atrarcurium besylate (Tracrium)

CLINICAL DIFFERENTIATION BETWEEN DEPOLARIZING AND NONDEPOLARIZING AGENTS

I. Depolarizing
  A. First transient muscle fasciculations caused by asynchronous depolarization
  B. Second paralysis due to prolonged depolarization of the motor endplate

TABLE 11-1

DOSE OF NMBA WITH SIDE EFFECTS AND CONTRAINDICATIONS

Agent	Species	Dose IV (mg/lb)	Duration of action (minutes)	Side effects	Contraindications in presence of:
Succinyl-choline chloride	Dog Cat Pig Horse	0.1 0.5 0.5 0.04	1-10 2-3 1-10	Little CV effect; muscarinic effect— bradycardia; nicotinic effect— hypertension, increased intraocular pressure, hyperpyrexia	Organophosphate anthelmintics, chronic liver disease, malnutrition, high K, glaucoma, pene-trating eye injury
Gallamine triethio-dide	Dog Cat Horse	0.5 1-2 0.5	15-20	Tachycardia, 10-20% in dogs due to antimuscarinic (atropine-like effect); transient decrease in arterial blood pressure in cats due to ganglionic blockade	Renal dysfunction
d-Tubo-curarine chloride	Dog Cat Pig	0.2 0.2 0.15	10-20	Hypotensive due to release of significant quantities of histamine; vagal blockade in dogs— therefore, not used routinely in veterinary medicine	Renal dysfunction
Pancuronium bromide	Dog Cat Pig	0.02 0.05	15-20	Negligible	Liver or kidney disease
Vecuronium*	Dog	0.006-0.01	10-15	Negligible	
Atracurium*	Cat	0.03-0.05	10-15	Negligible	

*Clinical pharmacodynamics and pharmacokinetics are not thoroughly described in animals.

    C. Paralysis is *not reversed* by anticholinesterase agents
    D. Paralysis is terminated by metabolism of the NMBA by pseudocholinesterase
II. Nondepolarizing
    A. No muscle fasciculation prior to muscle paralysis due to competitive inhi-bition of neurotransmitter at the motor endplate
    B. Effects *can be reversed* by anticholinesterase agents

DEPOLARIZING BLOCKING AGENTS

I. Mechanism of action
   A. Persistent depolarization alone may result in neuromuscular block because of Na^+ inactivation, which prevents AP generation
   B. Dual block: Prolonged exposure of ACh membrane receptors to large doses of depolarizing agents (ACh, succinylcholine, C-10) reduces the ability of these agents to cause conductance changes; the reason for this is uncertain

II. Indications
   A. Diagnostic or surgical procedures requiring a short duration of muscle relaxation
   B. Facilitation of endotracheal intubation in humans and primates
   C. Cesarean sections
   D. Fracture reductions if done early

III. Contraindications
   A. Patients with liver disease—pseudocholinesterase produced in the liver
   B. Chronic anemia—acetylcholinesterase partly located on RBC membrane
   C. Chronic malnutrition—reduced enzyme levels
   D. High K^+ (burns, massive muscle trauma, digitalis therapy) depolarizing blockers may exacerbate hyperkalemia
   E. Organophosphates (anthelmintics)—organophosphates are acetylcholinesterase inhibitors
   F. Glaucoma, penetrating eye injury—contraction of the extra-ocular muscles may result in expulsion of tissues within the globe

IV. Specific depolarizing agents
   A. Comparison of succinylcholine with acetylcholine (see Table 11-2)
   B. Adverse effects
      1. Muscle soreness: reason unknown, probably related to muscle fasciculations and K^+ release before paralysis
      2. Histamine release
      3. Cardiovascular effects
         a. Potential for bradycardia secondary to ganglionic stimulation
         b. The more common response is tachycardia and hypertension due to sympathetic stimulation
      4. Hyperkalemia: due to increased efflux of K^+ from endplate region of skeletal muscle
      5. Some patients have a deficiency of plasma cholinesterase; in these patients, neuromuscular block may be prolonged
      6. Genetic anomaly may be presented where plasma cholinesterase is replaced by an atypical cholinesterase with only low affinity for succinylcholine
      7. Differentiation is possible with dibucaine, which inhibits normal plasma cholinesterase 80% but atypical cholinesterase only 20%
      8. Malignant hyperpyrexia manifested by a severe, rapid rise in temperature, which may be accompanied by marked muscle ridigity

TABLE 11 - 2

COMPARISON OF SUCCINYLCHOLINE WITH ACETYLCHOLINE

	Succinylcholine	Acetylcholine
Duration of depolarization of motor endplate	1 to 10 minutes	Milliseconds
Hydrolyzed by enzyme	Pseudocholinesterase = plasmacholinesterase	Acetylcholinesterase = tissue cholinesterase = true cholinesterase
Split products	Succinylmonocholine chloride and succinic acid	Choline and acetate
Location of enzyme	Plasma (produced by liver)	Nerve, muscle, erythrocytes

      a. Usually seen when using succinylcholine and halothane together

      b. Treat with 100% O_2, rapid cooling, sodium bicarbonate to control acidosis, and dantrolene sodium (1-2 mg/lb)

   C. Suggestions to equine practitioners using succinylcholine

      1. Prior to use, get a good history of past illness and drugs administered to the horse. If any of the following agents were used in the last 30 days, do not administer succinylcholine: antibiotics ending in "mycin," procaine, organophosphate anthelmintics, insecticides

      2. The dose that gives good skeletal relaxation with minimal paralysis of the diaphragm is 0.04 mg/lb (4 mg/100 lb)

      3. Be prepared to give artificial respiration if apnea occurs

      4. Inform owner of danger of this form of chemical restraint (note: not analgetic)

      5. Be sure to have someone familiar with the horse holding the head; head trauma may result if the horse is not adequately restrained; the horse should be walked in a tight circle after injection to prevent it from going over backwards

      6. Keep vials refrigerated; hydrolyzes quickly at high temperatures

V. Decamethonium (C-10, Syncurine)

   A. Basically identical to succinylcholine except:

      1. No histamine release

      2. Not metabolized by plasma cholinesterase, thereby prolonging the duration of action

      3. No metabolism; excreted by the kidney unchanged; avoid use in renal disease

NONDEPOLARIZING BLOCKING AGENTS

I. Mechanism of action

   A. Competitive blocking agents: compete with ACh for postsynaptic receptors, thereby reducing the depolarization caused by a particular amount of ACh

II. Indications

    A. High-risk cases as part of a balanced anesthetic technique with narcotics, inhalation or other analgetic drugs

    B. Control of ventilation at any time

III. Specific nondepolarizing agents

    A. Tubocurarine

        1. Curare was used by South American Indians to poison the tips of arrows

        2. Poor oral absorption

          a. Usually administered IV

          b. Effective IM

        3. Ganglionic blockade only with high doses

          a. When used in clinical dosages, little ganglionic blockade is produced

          b. May partially account for hypotension observed with tubocurarine

        4. Releases histamine, which can cause

          a. Vasodilation and hypotension (probably main cause of hypotension with tubocurarine)

          b. Increased bronchial and salivary secretion

          c. Bronchospasm, which may precipitate an asthmatic attack

        5. Synergism

          a. Tubocurarine should be used carefully in the presence of streptomycin, neomycin, and polymyxin, which tend to block NM transmission

            (1) By a Mg^{++} type presynaptic block

            (2) By a curariform postsynaptic block

          b. High CO_2 enhances block

    B. Gallamine triethiodide (Flaxedil)

        1. No histamine release or ganglionic block in clinically effective dosages

        2. Selective blockade of parasympathetic innervation of the heart

          a. Questionable ganglionic block; questionable block of muscarinic receptors in heart

          b. Causes tachycardia and occasionally hypertension

    C. Pancuronium (Pavulon)

        1. No histamine release or ganglionic block

        2. Its action is increased by inhalation anesthetics

        3. Major portion is excreted unchanged in urine

        4. Tachycardia is occasionally seen following administration

    D. Vecuronium (Norcuron)

        1. Developed in an attempt to produce a competitive NMBA with short onset and duration times, and to eliminate the tachycardia seen occasionally with pancuronium

        2. In cats, 40% of dose is eliminated in bile, 15% through kidneys—potential advantage in patients with compromised renal function

        3. Minimal cardiovascular effects; no histamine release; no ganglionic block

    E. Atracurium (Tracrium)

        1. Developed as a rapid-onset and duration-competitive NMBA

TABLE 11-3

FACTORS ALTERING INTENSITY OF DEGREE AND DURATION OF
MUSCLE RELAXATION

Factor	Depolarizing agent	Nondepolarizing agent
Tranquilizers	↑	↑
Volatile anesthetic agents	↑	↑
Decreased body temperature	↑	↑
Decreased cardiac output/kg bodyweight	↓	↓ (Gallamine)
Increased age	↑	↑
Antibiotics:		
Streptomycin	↑	↑
Neomycin	↑	↑
Kanamycin	↑	↑
Organophosphates	↑	—

↑ = increase; ↓ = decrease; — = no effect

2. Under goes pH and temperature-dependent degradation (Hoffman elimination) once administered; therefore, a potential benefit is lack of requirement for biologically mediated metabolism and elimination via liver and kidney
3. Some histamine release at high dosages

FACTORS THAT MAY INFLUENCE NEUROMUSCULAR BLOCKADE

See Table 11-3
   I. Temperature
      A. Hyperthermia antagonizes competitive blockade, but enhances and prolongs depolarizing blockade
      B. Hypothermia prolongs nondepolarizing neuromuscular blocking drugs
  II. Acid-base balance (see Table 11-4)
      A. Respiratory acidosis augments nondepolarizing neuromuscular blockade
      B. Inadequate reversal of nondepolarizing agents causes depressed ventilation and respiratory acidosis, which enhances the blockade (vicious cycle)
 III. Fluid and electrolyte imbalance
      A. Hypokalemia and hypocalcemia potentiate nondepolarizing agents
      B. Dehydration increases the plasma concentration of a normal dose of a nondepolarizing agent, augmenting its effect
      C. High magnesium blood levels enhance both depolarizing and nondepolarizing neuromuscular blocking agents
  IV. Other drugs
      A. The following antibiotics potentiate nondepolarizing agents: neomycin, streptomycin, gentamicin, kanamycin, paromomycin, viomycin, polymyxin A and B, colistin, tetracycline, lincomycin, clindamycin

TABLE 11-4

THE EFFECT OF ALTERATIONS IN ACID-BASE BALANCE ON MAGNITUDE
AND DURATION OF NEUROMUSCULAR BLOCKADE

Acid-base	Succinylcholine	d-Tubocurarine	Gallamine	Pancuronium
Respiratory acidosis ($PaCO_2$ 60-170)	↓	↑	↓	↑ or —
Respiratory alkalosis ($PaCO_2$ 13-30)	↓	↓ or —	↑	↓ or —
Metabolic acidosis (pH 7.05-7.2)	↑	↑ or —	↓	ND
Metabolic alkalosis (pH 7.6-7.7)	—	↑ or ↓	↑	ND

↑ = increase; ↓ = decrease; — = no effect; ND = not determined

ANTICHOLINESTERASE AGENTS

I. Reversal of neuromuscular block

    A. Anticholinesterase drugs such as physostigmine, pyridostigmine, neostigmine, and edrophonium can be used together with or without atropine

        1. Atropine is used to block the undesirable muscarinic effects of anticholinesterase drugs. Muscarinic effects include increased bronchial and salivary secretions and bradycardia

        2. This regimen is ineffective against a depolarization block; in fact, it exacerbates the block because of additional depolarization by excess ACh

        3. This regimen may be effective when depolarizing blocking agent is producing a phase II block

    B. Reverse with 0.02 mg/lb neostigmine combined with 0.01 mg/lb atropine (average dose). Do not repeat the neostigmine dose more than three times

    C. Edrophonium dose is 0.25 mg/lb IV; may be repeated up to five times

    D. Complete reversal may take 5-45 minutes

II. Use in myasthenia gravis (MG)

    A. Reduced numbers of nicotinic receptors on motor endplates

        1. Reported as either a congenital disease or an acquired disease of autoimmune etiology

        2. Often a self-limiting disease in dogs

    B. Diagnosis

        1. Improvement in motor performance following IV administration of edrophonium (Tensilon); a short-acting anticholinesterase is practically diagnostic for MG

C. Treatment
  1. Neostigmine (Prostigmin) is often used
     a. Given orally
     b. Relatively short duration of action
  2. Pyridostigmine bromine (Mestinon) (0.1 mg/lb IV) and ambenonium chloride (Myetelase)
     a. Relatively longer duration of action
     b. Useful in some patients

CENTRALLY ACTING SKELETAL MUSCLE RELAXANTS

I. Guaifenesin
  A. Mechanism of action is poorly understood but probably relates to depression of transmission through spinal polysynaptic pathways, which normally maintain SM tone
  B. No effect on cerebral arousal
     1. Mild sedation
     2. Variable, mild analgesia
  C. Clinical usage is as a preanesthetic aid to induction of recumbency in horses and large ruminants
     1. Significantly reduces dose of induction agent required to produce recumbency
  D. Pharmacological effects
     1. SM relaxation
     2. Lacks significant adverse cardiovascular effects
     3. Signs of overdose
        a. Altered pattern of respiration (apneustic)
        b. SM rigidity
        c. Hypotension
  E. Dosage and route of administration
     1. 25 mg/lb or to ataxic effect by IV infusion
        50 mg/lb for recumbency by IV infusion
     2. Typically administered as a 5% solution
        a. Solutions greater than 7-8% may cause lysis of RBC in ruminants (greater than 15% in horses)
     3. Can be combined with a thiobarbiturate for simultaneous IV administration by infusion

II. Benzodiazepines
  A. Mechanism of SM relaxant activity is probably related to ability to enhance inhibitory neurotransmission mediated by glycine in the spinal cord
  B. See Chapter 3: Drugs used for Preanesthetic Medication for outline of the pharmacology of these drugs

CHAPTER TWELVE

Anesthesia for Cesarean Section

"The hand that rocks the cradle is the hand that rules the world."
WILLIAM ROSS WALLACE

OVERVIEW

Drugs used to produce chemical restraint and general anesthesia in pregnant animals will also affect the fetus. Generally, the depressant qualities of anesthetic drugs are more pronounced and longer-lasting in the fetus than when the mother. The rate at which drugs cross the placental membrane and enter the fetal circulation is a primary consideration when selecting drugs to produce anesthesia. Drugs that cross the placental barrier slowly, or not at all, are preferred. Some drugs promote premature delivery of the fetus, whereas others partially or totally inhibit uterine contractions and delay parturition. Drug effects may vary from animal to animal because of differences in pharmacologic responses to the same drug. This section describes the changes that occur in maternal physiology during advanced pregnancy and the effects of drugs used to produce chemical restraint and general anesthesia in pregnant animals.

GENERAL CONSIDERATIONS

I. Pregnancy, especially the immediate periparturient period, causes significant alterations in maternal physiology
  A. Altered pharmacokinetics and pharmacodynamics
II. Anesthetic drug and technique selection are based on:
  A. Providing optimal analgesia for surgery
  B. Minimizing fetal depression
  C. Minimizing postoperative maternal depression
  D. Neither inducing nor preventing uterine contractions

118

CHANGES IN MATERNAL PHYSIOLOGY IN ADVANCED PREGNANCY

I. Central nervous system
   A. Decreased inhalational anesthetic MAC due to increased progesterone concentration
   B. Decrease in size of epidural space due to epidural vessel vascular engorgement
   C. Significance of pregnancy on anesthesia
      1. Decreased requirement for inhalational anesthetics
      2. Decreased volume of local anesthetic for epidural anesthesia

II. Respiratory system
   A. Increased alveolar ventilation due to progesterone-induced respiratory center sensitivity to CO_2
   B. Decreased functional residual capacity due to anterior displacement of diaphragm
   C. Closure of small airways at higher lung volumes
   D. Significance
      1. Increased alveolar ventilation and decreased FRC result in a more rapid alveolar rate of rise of inhalational anesthetics
      2. Airway closure and decreased FRC result in greater ventilation perfusion mismatches, which result in decreased oxygenation

III. Cardiovascular system
   A. Increase in maternal blood volume is approximately 30%
   B. Packed cell volume and plasma protein concentration are decreased
   C. Cardiac output increases 30-50% due to increased stroke volume and heart rate
   D. Aortocaval compression in dorsal recumbency from weight of the gravid uterus
   E. Central venous pressure and systemic blood pressure remain relatively unchanged but may increase during labor
   F. Significance
      1. Cardiac reserves are decreased because of increased cardiac output and aortocaval compression
      2. Relative anemia means blood loss is not tolerated as well as in the nonpregnant patient
      3. Patients with a history of heart disease may decompensate

IV. Gastrointestinal system
   A. Increased gastric acidity secondary to placental gastrin secretion
   B. Cranial displacement of stomach and altered tone to the lower esophageal sphincter
   C. Significance
      1. Chance of regurgitation and severe aspiration pneumonia due to increased gastric acidity
      2. Necessity of properly fitting cuffed endotracheal tube

V. Miscellaneous
   A. Decreased plasma cholinesterase (pseudocholinesterase)

B. Significance
  1. Prolonged duration of action of succinylcholine
  2. Prolonged duration of action of ester local anesthetics

DRUG TRANSFER ACROSS THE PLACENTA

I. Factors influencing drug transfer
  A. Surface area available for diffusion and placental thickness
    1. Surface area of placenta is large and diffusion distance is small in all species, even with individual species variation in placental morphology
  B. Diffusion properties of drugs
    1. Lipid solubility: Most anesthetic drugs are extremely lipid-soluble. High lipid solubility = high diffusibility
    2. Molecular weight: Lower molecular weight = higher diffusibility
    3. Degree of ionization and protein binding: Decreased ionization and protein binding = greater diffusibility
  C. Relative maternal and fetal drug concentrations
    1. Discrete bolus doses of drugs result in rapid initial transfer to fetus but rapidly declining maternal concentrations
    2. Continuous infusion, repeated bolus administration, and inhalation anesthesia result in continuously high maternal drug concentration and continued drug transfer to the fetus

UTEROPLACENTAL CIRCULATION AND FETAL VIABILITY

I. Any condition resulting in decreased circulating maternal blood volume can potentially decrease placental perfusion, resulting in fetal hypoxia and acidosis. This includes maternal dehydration, hypovolemia, shock, and drug-induced hypotension
  A. Shock and hypovolemia
    1. Prolonged labor
    2. Anesthetic drugs
    3. Positioning: decrease venous return
    4. Endotoxic shock
  B. Hypovolemia
  C. Dehydration
    1. Prolonged labor
  D. Drugs
    1. Oxytocin: peripheral vasodilation and hypotension
    2. Ergot derivatives: vasoconstriction and hypertension

MATERNAL AND FETAL EFFECTS FROM VARIOUS INHALATION AGENTS

I. Activity
  A. All inhalation agents, because of their low molecular weight, lipid-solubility, and undissociative form, readily transfer across the placenta
  B. The degree of depression depends on the depth and duration of maternal anesthesia

    C. Due to changes in maternal respiratory physiology, minimum alveolar concentrations of inhalation agents are decreased at parturition

II. Nitrous oxide

    A. Rapid transfer across the placenta

    B. Administration exceeding 15-17 minutes may result in fetal depression

       1. Diffusion hypoxia may occur in the fetus. This can be circumvented with postparturient oxygen therapy

    C. When used in the mother, with adequate amounts of oxygen, there is minimal effect on the neonate; however, neonatal asphyxia at N_2O >75%

III. Halothane

    A. Present in the fetal circulation within 2 minutes

    B. A rapid and powerful uterine relaxant

       1. Inhibits uterine involution

       2. Increases the risk of uterine hemorrhage

    C. If used for cesarean section, the procedure should be performed as quickly as possible

       1. Neonatal depression should resolve rapidly if adequate ventilation is provided at birth

IV. Methoxyflurane

    A. Present in the fetal circulation within 2 minutes

    B. At analgesic levels of this agent, minimal depression in the newborn is noted

    C. Minimal uterine relaxation in analgesic dosages

    D. Neonatal depression may resolve slowly due to high blood/gas partition coefficient of methoxyflurane

V. Enflurane, isoflurane

    A. Present in fetal circulation within 2 minutes

    B. Both are rapid and powerful uterine relaxants

    C. If used for cesarean section, the procedure should be performed as quickly as possible

       1. There is no apparent correlation between maternal blood concentration and the degree of fetal depression

       2. Neonatal respiratory depression with enflurane may be severe, requiring postparturient ventilation

    D. Rapid elimination of these agents with ventilation may be an advantage

MATERNAL AND FETAL EFFECTS FROM VARIOUS DRUGS

I. Barbiturates

    A. Activity

       1. Barbiturates readily diffuse across the placenta into the fetal circulation

       2. Dose of barbiturates that does not produce anesthesia in the mother will completely inhibit fetal respiratory movements

       3. Barbiturates that depend on metabolism for their duration of action should be avoided because of reduced fetal ability to metabolize drugs

    B. Short-acting barbiturates

       1. Pentobarbital

        a. 30 mg/kg IV to dogs reaches equilibrium in 15 minutes

    2. Anesthetic recovery is prolonged, preventing newborn from feeding

    3. Respiratory depression in the newborn is the biggest problem and results in high mortality

    4. Should not be used if viable neonate is a goal

  C. Ultrashort-acting barbiturates

    1. Cross placenta readily and achieve equilibrium within 2-5 minutes

    2. A single dose of 4 mg/lb at induction allows only modest placental transfer and does not endanger the fetus significantly

        a. Additional dosing is discouraged

        b. Peak drug concentrations occur in the fetus in 10 minutes

    3. The use of small doses of ultrashort-acting barbiturates, because of their dependence on redistribution for their duration of action, has not been associated with a significant degree of fetal depression

II. Dissociogenic Agents (ketamine, Tiletamine)

  A. Activity

    1. Used to produce restraint and analgesia

    2. Poor muscle relaxation

    3. Relatively rapidly transferred across the placenta producing fetal depression within 5-10 minutes

  B. Ketamine

    1. Good restraint in queens with minimal fetal depression when used IV or IM in low dosages (1 mg/16 IV; 5 mg/16 IM)

    2. Poor muscle relaxation and questionable ability to block deep pain

  C. Telazol (Tiletamine-Zolazepam)

    1. Similar to ketamine but better muscle relaxation

III. Narcotics

  A. Activity

    1. Commonly used as preanesthetic medication for sedation and analgesia

    2. Narcotics are readily transferred across the placenta

    3. Concentrations of narcotics may be higher in the fetus than in the maternal circulation due to a lower fetal pH

    4. Moderate maternal doses will not produce serious depression in neonates. The depressant effect is potentially reversible by narcotic antagonists

    5. Narcotic antagonists may have a shorter duration of action than the narcotic used. This may required observation of neonates for several hours and redosing of the narcotic antagonist

  B. Meperidine (Demerol)

    1. Reaches the fetal circulation within 90 seconds after administration

    2. If birth is within the first hour after injection, no significant depression is apparent

  C. Morphine

    1. Clinical depression can be observed in the newborn

    2. Has a direct vasoconstrictor effect on placental vessels

    3. Nalorphine will antagonize the vasoconstrictor effect

D. Oxymorphone (Numorphan)
  1. Better analgesia and sedation than with meperidine
  2. Increased neonatal depression
E. Fentanyl (Sublimaze)
  1. 100 times more potent analgesic than morphine, with respiratory depression of shorter duration

IV. Sedatives/tranquilizers
  A. Activity: The use of these agents reduces the amount of potentially more dangerous anesthetic agents that might be used
    1. Phenothiazines (Acepromazine, Promazine)
      a. Appear in the blood of the fetus within 2 minutes and reach equilibrium in 4-5 minutes
      b. Little to no apparent effect on the newborn when used in clinical dosages
      c. α-adrenergic blockade may potentiate hypotension in stressed mother at parturition, resulting in decreased uterine blood flow and fetal hypoxia
    2. Benzodiazepines (Diazepam)
      a. Concentrates in fetal blood at a 2:1 ratio compared to maternal blood concentration
      b. Minimal respiratory and cardiovascular depression
      c. Duration of action is dependent on redistribution away from the CNS
    3. Xylazine hydrochloride (Rompun)
      a. Respiratory depression may be severe in both mother and fetus
      b. Use with caution in the equine. Contraindicated in small animal patients
      c. Increases intrauterine pressure in cattle; may be abortifacient. Effect in other species is unknown
    4. Ketamine
      a. May increase uterine tone and decrease uterine blood flow, leading to fetal hypoxia
      b. Fetal blood levels reach 70% of those found in the mother
      c. Little clinical depression is evident in the neonate

V. Muscle relaxants
  A. Activity
    1. Neuromuscular blocking agents (succinylcholine, pancuronium, atracurium, vecuronium)
      a. These compounds are highly ionized with a high molecular weight, resulting in little placental transfer
      b. In clinical doses there is no demonstrable effect on the newborn
      c. Succinylcholine metabolism is reduced due to decrease in pseudocholinesterase
  B. Guaifenesin
    1. Readily crosses the placental barrier
    2. Depression of the newborn has not been investigated but is believed to be minimal

TABLE 12 - 1

ANESTHETIC TECHNIQUES BY SPECIES

Species	Drug/technique	Dosage	Comments
Cow	*Local techniques:*		
	1. Standing; paravertebral analgesia, line block, inverted L block	2% lidocaine (see Chapter 5 for techniques)	Suitable for tractable animals without a sedative Suitable for animals in good physical condition
	2. Anterior epidural	2% lidocaine, 1ml/10lb at Cx_1-Cx_2 junction	Induces recumbency and sensory block anterior to umbilicus Watch for hypotension
	General:		
	3. Guaifenesin-ketamine-xylazine	500 mg ketamine 25 mg xylazine 500 ml and 5% guaifenesin + 0.25-0.5 mg/lb; to effect for maintenance	Intubate if possible
Horse	1. Premed: acepromazine or xylazine Induction: guaifenesin plus thiobarbiturate or ketamine Maintenance: halothane, isoflurane	Acepromazine: 0.02 mg/lb IV Xylazine: 0.1-0.3 mg/lb IV Guaifenesin: 25-50 mg/lb Thiobarbiturate: 1-2 mg/lb Ketamine: 0.7-1.0 mg/lb	Adjust dosage for physical condition of mother. Rely on guaifenesin to produce relaxation and to allow less thiobarbiturate or ketamine to be used
	1. Guaifenesin-ketamine	500 ml 5% guaifenesin containing 500 mg ketamine 0.25-1.0 mg/lb induction maintenance to effect	Intubate; copious salivation Moderate to poor muscle relaxation Can add 25 mg xylazine to mixture, but fetal depression is greater Use for induction to gas or as IV technique
Sheep, goat	2. Guaifenesin-thiobarbiturate induction or guaifenesin-ketamine induction; halothane, isoflurane	25 mg/lb Guaifenesin 1-2 mg/lb thiobarbiturate	Guaifenesin allows small bolus dose of thiobarbiturate
	3. Mask induction halothane or isoflurane	To effect	Useful in sick, toxic animals and fetal viability is of no concern

Species	Technique	Dose	Comments
Dog, cat	*Local techniques:*		
	1. Epidural with 2% lidocaine	1 ml/7.5 lb body weight	Requires assistant for physical restraint. Use sedative/tranquilizer in all but extremely tractable patients
	General techniques:		
	Induction:		
	2. Diazepam-ketamine induction	0.125 mg/lb diazepam plus 5.0 mg/lb ketamine combined	Single-bolus dose not depressant to fetus
	Telazol	1-3 mg/lb IM	Single administration causes minimal fetal depression
	Thiobarbiturate induction	4-8 mg/lb	Diazepam-ketamine good in depressed-shocky patients
	Maintenance:		
	Halothane or 50% isoflurane in N_2O plus muscle relaxant (atracurium, pancuronium)	see Chapter 11	Administer inhalation agent as late into procedure as possible
	Intractable animals:		
	3. Pre-med		
	Dogs: Innovar-Vet	1 ml/30-40 lb IM	Controlled ventilation necessary when using relaxants
	Acepromazine-oxymorphone	0.5 mg/lb of each maximum 4 mg of each	
	Cats: Ketamine induction	4 mg/lb IM	Sedative-hypnotics generally increase fetal depression; therefore, use sparingly
	Thiobarbiturate	1-3 mg/lb	
Pig	Maintenance:		
	Isoflurane or halothane		
	1. Epidural	2% lidocaine (see Chapter 5 for technique)	Restraint of sow's head and front legs necessary
	2. Innovar-Vet plus ketamine	1 ml/50-80 lb 3-5 mg/lb	Good chemical restraint; however, relatively more fetal depression than with epidural
	3. 500 mg ketamine plus 500 mg xylazine in 500 ml 5% guaifenesin	1 ml of mixture per lb; to effect for maintenance	Requires placement of IV catheter

VI. Anticholinergics
  A. Activity
    1. Both atropine and scopolamine pass placental barriers rapidly
      a. Fetal tachycardia noted within 10-15 minutes
      b. The effect of these drugs may vary
    2. There is reduced placental activity
    3. Glycopyrrolate does not readily cross the placenta due to its molecular size and charge
    4. Fetal disorientation or excitement may occur due to central action of atropine of scopolamine
VII. Local anesthetics
  A. Activity
    1. Local anesthetics administered by any route will cross the placental barrier
      a. Blood levels will depend on total dose, interval between final dose and delivery, and the presence of epinephrine
      b. Dosages of local anesthetics used clinically to produce regional anesthesia do not produce significant depression in the fetus
  B. Lidocaine
    1. Appears in umbilical venous blood of the fetus within 2-3 minutes with IV administration
    2. No correlation found between degree of neonatal depression and umbilical venous concentration of lidocaine
  C. Procaine
    1. Doses of 0.5-1.0 mg/lb did not produce demonstrable levels of drug in the fetus
    2. Procaine metabolism decreased due to decrease in pseudocholinesterase

ANESTHETIC TECHNIQUES

I. General principles
  A. Choice of a particular anesthetic regimen should be influenced by familiarity with the technique or drug
  B. Intubation is desirable in all patients induced to recumbency
  C. Majority of patient presurgical preparation should be done prior to administration of anesthetic drugs
  D. Excessive physical restraint is to be avoided
    1. Sedatives, tranquilizers, etc. are preferred over excessive physical force and subsequent maternal-fetal distress
  E. Avoid dorsal recumbency as much as possible. Left lateral recumbency may be safest
II. Anesthetic techniques by species (see Table 12-1)

CHAPTER THIRTEEN

Oxygen Toxicity, Anesthetic Toxicity, Waste Gas Scavenging, and Anesthetic-Drug Interactions

"Can we ever have too much of a good thing?"
DON QUIXOTE DE LA MANCHA

OVERVIEW

Inhalation anesthetic drug toxicity in patients and operating room personnel is cause for concern. All drugs that produce chemical restraint and anesthesia have the potential to produce cytotoxic effects. These toxic effects, if allowed to continue long enough or if sufficiently severe, can jeopardize the patient's life. Drug toxicity can occur because of unfamiliarity with the pharmacologic properties of a drug or insufficient knowledge regarding the means to counteract the drug's toxic effects. Occasionally, drug interactions occur, which emphasizes the importance of the preliminary physical examination and obtaining the patient's previous drug history. When inhalation anesthetics are used, scavenging of waste gases should be considered. All inhalation anesthetics are central nervous system depressants. Scavenging of anesthetic vapors and gases will help to minimize depression in operating room personnel, as well as other, more harmful, side effects.

GENERAL CONSIDERATIONS

I. All drugs used to produce chemical restraint and anesthesia are potentially toxic. Toxicity is caused by:
A. Inhibition of nervous system activity

B. Alteration of normal physiology and depression of cardiopulmonary function
C. Inhibition of enzyme systems
D. Direct cytotoxic effects
E. Differences in species' sensitivity to drugs
F. Idiosyncratic reactions

II. The toxic manifestations of drugs used to produce chemical restraint and anesthesia are generally reversible.

III. Many drugs used to produce chemical restraint and anesthesia can be antagonized.
A. Narcotics by narcotic antagonists such as naloxone
B. Xylazine by α_2 antagonists such as yohimbine, tolazoline, and idazoxan
C. Nondepolarizing muscle relaxants by acetylcholinesterase inhibitors such as neostigmine
D. General anesthetic–induced depression by analeptics, such as doxapram, 4-aminopyridine, and yohimbine

IV. Waste gas scavenging will minimize drug-related depression in operating room personnel and minimize the potential danger of drug-induced toxicity

V. Drug interactions may markedly potentiate or inhibit the actions of drugs used for chemical restraint and anesthesia

OXYGEN TOXICITY

I. Tolerance to oxygen
A. Exposure of animals to pure oxygen at atmospheric pressures for prolonged periods causes pulmonary dysfunction
1. Changes include decreases in vital capacity, minute ventilation, respiratory rate, pH, arterial oxygen partial pressure, total lung volume, and carbon dioxide–diffusing capacity
B. There is considerable variation in the susceptibility of animals to oxygen toxicity
C. The rate of onset of the disease process is proportional to the tension of oxygen and the duration of exposure
D. Reductions in vital capacity and pulmonary compliance are the best criteria for onset of toxicity

II. Lesions
A. Pulmonary responses to increased oxygen tension
1. Chronic type: Low doses of oxygen (25-60%) are associated with proliferative changes in endothelium and epithelium and permanent widening of the interstitium due to increased collagen and elastin fiber deposition
2. Acute type: Exposure to high concentrations (greater than 60%) of oxygen for more than 12 hours results in:
a. Atelectasis
b. Pulmonary capillary congestion and hyaline accumulation, type I epithelial cell death
c. Widening of the interstitium due to edema

      d. Capillary endothelial cell death

      e. Hemorrhage

III. Signs of toxicity

  A. Anorexia and lethargy

  B. Irregularity of respirations

  C. Coughing

  D. Gross difficulty in ventilation

  E. Death is from asphyxia and is preceded by cyanosis and apnea

IV. Mechanisms of pulmonary oxygen toxicity

  A. Oxygen is necessary for the production of energy and survival of all aerobic cells; it is also a cellular poison

  B. Studies of pulmonary surfactant, myocardial failure, inert gases, or carbon dioxide have provided no convincing evidence of the pathogenesis of the development of oxygen toxicity

  C. Absorption collapse

    1. Collapse of the lung when breathing oxygen is coincident with partial or complete occlusion of the airway

      a. Appears to be more a result than a cause of oxygen toxicity

    2. Collapse may occur more readily in the patient with pulmonary disease than in the normal patient

    3. Clinical management of absorption collapse

      a. Maintain patent airway

      b. Use high tidal volumes and positive end expiratory pressure (mixture of air and oxygen, 3:1)

      c. Promote coughing and periodic sighing

      d. General pulmonary care

  D. The formation of cytotoxic oxygen-free radicals may be a factor in oxygen toxicity, particularly when the period of hyperoxygenation is preceded by a period of hypoxia or ischemia

V. Endocrine system effects

  A. General rate of metabolism has been found to affect the responses to oxygen toxicity

  B. Hyperthyroidism and elevations of adrenocortical hormones hasten toxicity

  C. The depression of cellular activity by anesthesia decreases susceptibility to oxygen toxicity

  D. Sympathomimetic agents speed the onset of pulmonary damage; sympatholytic agents delay rate of toxicity

  E. Epinephrine augments the rate of toxicity

    1. Epinephrine toxicity is associated with pulmonary edema

IV. Recommendations

  A. *Do not* overreact to the use of oxygen

    1. Hypoxia is commonly associated with anesthesia and hypoventilation, and the damage it causes occurs rapidly

    2. Pulmonary injury from oxygen is uncommon, and onset is slow

B. There are no known contraindications to the use of pure oxygen for brief periods or in emergencies
  1. In the normal lung, no significant toxicity develops in breathing pure oxygen for 12 hours or less

VOLATILE ANESTHETICS

I. Volatile anesthetics are metabolized and thus are not completely biochemically inert. Metabolites are believed to be responsible for drug toxicity

II. Volatile anesthetics are amazingly uniform in distribution except in areas high in fat, in the thymus, and in the adrenal gland

III. Metabolism of inhalation anesthetics occurs primarily in the liver. Metabolites are excreted primarily by the kidneys

IV. The anesthetic molecule, per se, is nontoxic; however, the metabolites are potentially toxic. Chloride, bromide, and fluoride metabolites have been reported
  A. Toxic side effects occur when anesthetics and metabolites bind to the cell membrane

V. Binding of the anesthetic influences the amount and persistence of the anesthetic in the cell membrane
  A. Normal metabolic functions are affected as long as anesthetic is present

VI. At normal metabolic rates, there may be no toxic side effects. However, some individuals may have metabolic rates far below normal; thus toxic effects may be augmented
  A. Animals in shock
  B. Hypothermic animals

VII. Many inhalation anesthetic agents are teratogenic in mice. Further investigations are needed to clarify the importance of these findings in animals

VIII. Toxic impurities
  A. Cylinders of nitrogen oxide (N_2O) have contained nitrogen dioxide (NO_2)
  B. Improper storage can lead to decomposition of initially pure anesthetics
  C. Halogenated compounds are unstable in light
  D. Materials that are properly prepared, stored, and used have not led to any known catastrophes attributable to contaminants

TOXICOLOGY OF ANESTHETIC DRUGS

I. Halothane toxicity
  A. Patient response to halothane
    1. Many halogenated hydrocarbons are hepatotoxic
      a. Examples: chloroform and carbon tetrachloride
      b. Degree of halogenation increases the incidence of toxicity
      c. The liver is the organ most affected by these toxic side effects. Hepatic necrosis is believed to be due to the toxic effects of the fluoride or bromide molecules released after halothane metabolism by the liver

    B. Results of the National Halothane Study on Hepatic Necrosis concluded that:
       1. No unique or consistent lesion occurs following halothane administration
       3. Halothane sensitizes the heart to catecholamine-induced arrhythmias
       4. Halothane predisposes some animals to hyperpyrexia and malignant hyperthermia
    C. Toxicity to halothane
       1. Dose-related
       2. Increases with multiple use
       3. Thymol preservative in commercially prepared halothane is potentially toxic to both the liver and the kidney; however, it is present in very small quantities

II. Methoxyflurane toxicity
    A. Patient response to methoxyflurane
       1. Methoxyflurane is biodegraded
          a. Products of biodegradation
             (1) Carbon dioxide
             (2) Fluoride ion
             (3) Difluroacetic acid
             (4) Methoxyfluoroacetic acid
       2. There are elevated inorganic fluoride levels in all patients recovering from methoxyflurane anesthesia
          a. Fluoride ions are excreted via the kidney and are known nephrotoxins that can cause tubular injury
       3. Renal and liver failure may occur following methoxyflurane anesthesia in the dog, particularly if the animal is receiving other potentially nephrotoxic drugs (tetracyclines, aminoglycosides)
       4. Clinical studies in normal dogs have not proven renal dysfunction after clinical dosages of methoxyflurane
    B. Nephrotoxicity
       1. The degree of renal injury is dose-related
       2. Adequate fluid replacement should be provided to insure maximum excretion of fluoride ion
       3. Tetracycline antibiotics should not be administered coincidentally with methoxyflurane
          a. Tetracyclines may impair renal function, leading to renal failure
       4. Methoxyflurane should be avoided in the aged and markedly obese patient, especially those with impaired renal function
       5. Both high- and low-output forms of renal failure may occur

III. Enflurane and isoflurane toxicity
    A. The major toxic effects are due to decreased organ perfusion and resultant tissue hypoxia
    B. Teratogenic effects after long (many hours) exposures of mice to these agents

C. The clinical significance of these findings for single, short-term exposure (1-10 hours) is unknown
IV. Nitrous oxide toxicity
   A. Direct toxic effects of nitrous oxide appear after relatively long-term exposure (greater than 10 hours)
   B. More than 3 hours' exposure may be associated with neutropenia
   C. More than 10 hours' exposure may cause megaloblastic anemia
      1. Associated decrease in vitamin B_{12} and methionine synthetase
      2. Methionine synthetase activity declines within 30 minutes of nitrous oxide exposure
   D. Clinical use is not associated with any direct toxic effects
      1. Diffusion hypoxia and diffusion into closed cavity spaces are discussed in Chapter 10: Pharmacology of Inhalation Anesthetic Drugs
V. Barbiturate toxicity
   A. In general, clinical use of barbiturates is not known to display any direct cellular toxic manifestations
      1. Barbiturates stimulate liver microsomal enzymes and may alter the metabolism of other drugs
      2. Some seemingly normal animals appear to show a marked sensitivity to cardiorespiratory depressant effects of barbiturate anesthetics. This clinical observation is probably due to inadvertent overdosage but (although unlikely) may be due to idiosyncracy
      3. Acute tolerance to thiobarbiturates has been reported, although the cause is unknown
      4. Thiobarbiturates increase the susceptibility to the development of ventricular arrhythmias
VI. Local anesthetic toxicity
   A. In general, there are little or no deleterious effects to tissues caused by the proper administration of local anesthetics
   B. When overdosage occurs, it can cause:
      1. Hypotension
      2. Tremors
      3. Convulsions or severe depression
VII. Narcotic, ataractic, and cyclohexamine toxicity
   A. These drugs produce little or no toxic effects on the different organ tissues when administered in anesthetic dosages
   B. Deleterious side effects
      1. Narcotics
         a. The most common side effects produced by narcotics are hyperexcitability, respiratory depression, and bradycardia
         b. Blood dyscrasias, thrombocytopenia
      2. Ataractics
         a. Phenothiazine tranquilizers
            (1) Noted for their parasympatholytic and hypotensive effects
            (2) Rarely extrapyramidal behavioral changes and bradycardia

      b. Butyrophenone tranquilizers
        (1) Aggressive behavior and, rarely, excitement
      c. Diazepam
        (1) Propylene glycol, a preservative and dilutent for diazepam, may cause bradycardia and cardiac arrest
      d. Xylazine
        (1) Marked respiratory depression and bradycardia
    3. Cyclohexamines
      a. Produce an apneustic pattern of ventilation and increased arterial P_{CO_2}, resulting in respiratory acidosis
      b. Prolonged recovery from anesthesia may occur following the administration of Telazol to cats

WASTE GAS SCAVENGING

I. Problem: reports of increased incidence of abortion, congenital abnormalities, infertility, hepatic and renal disease, and CNS dysfunction in people exposed to chronic trace gas levels
    A. Anesthetics incriminated
      1. Nitrous oxide
      2. Halothane
      3. Methoxyflurane
      4. Enflurane
      5. Isoflurane
    B. Evidence
      1. Epidemiological studies, animal studies, and human volunteer studies reveal conflicting evidence; no one study has been able to conclusively prove cause and effect (see Occupational disease among operating room personnel, a national study. *Anesthesiology* 1974; 41: 321-340)
      2. Overall evidence implicates that trace anesthetic gases may affect human health
II. Recommendations
    A. Recommended acceptable levels (National Institute for Occupational Safety and Health [NIOSH])
      1. Volatile agents used alone: less than 2 ppm
      2. Volatile agents combined with nitrous oxide: less than 0.5 ppm volatile agent and less than 25 ppm nitrous oxide
      3. These are time-weighted averages over the span of a surgical procedure
    B. Waste gas scavenging
      1. The single most important method of eliminating waste gas
    C. Waste gas scavenging techniques (Fig. 13-1)
      1. Pop-off (pressure relief) valve fitted with gas collection assembly
      2. Transfer hose leading from gas collection assembly to scavenging interface and gas collection device
      3. Scavenging interface and gas collection device
        a. Connection to room ventilation system (past point of recirculation)

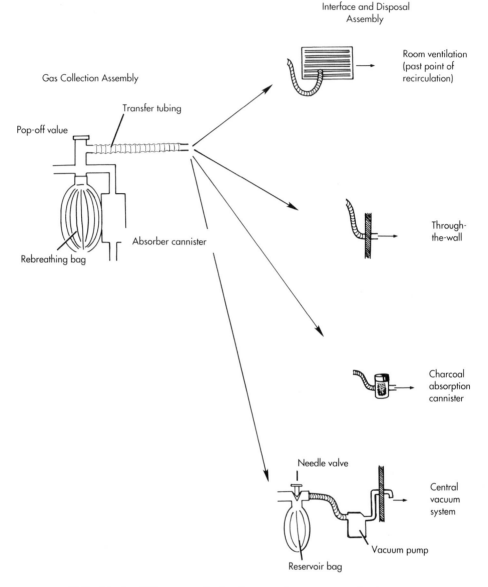

Interface and Disposal
Assembly

Gas Collection Assembly

Transfer tubing

Pop-off value

Room ventilation
(past point of
recirculation)

Through-
the-wall

Absorber cannister

Rebreathing bag

Charcoal
absorption
cannister

Needle valve

Central
vacuum
system

Vacuum pump

Reservoir bag

FIG. 13-1   Different methods of scavenging waste anesthetic gases.

  b. Pass scavenging tube from pop-off valve directly to and through an out-
     side wall; must be kept clear of debris, insects, rodents, etc. and directed
     away from wind currents
  c. Absorption device (activated charcoal) will not absorb nitrous oxide.
     Each cannister lasts 6-8 hours anesthetic time
  d. Central vacuum: expensive
 III. Other techniques to minimize trace gas concentrations
   A. Pressure-test all breathing circuits and machines for leaks

      1. Acceptable leakage is less than 100 ml/min at system pressure of 30 cm water
  B. Fill vaporizers carefully to avoid spillage. Fill at end of work day when less people are present
  C. Use low-flow or closed-system techniques when possible
  D. Recover patients in well-ventilated area, and remain at least 3 feet from patient's head
  E. Do not turn on gas flow until patient is connected to the machine
  F. When disconnecting patient from breathing circuit, occlude Y piece, turn off flowmeter, and evacuate remaining gas in system into scavenger
  G. Avoid chamber and mask inductions
  H. Inform all employees of potential risks of trace gas exposure and steps necessary to reduce exposure
      1. There are indications of an increased risk of abortion in women exposed during first trimester of pregnancy or exposed to trace gas concentrations within a year prior to pregnancy

ANESTHETIC DRUG INTERACTIONS

I. Types of interactions
  A. Physicochemical: Combining two or more drugs in a solution may result in a chemical incompatibility. Unless you are certain there is no incompatibility, don't combine drugs
  B. Some known incompatibilities
      1. Blood or blood products with any solution other than saline
      2. Acidic drug with basic drug
         a. Thiobarbiturate plus lidocaine
         b. Sodium bicarbonate with calcium-containing solutions
  C. Pharmacokinetic interactions: interactions affecting absorption, distribution, or elimination of a drug
      1. Protein binding effects
         a. Phenylbutazone displacing thiobarbiturates from binding sites, resulting in relative barbiturate overdosage
         b. Decreased protein binding due to hemodilution of intravenous fluid administration
      2. Alterations in biotransformation
         a. Phenobarbital enhances liver microsomal enzyme activity
         b. Organophosphates inhibit plasma cholinesterase, prolonging duration of action of ester-linked local anesthetics and depolarizing muscle relaxants
         c. Cimetidine and chloramphenicol reduce hepatic microsomal enzyme activity, thus prolonging duration of action of some drugs
         d. Epinephrine prolongs local anesthetic duration of action and hyaluronidase increases area of local anesthetic spread
  D. Pharmacodynamic interactions: The actions of a drug on a particular organ system or on the body as a whole can be altered by concurrently administered drugs

1. Agonist-antagonist interactions
    a. Narcotic agonists-antagonists
    b. Xylazine-yohimbine/tolazoline
    c. Nondepolarizing muscle relaxants–cholinesterase inhibitors
    d. Autonomic receptor agonists-antagonists
2. Other alterations in pharmacodynamics
    a. Arrhythmogenicity of halothane in presence of catecholamines
    b. Enhancement of halothane-catecholamine arrhythmias by certain drugs, such as barbiturate, xylazine, or ketamine
    c. Decrease in digitalis-induced arrhythmias by halothane
    d. Acepromazine and epinephrine reversal
    e. Aminoglycoside antibiotics prolong effects of muscle relaxants
    f. Tetracyclines enhance nephrotoxicity of methoxyflurane

CHAPTER FOURTEEN

Anesthetic Equipment and Maintenance

"Give the tools to him that can handle them."

NAPOLEON BONAPARTE

OVERVIEW

A wide variety of equipment is needed to administer inhalation anesthetic drugs. Volatilizing the anesthetic, delivering it safely to the patient, and minimizing environmental pollution requires the use of relatively sophisticated and, at times, cumbersome devices. Regardless of their seeming complexity, most inhalation anesthetic delivery systems have similar designs, many common features, and the same ultimate goal—the delivery and maintenance of safe anesthetic concentrations to the patient. This chapter outlines approaches to the delivery of inhalation anesthetics to animals.

GENERAL CONSIDERATIONS

I. The safe delivery of inhaled anesthetics to patients requires:
   A. A source of compressed gas
   B. Pressure-reducing valves and associated high-pressure tubing
   C. Flowmeters, vaporizers, and patient connecting tubing
   D. Endotracheal tubes
II. Methods by which inhalation anesthetics are delivered conform to:
   A. Open insufflation
   B. Semiopen with rebreathing
   C. Semiopen without rebreathing

TABLE 14-1

COMPRESSED GASES

Agent	Color	Cylinder specifications (liters, STP)			Filling pressure (psi)
		E (4" × 30")	G (8" × 55")	H (9" × 55")	
Oxygen	Green	655	5,290	6,910	2,200
Nitrous oxide	Blue	1,590	12,110	14,520	750
Carbon dioxide	Gray	1,590	4,160		800
Helium	Brown	500	4,350	5,930	1,650

    D. Semiclosed

    E. Closed

III. Selection of the appropriate anesthetic system is dependent on:

    A. Species

    B. Patient size and weight

    C. Patient's physical status

    D. Familiarity of the personnel with the equipment

IV. All anesthetic equipment requires routine maintenance. This is particularly true of anesthetic vaporizers, which should be recalibrated at least once every 2 years

V. Carbon dioxide–absorbent material should always be visible and should be changed at the first sign of color change

VI. Rebreathing tubing and reservoir bags should be thoroughly cleaned daily in order to avoid the possibility of spreading infection

ANESTHETIC EQUIPMENT

I. Compressed gases

    A. Supplied in color-coded tanks of varying size (see Table 14-1)

        1. Tanks should be handled carefully

            a. Never leave an unattended tank sitting upright

            b. Due to high pressure, a tank may explode if dropped

            c. Open valves slowly and completely

            d. Crack tank (open and shut quickly) before attaching to machine to remove dust from attachments

        2. Hanger yokes are keyed with pegs to prevent inadvertent connection of the wrong gas (pin index safety system)

            a. Use a fresh gasket for each cylinder

            b. Lubricate with small amount of silicon (no oil) if not prelubicated

    B. Centralized oxygen sources usually use G or H cylinders (more economical)

C. Separate pressure regulators are necessary for oxygen and nitrous oxide (thread size and connection coded for different types of gas)

D. There is frequently an adapter on the anesthetic machine for connection to a central-supply gas source (special high-pressure hosing necessary)

II. Pressure-reducing valves

    A. Valves function to reduce the pressure of the gas to approximately 50 psi, thus providing a constant pressure at the outlet over a wide range of flows

        1. Provides constant pressure at the flowmeter

        2. Allows a wider range of flowmeter settings (increased sensitivity)

        3. Flowmeter does not have to operate at dangerously high pressures

        4. Most anesthetic machines have pressure regulators built in

III. Flowmeters

    A. Flowmeters control the amount of a particular gas entering the anesthetic system

    B. Long tubes (10-12 inches in length) with a nearly uniform taper give more accurate readings

        1. Rotameters most commonly used

    C. Ideally, the oxygen flowmeter should be the last in a series of flowmeters (prevents dilution of oxygen by a crack in another flowmeter)

    D. Avoid excessive torque when closing flowmeters; the valve seat may be scored

IV. Oxygen flush valve

    A. Set to deliver oxygen into the system at 50 L/min

    B. Generally bypass the vaporizer

    C. Serve to dilute the anesthetic gases in the system

V. Anesthetic vaporizers

    A. Vaporizers used out of the circle (VOC)

        1. Precision-type instruments

        2. Thermocompensated or thermostable (vaporization chamber temperature changes slowly)

        3. Deliver precise anesthetic concentrations for long periods of time independent of temperature and semi-independent of flow rate

            a. Be sure to check vaporizer specifications concerning accuracy at different flow rates

        4. Anesthetic concentration can be changed relatively rapidly

        5. Expensive

    B. Specific out-of-circle vaporizers

        1. Halothane vaporizers

            a. Fluotec Mark II, III, and IV (Cyprane, serviced by Fraser Harlake)

            b. Fluomatic (Foregger)

            c. Vapor and Vapor 19.1-Halothane (Drager)

            d. Ohio Vaporizer for Halothane (Ohmeda)

        2. Methoxyflurane vaporizers

            a. Pentec Mark II (Cyprane, serviced by Fraser Harlake)

      b. Pentomatic (Foregger)

      c. Vapor-Methoxyflurane (Drager)

      d. Metomatic (Pitman-Moore): measured flow (Vernitrol)

    3. Enflurane vaporizer

      a. Enfluratec (Cyprane, serviced by Fraser Harlake)

      b. Enflurane Vapor 19.1 (Drager)

      c. Ohio Vaporizer for Enflurane (Ohmeda)

    4. Isoflurane vaporizers

      a. Ohio Vaporizer for Isoflurane (Ohmeda)

      b. Vapor 19.1 (Drager)

      c. Fortec and Fortec 4 (Cyprane, serviced by Fraser Harlake)

      d. Isoflurane can be used in halothane vaporizers, provided vaporizer is completely drained and wick is thoroughly dried

    5. Vaporizers used for various inhalation agents (measured-flow, non-agent-specific)

      a. Vernitrol (Ohio Medical)

      b. Copper Kettle (Foregger)

      c. A separate flowmeter controls carrier gas flow through vaporizer

      d. A slide rule is provided by the manufacturer to calculate flow rate through the vaporizer

    6. Maintenance

      a. Fluotec

     (1) May be cleaned by bubbling diethyl ether through the vaporizer

     (2) Should be drained completely once every week

     (3) Should be sent to the factory every 2 years for cleaning and recalibration

  C. Vaporizers in the circle (VIC)

    1. Less precise and less efficient

    2. Variation in respiration alters flow through the vaporizer, thus affecting the concentration of anesthetic delivery

    3. Calibration marks on top of vaporizer are not synonymous with percentage

    4. Relatively inexpensive

    5. Types

      a. Ohio #8 Vaporizer for Methoxyflurane (Pitman-Moore)

      b. Stevens Universal, Komesaroff, multiagent

      c. Snyder, methoxyflurane

      d. Modified Goldman, halothane or methoxyflurane

    6. Maintenance

      a. Wick should be cleaned with ether every 3-6 months depending on use

      b. Wick should be allowed to dry each night to rid system of excess water vapor

VI. Rebreathing bag

  A. Capacity should be five to six times animal's tidal volume

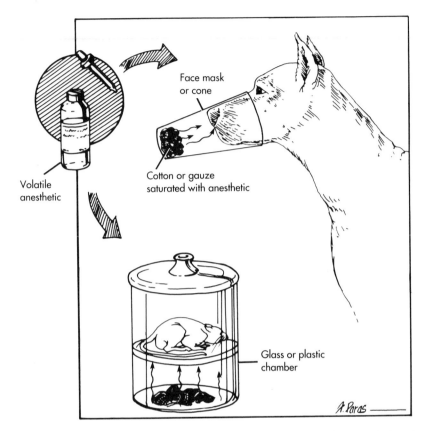

FIG.14-1 Open system: Gauze or cotton is saturated with anesthetic and placed in a cone or chamber from which the animal breathes.

VII. Pressure manometers
   A. Indicate pressure within the system
   B. Calibrated in cm of water or mm of mercury

ANESTHETIC SYSTEMS

   I. Purpose
      A. Delivery of anesthetic gases safely, inexpensively, and with adequate oxygen
      B. Removal of carbon dioxide by one of three methods
         1. Dilution
         2. Nonrebreathing valves
         3. Carbon dioxide absorbents
   II. Classification of systems
      A. Open (nonrebreathing)
         1. Examples
            a. Open drop or cone (Fig. 14-1)

TABLE 14-2

RECOMMENDED OXYGEN FLOW RATES FOR ANESTHESIC SYSTEMS

Closed circle	2-5 ml/lb/min O_2*
Semiclosed circle	10-20 ml/lb/min O_2**
Systems with nonrebreathing valves	
Digby-Leigh and Stephen-Slater	Equal to minute ventilation
Mapleson systems	
Magill system	Equal to minute ventilation (spontaneous respiration only)
Ayre's T piece	
Kuhn system	2-4 L/min***
Norman elbow	(> 1.5 × minute ventilation)
Bain circuit	

*Cannot use nitrous oxide in a closed circle
**If using nitrous oxide, add to the O_2 flow
***Indicates total flow rate for nonrebreathing

   b. Insufflation
   c. Ayre's T piece without reservoir
   d. Induction chamber
2. Identification by:
   a. No reservoir
   b. No or slight rebreathing of expired gases
   c. Carbon dioxide removal by dilution with room air
3. Advantages
   a. Low cost of equipment
   b. Minimal or no rebreathing of expired gases by patient
   c. Minimal resistance to breathing
4. Disadvantages
   a. Wastes anesthetic: no control of anesthetic being vaporized
   b. Difficult to control anesthetic concentration delivered
   c. No method to support ventilation
   d. Difficult or impossible to scavenge waste gas
   e. Vaporization of anesthetic dependent on room temperature
5. Hazards and precautions
   a. Difficulty of maintaining a stable anesthetic plane—use high flow rates (see Table 14-2)
   b. Dilution of anesthetic by room air—use high flow rates (see Table 14-2)
B. Semiopen
1. Mapleson systems
   a. Rees modification of Ayre's T piece (Fig. 14-2)
   b. Norman mask elbow (Fig. 14-3)
   c. Kuhn system (Fig. 14-4)
   d. Bain circuit (Fig. 14-5)
   e. Magill system (Fig. 14-6)

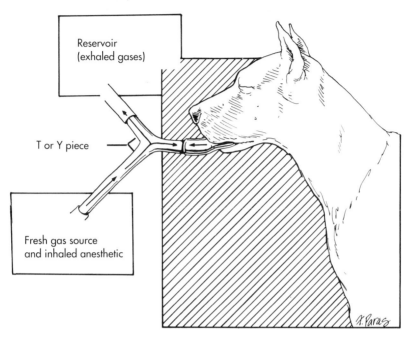

FIG. 14-2 T or Y piece: a low-resistance method of delivering vaporized anesthetic and gas (O_2, N_2O) to patients. High flow rates are used to minimize or prevent rebreathing.

Norman Elbow System

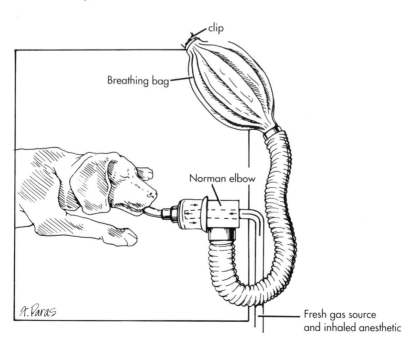

FIG. 14-3 Norman elbow: a modified T piece that minimizes equipment dead space.

Kuhn System

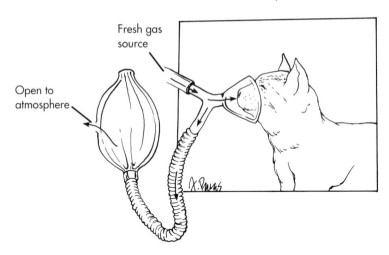

FIG. 14-4 Kuhn system: a modified T piece that allows exhaled gas to escape from the side of the bag, facilitating its occlusion and manual support of ventilation.

Bain Circuit

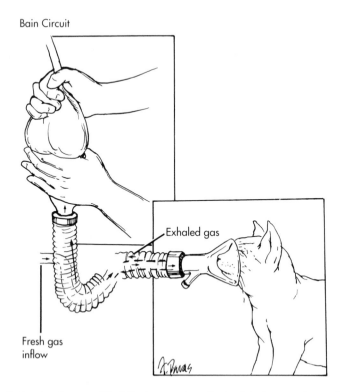

FIG. 14-5 Bain circuit: a modified T piece system that minimizes equipment dead space and facilitates warming of the inspired gases.

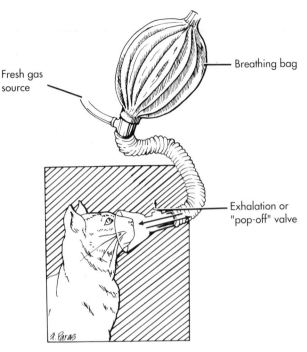

FIG. 14-6 Magill system: a modified T piece that utilizes the use of low flow rates of O_2 and N_2O because of the presence of a pop-off valve.

2. Systems employing nonrebreathing valves
   a. Stephen-Slater (Fig. 14-7, *A*)
   b. Fink modification of Stephen-Slater (Fig. 14-7, *B)*
   c. Digby-Leigh
3. Identification by
   a. Reservoir (e.g., rebreathing bag)
   b. No or minimal rebreathing of expired gases
   c. Carbon dioxide removal by dilution or nonrebreathing valves
4. Advantages
   a. Resistance to breathing is minimal
   b. Dead space is minimal
   c. Inspired concentrations are held constant and can be rapidly changed
   d. Efficient elimination of carbon dioxide
   e. Reservoir bag permits assisted or controlled ventilation
   f. Reservoir permits visual and tactile impression of depth, rate, and rhythm of respiration
5. Disadvantages
   a. High flow rates are suggested to prevent rebreathing of expired gases. Useful only in small patients (<15 pounds)

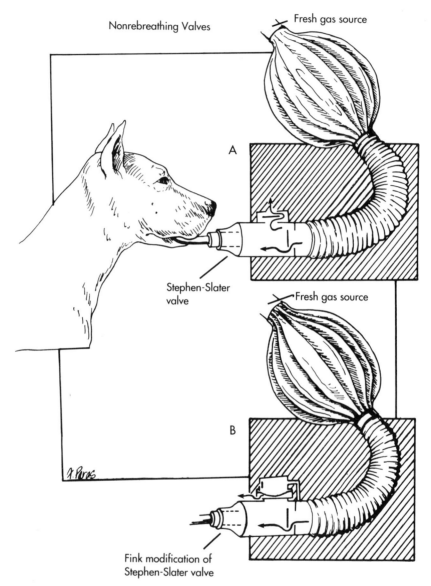

FIG. 14-7 Nonrebreathing valve: The Stephen-Slater valve (*A*) prevents rebreathing of exhaled gas. The Fink modification of the Stephen-Slater valve (*B*) prevents rebreathing and permits manual ventilation.

  b. Loss of heat
  c. Loss of humidity
  d. Less economical on a day-to-day basis than closed or semiclosed systems
  e. Nonrebreathing valves may stick

6. Hazards and precautions
   a. Rebreathing at low flow rates—see Table 14-2 for recommended oxygen flow rates
   b. Improper valve functioning—check valves for stickiness and foreign material before use
   c. Excessive inflation of lungs by inflow—watch flow rates and avoid kinking of the system (reservoir bag)
C. Semiclosed (partial rebreathing)
   1. Circle system with pop-off valve *open*
   2. To-and-fro systems
   3. Components
      a. Pop-off (pressure relief) valves
         (1) Allow the release of excess pressure from the system
         (2) Spring-loaded or variable orifice
         (3) Fitted with orifice for scavenging
      b. Carbon dioxide absorbent
         (1) Removes carbon dioxide from the expired gases
         (2) Capacity should be one to two times tidal volume (5 ml/lb)
         (3) Absorbent used is either soda lime or barium hydroxide lime
         (4) Use 4-8 mesh granule-size soda lime
         (5) Absorbent has a color indicator that turns blue on consumption. The indicator may revert to original color when allowed to rest. Should be changed after 2-8 hours of use, dependent on fresh gas flow rates
      c. Unidirectional flow valves
         (1) Two used in circle system
         (2) Also a component of some nonrebreathing systems
      d. Vaporizer (in or out of the circle; see Figs. 14-8, 14-9)
      e. Rebreathing bag
   4. Oxygen flow rate depends on patient's needs and denitrogenation of the system. Denitrogenation takes approximately 15 minutes using high (at least 10-20 ml/lb/min) flow rates
      (*Note:* Some vaporizers have minimal flow requirements to deliver accurate concentrations)
   5. Portion of expired gases are eliminated by means of a pop-off valve
   6. Advantages
      a. Low gas flow rate is economical
      b. Carbon dioxide—absorbent cannister is away from patient
      c. Ventilation is readily observed and controlled
      d. Minimal heat loss and drying
      e. Absence of abrupt fluctuations in anesthetic depth
   7. Disadvantages
      a. System is bulky
      b. Many parts may be disarranged or may malfunction
      c. Resistance to gas flow is greater than with semiopen systems

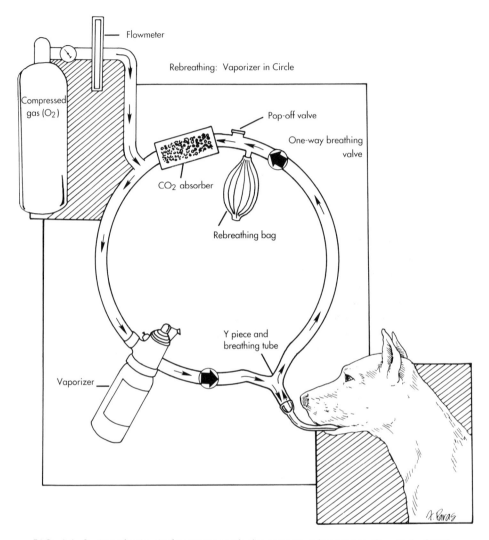

FIG. 14-8 Anesthetic circle system with the vaporizer located in the circle (VIC).

    d. Some components are difficult to clean

    e. Potential cross-infection of patients

  8. Hazards and precautions

    a. Valve systems can be accidentally bypassed or omitted—routinely check machine before use

    b. Incompetent valves—routinely check and clean valves, use nonwetting valves

    c. Channeling of gases in carbon dioxide cannister—uniformly pack absorbent cannister and position straight up; fill to within 1 inch of top

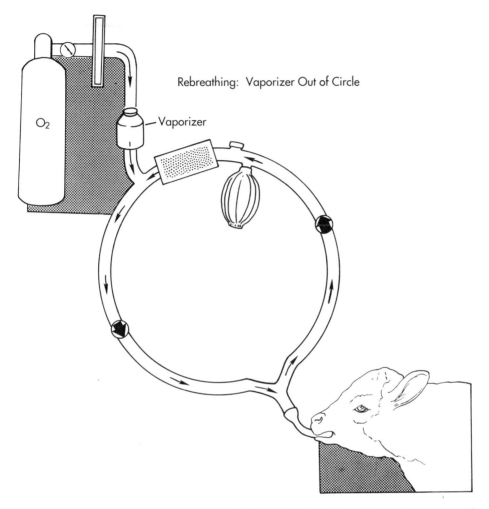

FIG. 14-9 Anesthetic circle system with the vaporizer located out of the circle (VOC).

  d. Inhalation of soda lime dust in to-and fro-systems—avoid use of crumbly soda lime
  e. Accumulation of moisture occluding expiratory limb—empty water-filled tubings after long anesthetic procedures
 D. Closed
  1. Circle systems with pop-off valve closed
  2. Components are similar to semiclosed system
   a. Circle systems with the vaporizer in the circle (VIC) (Fig. 14-8) and vaporizer out of the circle (VOC) (Fig. 14-9)
   b. Komesaroff and Stephens anesthesia machines
    (1) Isoflurane, halothane, or methoxyflurane can be administered by in-the-circle vaporizers
    (2) Halothane vaporizer should be turned off if controlled ven-

Closed (To and Fro) Rebreathing

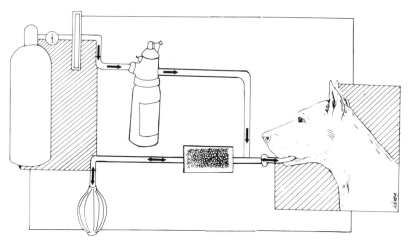

FIG.14-10 The to-and-fro anesthetic system maximizes carbon dioxide removal and aids in the maintenance of body temperature.

   tilation is used because excessively high concentrations may develop
      (3) Higher percentages of each anesthetic may be required for maintenance
   3. Advantages of using a closed over a semiclosed system
      a. More economical
      b. Minimal gas flows needed, depending on patient's metabolic needs (range: 2-5 ml/lb)
      c. Less pollution
      d. Body temperature more easily maintained
   4. Disadvantages of using a closed over a semiclosed system
      a. Requires close monitoring of anesthetic circuit (e.g., oxygen content, anesthetic content, attention to leaks)
      b. Difficult to rapidly change anesthetic concentration in circuit
   5. Hazards and precautions
      a. Similar to semiclosed systems
      b. Virtually no gas escapes from the system; the pop-off valve, if present, remains closed—watch pressure manometer for pressure buildup
      c. Nitrous oxide should *not* be used in closed systems unless an oxygen analyzer is incorporated in the system to assure adequate oxygen levels
III. To-and-fro systems (Fig. 14-10) are not commonly used
   A. Heat accumulates in the system because the carbon dioxide cannister is attached directly to the endotracheal tube

B. Alkaline dust from carbon dioxide absorbent may be inhaled
C. Cannister dead space may increase due to exhaustion of absorbent activity
D. Advantages include low resistance and efficient carbon dioxide absorption

IV. Anesthetic machines in common use
   A. Foregger compact 50
   B. Dupaco Compact 78
   C. Fraser Harlake VMS (small and large animal)
   D. Narkovet and Narkovet Deluxe (small and large animal)
   E. Pitman-Moore 970, 980, and Vetaflex-5
   F. Ohio Medical Products Vernitrol
   G. Bird anesthesia ventilator (JD Medical) (large animal)
   H. Snyder (small and large animal)
   I. Komesaroff

CARE OF RUBBER ARTICLES

I. Rubber articles absorb anesthetics and may become brittle or tacky
II. Remove metal connections immediately after use
III. Wash with soap and water; do not use detergents or soap containing creosol or unreactive hydrocarbon solvents
IV. Powdering to prevent tackiness may be done for articles stored or steam-sterilized in close contact
V. Sterilize and store in sterile or dry containers
VI. Soaking in alcohol or bichloride solutions is not as effective
VII. Avoid contact with animal or vegetable oils
VIII. If contaminated, wash with acetone and then soap and water
IX. Avoid contact with aerosols, phenols, terpenes, hydrocarbon solvents, esters, chlorinated hydrocarbons, and oxidizing acids
X. Store in the dark away from electric motors

TROUBLESHOOTING ANESTHETIC EQUIPMENT PROBLEMS

I. Rebreathing bag empty
   A. Flow rate too low
   B. System leak
      1. Gasket on carbon dioxide cannister improperly installed
      2. Hole in rebreathing bag or tubing
      3. Leak in endotracheal tube cuff
      4. Waste gas scavenging system employing active suction improperly regulated
      5. Water drain near carbon dioxide absorbent cannisters is open
II. Rebreathing bag overly distended (positive pressure in circuit)
   A. Pop-off valve inadvertently left closed
   B. Flow rate too high in closed system
   C. Waste gas scavenging system improperly regulated
III. Patient seems "light"
   A. Vaporizer empty

B. Excessive carbon dioxide buildup
   1. Exhausted carbon dioxide absorbent
   2. Sticky unidirectional valve
C. Vaporizer needs service
   1. Water buildup on wick
   2. Recalibration necessary
D. Patient receiving hypoxic gas mixture
   1. Nitrous oxide flowmeter set too high relative to oxygen flow

CHAPTER FIFTEEN

Ventilation and
Mechanical Assist Devices

"You don't need a weatherman to know which way the wind blows."

Bob Dylan

OVERVIEW

One of the most crucial aspects of providing safe general anesthesia is the maintenance of normal ventilation. Normal ventilation is defined as the ability to maintain arterial carbon dioxide levels within normal limits (35-40 mm Hg). Generally, respiratory effort can be visualized by observing the patient's chest and abdominal wall movement. Although these movements may be regular and give the appearance of satisfactory gas exchange, they do not ensure adequate movement of air in and out of the lungs. Adequate gas exchange can be provided by inflating the lungs to a predetermined pressure or predetermined volume by manually squeezing a rebreathing bag on an anesthetic machine or utilizing a mechanical ventilatory-assist device. High-frequency ventilation is a unique technique for ventilating patients. This technique utilizes the principle that diffusion is the primary means by which fresh gases are delivered to peripheral airways and gas exchange sites.

GENERAL CONSIDERATIONS

I. Artificial ventilation can do more harm than good if improperly used
II. Anyone attempting artificial ventilation should be thoroughly familiar with normal cardiopulmonary physiology and blood gas interpretation
III. Generally speaking, mechanical ventilatory-assist devices do no more than compress a rebreathing bag to inflate the lungs; they are an extra pair of hands

153

IV. The use of artificial ventilation should be considered in those patients who are not breathing adequately

V. Blood gas determinations are the only valid tests of ventilatory adequacy

SOURCES OF RESPIRATORY INADEQUACY

I. Depression of respiratory centers
  A. Drug-induced
    1. Anesthetic
    2. Neuromuscular blocking agents
    3. Drug toxicities
  B. Metabolic
    1. Acidosis
    2. Coma
    3. Toxic metabolites (endotoxins)
  C. Physical
    1. Head trauma (increased intracranial pressure)
    2. Chest trauma
    3. Severance of nerves
    4. Nerve trauma (edema)

II. Inability to adequately expand the thorax
  A. Pain (splinting of chest)
  B. Chest trauma
  C. Thoracic surgery
  D. Abdominal distention
  E. Muscle weakness
  F. Obesity
  G. Bony deformities of the chest wall
  H. Positioning
    1. Weight of viscera may impede expansion
    2. Abdominal compression may impede expansion

III. Inability to adequately expand the lungs
  A. Pneumothorax (especially tension pneumothorax)
  B. Pleural fluid
  C. Diaphragmatic hernia
  D. Thoracic surgery
  E. Neoplasia
  F. Pneumonia
  G. Atelectasis

IV. Acute cardiopulmonary arrest

V. Pulmonary edema or insufficiency

MANAGEMENT OF VENTILATION IN ANESTHESIA

I. Anesthetics are respiratory depressants; thus ventilation may need to be assisted if hypoventilation occurs

II. Special indications for artificial ventilation in anesthesia
  A. Thoracic surgery

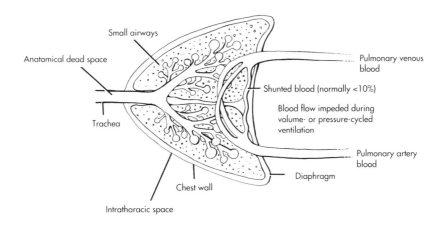

FIG. 15-1 Lung volume and airway pressure can augment or impede blood flow through the lung.

1. Controlled respiration minimizes extraneous chest wall movements, thus aiding the surgeon
2. With the chest open, the patient cannot adequately expand the lungs (pneumothorax)
   B. Neuromuscular blockers
   1. Clinical doses of neuromuscular blocking drugs, which produce muscular relaxation, also paralyze the diaphragm and intercostal muscles
   C. Prolonged anesthesia (>90 minutes), especially in the horse
   D. Trauma
   E. CNS trauma
   F. Drug overdose

PHYSIOLOGIC CONSIDERATIONS

I. Pulmonary system
   A. Normal lungs are well ventilated by a variety of different pressures, volumes, and flow rates (see Fig. 15-1)
   B. During spontaneous ventilation, the portions of the lung in closest contact with moving surfaces, i.e., the peripheral lung field, receive the greater volume of the inspired gases
   C. During artificial ventilation, preferential inflation of the peribronchial and mediastinal areas of the lung occurs due to the pressure gradient induced. The peripheral segments remain relatively hypoventilated
   1. Pressure or volume ventilation may increase anatomical dead space due to increases in airway diameter, further reducing alveolar ventilation
   D. Positive pressure ventilation results in a marked reduction in lung compliance

and a progressive decline in lung volume, which can lead to atelectasis and hypoxemia

1. Airway closure can occur
2. Increased lung water reduces compliance
3. Distribution of ventilation is altered
4. Volume-cycled ventilators compensate to a greater degree for worsening of lung mechanics than do pressure-cycled ventilators (by insuring delivery of a constant volume)
   a. Pressure-cycled ventilators must be reset to compensate for stiffened lungs

II. Cardiovascular systems (Table 15-1)
   A. During spontaneous ventilation, the subatmospheric pressure within the thorax augments venous return. This subatmospheric pressure is made more negative during inspiration by downward movement of the diaphragm
   B. During artificial ventilation, the pressure in the trachea and lung is transmitted to the thoracic cavity, thus impeding venous return and potentially decreasing cardiac output (see Figs. 15-1, 15-2)
   C. Artificial ventilation will decrease arterial blood pressure due to decreased cardiac output in any of the following instances
      1. Average airway pressure consistently exceeds 10 mm mercury
      2. Circulating blood volume is low (dehydration, anemia, blood loss)
      3. Sympathetic nervous system activity is impaired (anesthesia, local anesthetics, shock)
   D. Artificial ventilation decreases pulmonary blood flow and therefore may lead to ventilation/perfusion abnormalities
   E. All circulatory changes caused by artificial ventilation are due to or are the result of prolonged increases in mean airway pressure

III. Important normal values to remember
   A. Tidal volume (V_T): the amount of gas exchanged in one respiratory cycle
      1. 5 ml/lb in small animals (less than 400 pounds)
      2. 3-4 ml/lb in large animals (more than 400 pounds)
      3. V_T is usually increased by 1-2 ml/lb in calculating the volume needed during IPPV in order to compensate for the added compliance of the anesthetic or respiratory equipment
   B. Minute volume ($\dot{V}$): the volume of gas exchanged in one minute
      1. Dependent on tidal volume (V_T) and breaths per minute (BPM): $V_T \times BPM = \dot{V}$
   C. Adequate inflation of a normal animal's lungs requires approximately 20 cm H_2O pressure
      1. Lung compliance (volume/pressure/kg) is important in determining the pressure required to inflate the lung
   D. The spontaneous ventilatory cycle
      1. Inspiration (I) is active
         a. 1 second in small animals
         b. 1.5-3 seconds in large animals

TABLE 15-1

CARDIOVASCULAR SYSTEM

	Phase of cycle	Intrathoracic pressure	Right ventricle filling	Right ventricle cardiac output	Total thoracic blood volume	Left ventricle filling	Left ventricle cardiac output
Normal breathing	Inspiration active	↓ (5 cm H$_2$O) active	↑	↑	↑	→	→
	Expiration passive	↑ (−2 cm H$_2$O)	↓ When compared to normal inspiration	↓	→	↑ Due to venous return from lung	↑
IPPV	Inspiration passive	↑ (15-20 cm H$_2$O)	↓ (Peripheral venous pressure ↑)	↓	→	↑ (for a few beats only [3-5], then ↓)	↑ (↓ if IPP prolonged
	Expiration generally passive	↓ To atmospheric pressure	↓ When compared to previous positive pressure inspiration	↑ (If expiration long enough that is ≥ inspiration	↑	↓	→

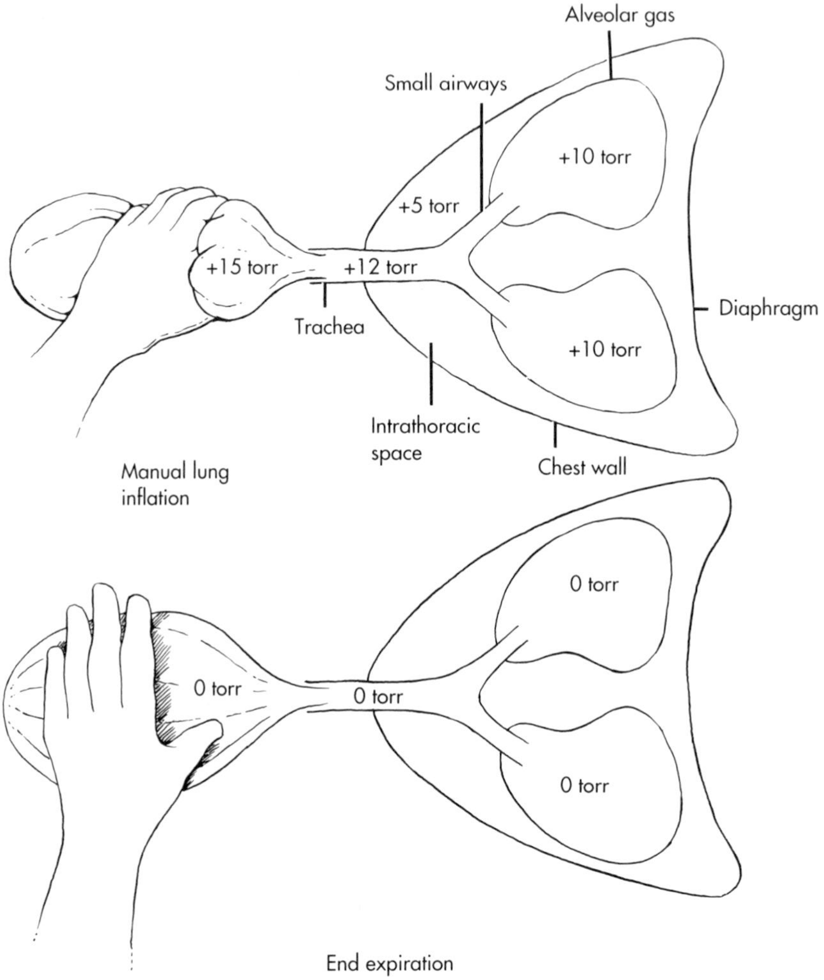

FIG. 15-2 Manual lung inflation produces a positive pressure in the lung and thoracic cavity, which impedes lung blood flow and lowers cardiac output.

   E. Guides to adequate mechanical artificial ventilation in the normal patient
      1. V_T (under normal conditions)
        a. Up to 7 ml/lb in small animals
        b. Up to 6-7 ml/lb in large animals
      2. Pressures
        a. 20-25 cm H_2O in both large and small animal species with normal lungs
        b. During open chest procedures or in the presence of stiff or mechanically inhibited lungs, pressure must be increased
      3. I/E ratios

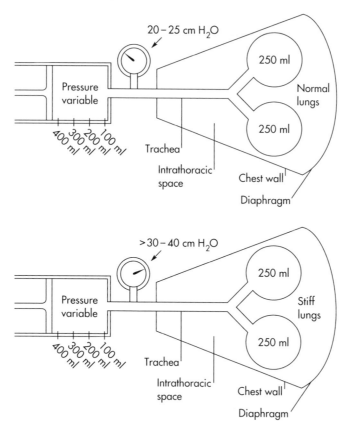

FIG. 15-3 Volume-cycled ventilators deliver a predetermined volume irrespective of the pressure developed.

    a. 1:2, 1:3 in small animals
    b. 1:1, 1:2 in large animals
  4. Inspiratory times
    a. Less than 1.5 seconds in small animals
    b. Less than 3 seconds in large animals
  5. Visualization of chest wall movements
    a. Helpful indication of lung inflation

CLASSIFICATION OF VENTILATORS

I. Volume-cycled (Fig. 15-3)
  A. A gas or gas mixture is delivered in a preset volume by the ventilatory-assist device
  B. Advantages
    1. Delivers a known V_T regardless of the pressure imposed

      a. Most volume-cycled ventilators are equipped with a blow-off safety valve to prevent the development of extremely high pressure (>60 cm H_2O)

      b. Delivers a constant volume despite stiffening of the lungs during anesthesia

    2. Relatively simple machine

  C. Disadvantages

    1. High airway pressures may develop

    2. Volume ventilators do not compensate for small leaks in the system; they require an airtight system. A major leak will prevent the patient from receiving an adequate V_T

  D. Types

    1. Piston or bellows type

      a. A predetermined volume is delivered

    2. Time-flow type

      a. Volume is delivered in a preset basic flow rate of gas for a specific amount of time

II. Pressure-cycled (Fig. 15-4)

  A. A gas or gas mixture is delivered by a ventilatory-assist device during the inspiratory phase until the system reaches a preset pressure

  B. Advantages

    1. High safety factor. A high pressure will not develop unless preset by the operator

    2. Small leaks are compensated for. Large leaks cause the prolongation of inspiratory time

  C. Disadvantages

    1. The volume delivered is variable and is dependent on the following

      a. Lung compliance

      b. Airway resistance

      c. Number of functional alveoli

      d. Pressure within the thorax

    2. Measurement of tidal volume may be difficult if the ventilator is not equipped with a bellows

    3. Pressure may need to be increased during a procedure to maintain adequate tidal volume

III. Tank ventilator (iron lung)

  A. Delivers a negative pressure to the body

  B. Advantages

    1. Improves cardiovascular hemodynamics by producing a negative pressure in the chest during inspiration

    2. Minimal reduction in lung compliance

  C. Disadvantages

    1. Access to the patient is limited

    2. Environment within the chamber must be controlled (temperature, humidity)

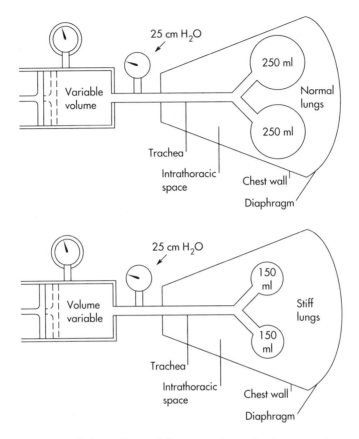

FIG.15-4 Pressure-cycled ventilators deliver a predetermined pressure irrespective of the volume delivered.

MODES OF OPERATION OF VENTILATORY-ASSIST DEVICES

I. Assist mode

    A. Patient triggers the ventilatory device by initiating an inspiratory effort

II. Controlled mode

    A. The ventilator is insensitive to the patient's inspiratory efforts

    B. If the patient resists controlled ventilation ("bucks" the ventilator), severe cardiopulmonary embarrassment may occur

III. Assist-controlled mode

    A. A minimal respiratory rate is set by the operator, which the patient may override by initiating spontaneous ventilatory efforts at a faster rate

TERMS USED FOR VARIABLE MODES OF OPERATION
DURING MECHANICAL VENTILATION

I. IPPV (intermittent positive-pressure ventilation): positive pressure maintained only during inspiration

II. CPPV (continuous positive-pressure ventilation): positive pressure maintained during inspiration and expiration

III. PNPV (positive/negative-pressure ventilation): positive pressure during inspiration and negative pressure during expiration

IV. PEEP (positive end-expiratory pressure): used to open small airways following lung trauma or pulmonary edema

V. ZEEP (zero end-expiratory pressure): normal passive expiration

VI. NEEP (negative end-expiratory pressure): used to hasten expiration

VII. CPAP (continuous positive airway pressure)

VIII. IMPV (intermittent mandatory positive-pressure ventilation)

VENTILATORS COMMONLY USED IN VETERINARY MEDICINE

I. North American-Drager Large and Small Animal Anesthetic Machine and Ventilator
  A. Volume-cycled/flow-regulated
    1. Volume adjusted by raising and lowering bellows support to appropriate level
    2. pressure manometer indicates the pressure within the system
  B. Controls
    1. On/off switch
    2. Frequency (respiratory rate)
      a. Adjusted to BPM
      b. Usually maintain 6-10 BPM in the horse
    3. Flow
      a. Inspiratory flow rate; determines inspiratory time
    4. I/E ratio: adjustable from 1:1 to 1:4.5
  C. Pop-off valve
    1. Manual pop-off valve must be closed during ventilator use
    2. Automatic pop-off closes with the inspiratory cycle

II. Bag-in-a-barrel type ventilator, generally powered by a Bird pressure-cycled ventilator
  A. Controlled by a modified Bird Mark 7 or Mark 9 ventilator
  B. L.A. Ventilator
    1. Driven by a modified Bird Mark 7 ventilator
  C. Pressure-cycled
    1. Volume indicated on the chamber encasing the bellows
    2. Can adjust the pressure to give the desired volume
  D. Mode
    1. Assisted
      a. Adjust sensitivity so the patient can trigger the machine
    2. Controlled
      a. Increase value of sensitivity so patient cannot trigger the machine
    3. Assist-controlled
  E. Controls
    1. Inspiratory pressure

        a. Usually set at 20-30 cm water

        b. Adjusted to give the desired tidal volume

    2. Expiratory time

        a. Controls respiratory rate by controlling time between breaths

        b. Rate usually set at 6-10 BPM for the horse

    3. Flow rate

        a. Adjust to an inspiratory time of 3 seconds for the horse

    4. Air mix

        a. Set at 50% oxygen to conserve oxygen

        b. *Does not* affect oxygen supply to the animal

    5. Sensitivity

        a. Governs ability of the animal to trigger the ventilator

        b. Numbers are merely a rough guide to indicator of position

III. Metomatic veterinary ventilator (small animal patients only)

    A. Volume-cycled ventilator

        1. Pressure limited

        2. Accessories include a manometer to measure pressure

    B. Controls

        1. Tidal volume

            a. Controlled by adjustable knob

            b. Indicated on the front of the bellows

        2. Inspiratory flow rate

            a. Controls inspiratory times

            b. Adjusted to be equal to or less than expiratory time

        3. Expiratory time

            a. Controls rate by controlling length of expiration

            b. Usually 6-12 BPM

        4. Inspiratory hold

            a. Holds ventilator at peak pressure; used to eliminate atelectasis

            b. Can cause cardiovascular embarrassment if the chest is closed

        5. Inspiratory pressure

            a. Governs maximal pressure

            b. Reduces possibility of an extreme pressure being placed on the chest

        6. Inspiratory trigger effort

            a. Governs ability of animal to initiate inspiration

        7. Expiratory flow rate

            a. Governs rate of fall of the bag and, therefore, expiration

            b. Adjusted to regulate impedance to expiration

IV. Bird Mark 7 and Mark 9 ventilators

    A. Pressure-cycled

        1. Volume delivered is controlled by the pressure developed unless equipped with a bellows

    B. Bird must be equipped with a bag-in-a-barrel or a bellows to be used as an anesthetic system

    C. Controls

1. Inspiratory pressure
   a. Controls peak pressure
   b. Normally set at 20-30 cm water
2. Sensitivity
   a. Controls ability of animal to trigger the machine
   b. Low numbers; easily triggered
   c. High numbers; difficult to trigger
3. Inspiratory flow rate
   a. Controls inspiratory time
   b. Set equal to or less than expiratory time
4. Expiratory time
   a. Controls respiratory rate by controlling expiratory time
   b. Respiratory rate normally 6-12 BPM
5. Air mix
   a. Varies percentage of inspired oxygen from 50% to 100%
   b. Negative pressure (Bird Mark 9 only)
      (1) The Bird Mark 9 allows the operator to produce NEEP
6. Weaning the patient off the ventilator
   a. The initiation of spontaneous respirations following controlled venti-
      lation can be hastened by:
      (1) Decreasing the rate of controlled respiratory frequency
      (2) Physical manipulation—rolling the patient, twisting an ear, toe
          pinch
      (3) Respiratory stimulants: doxapram administration, 0.1-0.3 mg/lb IV

HIGH-FREQUENCY VENTILATION (HFV)

I. High-frequency ventilation is a relatively new form of mechanical ventilation
in which respiratory rate (f) > 1 Hz (cycle/sec) and tidal volume (V_T) $<$
anatomical dead space. Generally, one of three modes is used:
  A. High-frequency positive-pressure ventilation: f $=$ 1-2 Hz; positive pressure
     maintained throughout the respiratory cycle
  B. High-frequency jet ventilation: f $=$ 2-7 Hz; a small cannula is used to deliver
     jets of gas into the airway
  C. High-frequency oscillating ventilation: f $=$ 6-40 Hz; bias flow of fresh gas
     entrained by oscillating column of gas
II. Potential uses include acute respiratory distress syndrome (ARDS), hyalin mem-
brane disease, bronchopleural fistula, pulmonary contusion

CHAPTER SIXTEEN

Patient Monitoring During Anesthesia

*"You see only what you look for,
You recognize only what you know."*

MERRIL C. SOSMAN

OVERVIEW

The effects of chemical restraint and anesthesia need to be monitored. A variety of sophisticated and complex technical equipment is available for determining the patient's status following chemical restraint and anesthesia. This instrumentation facilitates the recording and interpretation of the electroencephalogram, the electrocardiogram, and the electromyogram. Other monitoring methods include the measurement of arterial and central venous blood pressure, recording and audio transmission of heart sounds, and the measurement of arterial and venous oxygen and carbon dioxide tensions. End-expired samples of respiratory gases can be measured for oxygen/carbon dioxide content as well as inhalation anesthetic concentration.

GENERAL CONSIDERATIONS

I. Physiological homeostatic mechanisms are altered by drugs used during anesthesia and by the pathophysiological processes of disease
II. Intraoperative physiological monitoring optimizes patient status for successful anesthetic procedures
   A. Allows for informed, flexible responses to changes in patient status

**PATIENT
MONITORING
NONINVASIVE AND
INVASIVE TECHNIQUES**

166

Veterinary Anesthesia

  B. Provides data base for any subsequent anesthetic procedures on the same animal

III. Prerequisites for intraoperative monitoring

  A. Knowledge of pharmacodynamics, toxicity, and pharmacokinetics of anesthetic drugs and adjuncts

  B. Complete understanding of normal physiology and pathophysiology

  C. Thorough, accurate knowledge of the patient's preoperative physiologic status

BASIC PRINCIPLES

  I. Monitor the functions of body systems that are known to change

  A. Formulate monitoring plan based on preoperative assessment of the case

    1. Specific procedure
    2. Specific disease
    3. Anticipated duration of anesthesia

  B. Intraoperative decisions are based on comparisons of observed responses to predicted responses; i.e., are observed responses qualitatively and/or quantitatively appropriate to the case?

  II. Monitor more than one body system and more than one parameter per body system if possible

  A. Consideration of integrated responses rather than fragments of information increases likelihood of correct assessment

  B. Intraoperative therapeutic techniques and/or drug administration will often affect more than one body system

  III. Use monitoring techniques that are specific, accurate, and complementary

  A. Use simple, reliable techniques

    1. Visual inspection, palpation, auscultation

  B. Continually check instrument calibrations

    1. Instruments may provide specific data, but inaccurate information may be confusing, distracting, and misleading

  IV. Noninvasive vs. invasive techniques

  A. Noninvasive

    1. Information gathered by observing readily apparent variables (e.g., counting respiratory rate) and/or transducing events from the body surface without entering the body (e.g., ECG)

    2. Advantages

      a. Most techniques are simple, reliable, and informative
      b. Patient not placed at risk for serious problems secondary to monitoring techniques

    3. Disadvantages

      a. Certain potentially useful physiological variables cannot be monitored noninvasively
      b. Inaccurate information is sometimes gathered when noninvasive techniques are substituted for more invasive procedures used to monitor the identical parameter (e.g., blood pressure)

  B. Invasive

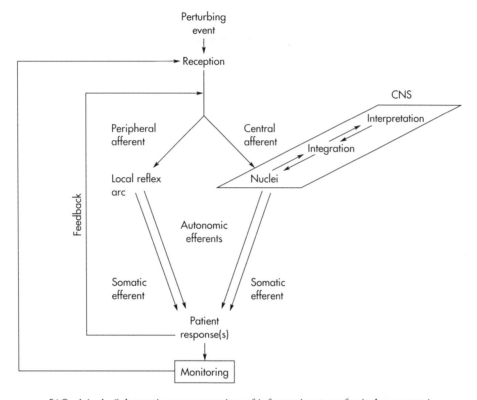

FIG.16-1 Schematic representation of information transfer in homeostasis.

1. Information gathered via placement of appropriate equipment inside the
   body (e.g., pressure catheters)
2. Advantages
   a. Increases physiological data base
   b. Many techniques are simple to perform and are reliable
   c. Often provides a direct measurement of a physiological variable rather
      than a derived value
3. Disadvantages
   a. Patient at risk of secondary complications; depending on technique,
      these may include:
      (1) Sepsis
      (2) Direct tissue damage
      (3) Inflammation with subsequent tissue damage
      (4) Acute perturbation of tissue function (e.g., cardiac dysrhythmias)
   b. Some techniques require elaborate or expensive instrumentation

PHYSIOLOGICAL CONSIDERATIONS

I. Homeostasis
   A. Schematic representation (Fig. 16-1)

TABLE 16-1

NORMAL HEART AND RESPIRATORY RATES IN CONSCIOUS ANIMALS

	Dog	Cat	Horse	Cow	Goat/ sheep	Pig
Heart rate*	70-180	145-200	30-45	60-80	60-90	60-90
Respiratory rate**	20-40	20-40	20-40	20-40	20-40	20-40

* May be altered by drugs that directly or reflexly change autonomic nervous system tone (e.g., xylazine-induced bradycardia)
** Respiratory rate and pattern may be influenced by drugs (e.g., ketamine-induced apneustic breathing)

   B. Monitoring
      1. Responses are observed
         a. Individual organ systems
         b. Integrated responses
      2. Invasive monitoring techniques may themselves be events that evoke responses
II. Individual organ systems
   A. Central nervous system
      1. Observe reflex activity to monitor degree of CNS depression
         a. Eye reflexes
            (1) Palpebral
            (2) Corneal
            (3) Nystagmus
            (4) Lacrimation
         b. Jaw tone
         c. Anal reflex
         d. Pedal reflex
   B. Cardiovascular system (see Table 16-1)
      1. Noninvasive
         a. Auscultation of heart rate and rhythm
         b. Palpation of pulse
         c. Evaluation of mucous membrane color and refill time
         d. Electrocardiogram
         e. Indirect measurement of arterial blood pressure
            (1) Oscillometric device
               (a) Cuff placed around limb over peripheral artery is automatically inflated and deflated by machine
               (b) Oscillations in artery beneath cuff transduced to digital display of heart rate and systolic, diastolic, and mean arterial blood pressure
               (c) Accuracy of readings dependent on many factors, including selection of appropriate cuff size
               (d) Useful in small and large animals

(e) Difficult to adapt to small animals
    (2) Doppler device
        (a) Ultrasound emitted by probe placed over peripheral artery is echoed off of red blood cells in vessel
        (b) Cuff placed over artery and inflated to occluding pressure measured on a manometer
        (c) Systolic arterial blood pressure is read from manometer as pressure when echo is first detected during slow release of cuff pressure
        (d) Useful in most species
        (e) Gives an estimate of systolic arterial pressure only
1. Invasive
    a. Direct arterial blood pressure determination
        (1) Placement of indwelling arterial catheter
            (a) Percutaneous
            (b) Surgical cutdown
        (2) Interface catheter with an external transducer coupled to an electronic meter
        (3) Multiple peripheral arteries available in horses, ruminants, and some exotic species
        (4) Limited sites for catheter placement in dogs and cats (e.g., femoral, dorsal pedal arteries)
    b. Direct measurement of right atrial (central venous) pressure, pulmonary arterial pressure, or pulmonary capillary wedge pressure
        (1) Venous catheterization
    c. Measurement of cardiac output
        (1) Thermodilution
        (2) Dye dilution
C. Respiratory system (see Table 16-1)
    1. Noninvasive
        a. Respiratory frequency
        b. Respiratory pattern
        c. Subjective estimate of changes in tidal volume by observation of thorax and rebreathing bag
        d. Analysis of inspired oxygen concentration
        e. Analysis of inspired or expired carbon dioxide concentration
        f. Spirometry
    2. Invasive
        a. Hematocrit (packed cell volume percentage) and/or hemoglobin concentration
        b. Arterial and/or venous blood gas analysis
        c. Blood pH analysis
D. Musculoskeletal system
    1. Skeletal muscle tone
    2. Quality of elicited reflexes

3. Peripheral nerve stimulation
   a. Used to assess quality of skeletal muscle responses during onset and reversal of neuromuscular blocking agents
      (1) Observed reversal responses may not correlate well with actual return of functional muscle strength

III. Thermoregulation
   A. Body temperature regulation is an integrated process involving the following body systems or organs
      1. CNS
      2. Cardiovascular system
      3. Musculoskeletal system
      4. Respiratory system
      5. The liver
   B. Abnormalities of thermoregulation during anesthesia
      1. Hypothermia
         a. Heat loss in excess of production
         b. Most often encountered in small animals due to their larger surface area to body mass ratio
         c. Potential causes
            (1) CNS depression
            (2) Vasodilation
            (3) Reduced heat production by skeletal muscle
            (4) Other iatrogenic causes
               (a) Cold IV fluids
               (b) Open body cavities
      3. Hyperthermia
         a. Heat production exceeding loss
         b. Iatrogenically produced in response to specific drug combinations in certain species
            (1) Drugs
               (a) Halothane, succinylcholine, and ketamine
            (2) Species
               (a) True malignant hyperthermia syndrome occurs in humans, pigs, and dogs
               (b) Isolated reports of increased body temperature during anesthesia also reported in horses and cats
   C. Body temperature monitoring during the anesthesia and postoperative periods should be considered an integrated response involving the specific species, drugs, and each of the body systems listed

IV. Integrated responses (see Table 16-2)
   A. Body systems do not exist as separate entities in vivo
   B. Observed responses represent the outcome of a series of events involving simultaneous input and output of many systems, leading to combined autonomic and somatic responses (see Fig. 16-1)
   C. Integrated responses to diseases, surgical stress, and anesthetic-induced

TABLE 16-2

COMMONLY MONITORED PARAMETERS AND POTENTIAL CAUSES OF ABNORMAL RESPONSES

Heart rate

Tachycardia	Pain, hypotension, hypoxemia, hypercarbia, ischemia, acute anaphylactoid reactions, anemia, drug effects (e.g., thiobarbiturates, ketamine, catecholamines), fever
Bradycardia	Hypertension, elevated intracranial pressure, surgically induced vagal reflexes (e.g., visceral stretch responses), hypothermia, hyperkalemia, myocardial ischemia/anoxia, drug effects (e.g., xylazine, narcotics)

Respiratory rate and pattern

Tachypnea	Pain, hypoxemia, hypercarbia, hyperthermia, true or paradoxical CSF acidosis, drugs effects (e.g., doxapram)
Apnea	Hypothermia, recent hyperventilation (especially while breathing O_2-enriched gases), musculoskeletal paralysis (pathological or pharmacological), drug effects (e.g., ketamine, thiobarbiturates)

Arterial blood pressure

Hypotension	Relative or absolute hypovolemia, sepsis, shock, drug effects (e.g., thiobarbiturate boluses, inhalation anesthetics)
Hypertension	Pain, hypercarbia, fever, drug effects (e.g., catecholamines, ketamine)

Corneal reflexes*

Hyperactive	Pain, hypotension, hypoxemia, hypercarbia, drug effects (ketamine)
Hypoactive	CNS depression, e.g., excessively deep anesthesia, acidosis, hypotension

*Pertains to horses and ruminants only; not very useful in pigs, dogs, and cats

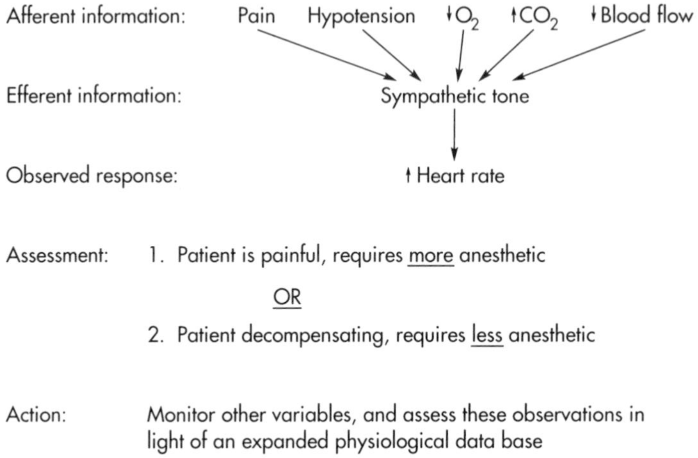

Afferent information: Pain   Hypotension $\downarrow O_2$ $\uparrow CO_2$ $\downarrow$ Blood flow

Efferent information: Sympathetic tone

Observed response: $\uparrow$ Heart rate

Assessment: 1. Patient is painful, requires <u>more</u> anesthetic

                              OR

                  2. Patient decompensating, requires <u>less</u> anesthetic

Action: Monitor other variables, and assess these observations in
                  light of an expanded physiological data base

FIG. 16-2 An action plan requires a knowledge of the cause for change (pain, hypotension, decreased O_2, increased CO_2, decreased blood flow).

  depression of certain functions are modulated by the autonomic nervous
  system and the adrenal medulla
  1. Sympathetic tone mediates "fight-or-flight" responses to any stress
     a. Causes of increased sympathetic tone
        (1) Pain
        (2) Hypotension
        (3) Hypoxemia
        (4) Hypercarbia
        (5) Ischemia
  2. Parasympathetic tone may change as part of an integrated reflex
     a. Vagovagal
     b. Vagophrenic
     c. Vagal efferent (baroreceptor)
  D. Correct interpretation of an isolated response requires understanding of
     integration and ability to work backwards from the observation to its probable cause (see Fig. 16-2)
  E. Acute intervention in the care of anesthetized patients should be justified
     on the basis of:
     1. A set of monitored observations
     2. Rational selection of alternative approaches to achieve desired physiological goals
     3. The anticipated patient responses to the procedure

CHAPTER SEVENTEEN

Hemodynamic Monitoring

"Diligence is the mother of good fortune."

MIGUEL DE CERVANTES

OVERVIEW

Careful hemodynamic monitoring is one of the most important and sensitive means of determining a patient's well being. Techniques used to monitor the hemodynamic status of a patient range from simple to complex and are either indirect (noninvasive) or direct (invasive). Direct methods usually involve entering a body cavity, such as the vascular channels. Relatively simple methods can be used to evaluate a patient's cardiovascular status, including such observations as the patient's color, capillary refill time, peripheral pulse pressure, and pulse rate. A pale grey or bluish discoloration (cyanosis), prolonged capillary refill time (>2-3 seconds), and weak peripheral pulse pressure are general indications of too great a depth of anesthesia and poor cardiovascular function. More sophisticated means to monitor the cardiovascular system include the recording and amplification of heart sounds, measurement of the esophageal or surface electrocardiogram, and the indirect or direct measurement of arterial blood pressure. All of these are useful in assessing patient status and in determining an appropriate approach to therapy, if required. New technology has resulted in the development of more accurate, indirect methods of assessing cardiovascular function. The continuous measurement of blood flow and cardiac output by Doppler-echocardiography are the most recent developments.

GENERAL CONSIDERATIONS

I. Hemodynamic monitoring is mandatory in order to:
   A. Assess anesthetic depth
   B. Determine trends

    C. Evaluate and institute a change in anesthetic plan and subsequent drug therapy

    D. Assess patient status

II. A variety of indirect and direct methods are available for monitoring the cardiovascular system. These are based on:

    A. Visual inspection

    B. Sound

    C. Palpation of vessels

    D. Electrical activity

    E. Pressure and flow measurements

III. Direct methods of measurement, although often invasive, are more sensitive to real changes than indirect methods

IV. More information can usually be derived from direct measurements

V. All the monitoring equipment in the world cannot replace an educated, attentive anesthetist

NONINVASIVE HEMODYNAMIC MONITORING

I. Heart rate

    A. Range of normal values, by species

        1. Dog: 70-180

        2. Cat: 145-200

        3. Cow: 60-80

        4. Horse: 30-45; foal up to 80

        5. Sheep, goat: 70-90

        6. Pig: 60-100

    B. Limits during anesthesia (BPM) (values outside these limits indicate cardiovascular function may be impaired)

        1. Dog: <60, >200

        2. Cat: <100, >260

        3. Cow: <48

        4. Horse: <28

        5. Sheep, goat: <60

II. Techniques for monitoring heart rate

    A. Direct palpation

        1. Dog: femoral a., dorsal pedal a., digital a., lingual a., precordium

        2. Cat: femoral a., precordium

        3. Cow, sheep, and goat: auricular a., digital a., coccygeal a., dorsal metatarsal a.

        4. Horse: facial a., transverse facial a., dorsal metatarsal a., palatine a.

        5. Pig: femoral a.

    B. Indirect methods

        1. Esophageal stethoscope (see Figs. 17-1 and 17-2)

           a. Coupled to earpieces or to electronic amplifier

           b. Advantages: inexpensive; can detect abnormalities in rhythm as well as rate; can monitor breath sounds

           c. Disadvantages: difficult to use for surgeries involving the head

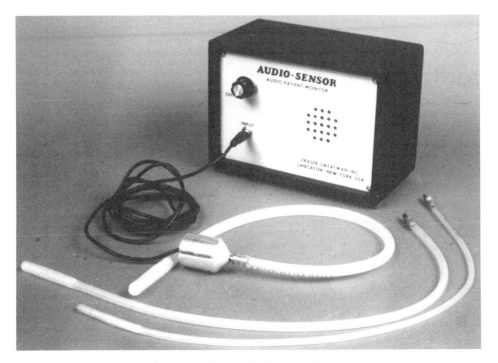

FIG. 17-1 Esophageal catheters can be attached to a stethoscope or audio monitor in order to hear heart sounds.

2. Peripheral pulse amplifiers
   a. Applied over peripheral pulse; audible beep heard with each pulse
   b. Advantages: inexpensive
   c. Disadvantages: prone to electrical interference; difficult to keep in place
3. Ultrasonic Doppler device
   a. Doppler crystal applied over peripheral pulse; sound of blood flow amplified
   b. Advantages: can also be used to estimate systolic blood pressure; detects abnormalities in rhythm as well as rate
   c. Disadvantages: expensive
4. Electrocardiogram and ECG-R wave amplifier
   a. Direct visualization of ECG, or sound amplifier that beeps with each R wave
   b. Advantages: direct visualization of ECG allows interpretation of cardiac rhythm
   c. Disadvantages: ECG monitors can be expensive; ECG activity can continue to look and sound normal in absence of mechanical activity (electromechanical dissociation)

III. Reasons for abnormal heart rates
   A. Bradycardia

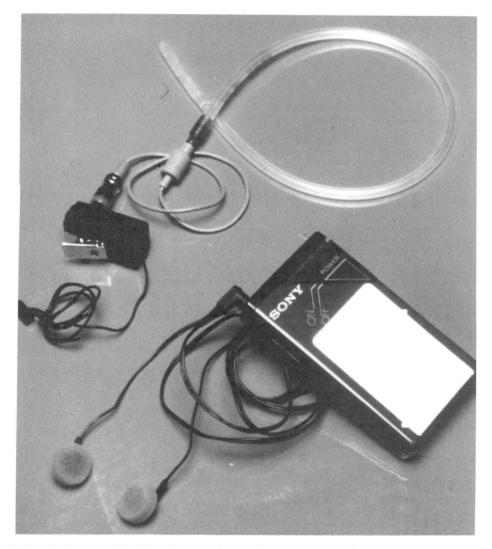

FIG. 17-2 An esophageal catheter can be coupled to a transmitter for transmission of heart sounds to a remote receiver.

1. Drugs: narcotics, xylazine, anticholinesterases
2. Excessive anesthetic depth
3. Hyperkalemia
4. Pre-existing heart disease
5. Vagal reflex (intubation, oculocardiac reflex)
6. Visceral manipulation or traction
7. Terminal stages or hypoxemia
8. Hypothermia

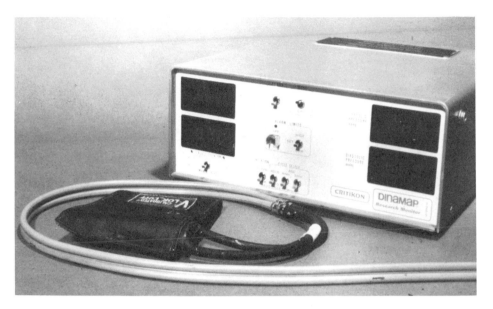

FIG. 17-3 Oscillometric peripheral pulse monitor can be used to monitor pulse rate and blood pressure.

    B. Tachycardia
        1. Drugs: ketamine, thiobarbiturates, anticholinergics, sympathomimetics, pancuronium, gallamine
        2. Hypokalemia
        3. Hyperthermia
        4. Inadequate anesthetic depth
        5. Hypercarbia and hypoxemia
        6. Anemia, hypovolemia
        7. Hyperthyroidism, pheochromocytoma
        8. Anaphylaxis
IV. Perfusion
    A. A function of arterial-venous blood pressure difference and local vasomotor tone
    B. Assessment
        1. Capillary refill time
            a. Normal: <1-2 seconds
            b. Assess on oral or vulvar mucous membranes
        2. Urine production
            a. Palpation of bladder
            b. Urinary catheterization
            c. Dog and cat: 1-2 ml/kg/hr
  V. Blood pressure
    A. Oscillometric method (see Fig. 17-3)

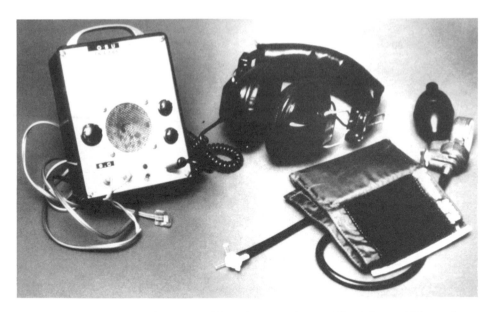

FIG. 17-4 An electronically activated Doppler crystal senses blood flow, which can be audibly broadcast and used to monitor blood pressure.

1. Air-filled cuff is placed around peripheral limb (small animal, foal) or base of tail (large animal). Air is gradually released from the cuff, and changes in oscillations at systolic, mean, and diastolic pressures are detected and electronically displayed

2. Advantages: easy to use; determines heart rate as well as systolic, mean, and diastolic blood pressure

3. Disadvantages: may not be absolutely accurate but will accurately reflect trends; expensive

B. Ultrasonic Doppler apparatus (see Fig. 17-4)

1. Doppler crystal placed over peripheral artery
   a. Dog: digital, dorsal pedal
   b. Horse: coccygeal

2. Inflatable cuff with aneroid gauge placed proximal to Doppler crystal. Cuff is inflated until pulse sound stops, then slowly deflated until pulse is first heard. This corresponds to systolic blood pressure as displayed on aneroid gauge

3. Advantages: relatively inexpensive; can count pulse rate and detect abnormalities in pulse rhythm

4. Disadvantages: accuracy related to many factors; cuff size must be matched to limb circumference; systolic pressure only

NONINVASIVE MONITORING OF SYSTEMIC OXYGENATION

I. Pulse oximetry: a spectrophotoelectric device applied directly to nonhaired skin over a pulsating vascular bed. Light absorbance of oxygenated vs. reduced

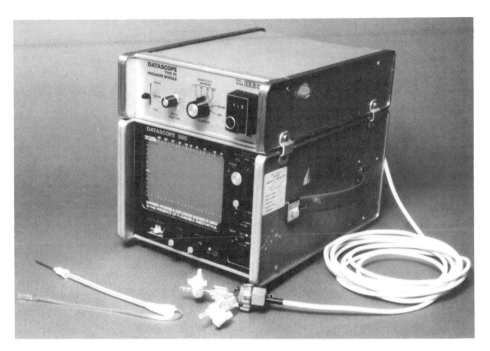

FIG. 17-5 Oscilloscope used to display and monitor the electrocardiogram (ECG) and blood pressure via an intravenous catheter.

hemoglobin detected and percentage of saturated hemoglobin displayed numerically

    A. Inaccurate in presence of carboxyhemoglobin

    B. Not yet fully evaluated in all domestic species

II. Transcutaneous oxygen measurement: small probe with Clark-type oxygen electrode attached to nonhaired skin. Skin under probe heated to constant temperature and oxygen partial pressure of blood below probe is measured and numerically displayed

    A. PaO_2 values will depend on arterial oxygenation and peripheral perfusion

    B. Not yet fully evaluated in all domestic species

    C. Inhalation anesthetic drugs may interfere with accurate recording

CENTRAL VENOUS PRESSURE (CVP)

I. Central venous pressure is obtained by measuring the mean right atrial pressure. Awareness of the CVP value and monitoring its changes can be important in some clinical situations (see Fig. 17-5)

    A. Range of normal values

        1. -3.0-4.0 cm H_2O standing, awake animals

        2. 2.0-7.0 cm H_2O anesthetized small animals

        3. 15-25 cm H_2O anesthetized large animals

    B. Indications

        1. Monitoring fluid therapy

    2. Assessing cardiac output
      a. Shock
      b. Heart failure
      c. Anesthesia

II. Physiological significance
  A. Right atrial pressure is a balance between:
    1. Cardiac output—ability of the heart to pump blood out of the right atrium
    2. Venous return—tendency for blood to flow from the peripheral veins back into the right atrium

III. Primary factors affecting CVP
  A. Blood volume
    1. Increase in circulating blood volume may cause an increase in CVP
      a. Renal retention of fluid in chronic heart failure
      b. Overzealous intravenous fluid administration
    2. Decrease in effective circulating blood volume may cause a decrease in CVP
      a. Acute hemorrhage
      b. Dehydration
      c. Strangulation, obstructive lesions causing vascular congestion and sequestration of blood or body fluids
        (1) Cat—intussusception of small bowel
        (2) Dog—gastric dilatation/volvulus
        (3) Horse—large colon torsion
        (4) Cow—abomasal torsion
  B. Vascular tone
    1. Regulated by the sympathetic nervous system and local tissue factors
    2. Markedly altered by various anesthetic agents
    3. Venous dilatation may result in a decrease in CVP due to peripheral pooling of blood and decreased venous return
    4. Arteriolar dilatation may result in increased CVP due to decrease in total peripheral resistance to cardiac output, allowing more rapid flow of blood from arterial to venous side of circulation
  C. Contractility
    1. Regulated by the autonomic nervous system
    2. Affected by venous return; increased venoconstriction increases contractility
    3. Usually decreased by most anesthetic agents
    4. Decreases in contractility may result in an increased CVP due to the decrease in effectiveness of the heart as a pump
  D. Heart rate
    1. Regulated by the autonomic nervous system
    2. CVP may decrease acutely with sudden elevation of the heart rate
    3. CVP may increase with sustained extreme tachycardias due to inadequate cardiac filling during shortened diastole

      4. Severe bradycardia, A-V conduction disturbances, and arrhythmia may result in an increased CVP due to the decrease in cardiac output

  E. External cardiac factors

    1. Intrathoracic pressure

      a. Elevations in intrathoracic pressure will impede venous return. Decreases in intrathoracic pressure will facilitate venous return to the heart

      b. An elevation in intrathoracic pressure is accompanied by an elevation in central venous pressure, impediment of venous return, and lowered cardiac output (CO)

      c. Factors affecting intrathoracic pressure

        (1) Cyclic changes during normal respiration

        (2) Positive-pressure ventilation

        (3) Pneumothorax

        (4) Opening thoracic cage to the atmosphere

        (5) Diaphragmatic hernia

        (6) Thoracic neoplasia or pulmonary disease

        (7) Fluid in the thorax

    2. Intrapericardial pressure

      a. Cardiac tamponade

      b. Congenital pericardial herniation

    3. Body position

      a. Alterations in body position can cause changes in vascular hydrostatic pressure

      b. Primarily a factor in large animal species

        (1) CVP may drop 10-15 cm H_2O when a horse is rolled from dorsal to lateral recumbency

IV. Clinical values of central venous pressure

  A. Three common clinical situations to be considered

    1. Reduced blood volume, cardiac function normal: ↓ CVP   ↓ CO

    2. Expanded blood volume, cardiac function normal: ↑ CVP   ↑ CO

    3. Normovolemic patient, cardiac function decreased: ↑ CVP   ↓ CO

  B. Clinical approach to low central venous pressure

    1. Reduced effective circulating blood volume

    2. Patients in whom there is a relative or absolute hypovolemia should receive appropriate intravenous fluid until the CVP approaches the upper limit of normal range

      a. If the fluid administration is accompanied by signs of adequate peripheral perfusion, the function of the heart can be assumed to be adequate

        (1) Urine output

        (2) Strong pulses

        (3) Pink mucous membranes

        (4) Capillary refill <2.5 seconds

      b. If fluid administration is accompanied by signs of inadequate perfusion, increasing metabolic acidosis, and pulmonary edema, further treatment should be directed toward improving cardiac function

C. Clinical approach to elevated CVP
1. Generally indicates hypervolemia or myocardial depression/heart failure
   a. Danger of development of pulmonary edema exists
   b. Metabolic acidosis due to underperfusion of peripheral tissues may result due to heart failure
2. Clinical history may give indication of cause of elevated CVP
   a. Iatrogenic due to excessive fluid administration
   b. Primary cardiac disease
   c. Generalized drug-induced myocardial depression
3. Treat the patient with one or more of the following
   a. Decrease or stop IV fluid administration
   b. Administer drugs to improve cardiac function (dobutamine)
   c. Diuresis (furosemide)

V. Hazards of central venous pressure measurement
A. Impaired blood clotting due to excessive heparinization of the fluid-filled catheter
B. Thrombophlebitis
C. Septicemia
D. Air embolism
E. Vascular endothelial damage or puncture
1. Extravascular migration
2. Cardiac tamponade
F. Improper placement
1. Inaccurate data collection

VI. Equipment
A. Intravenous catheter of sufficient length to reach the great veins in the chest (preferably the right atrium)
B. Central venous pressure manometer kit (see Fig. 17-6)
1. Homemade
   a. Three-way stopcock
   b. Graduated cylinder or pipette
   c. Connecting tubes
2. Commercially available
   a. Baxter
   b. Abbott
3. Appropriate fluids and a fluid administration set

VII. Procedure (see Fig. 17-6)
A. Thread a fluid-filled intravenous catheter into the right jugular vein (toward the heart)
B. Flush the catheter with saline
C. Attach fluid connecting tubes to the intravenous catheter
D. Attach a three-way stopcock and graduated cylinder

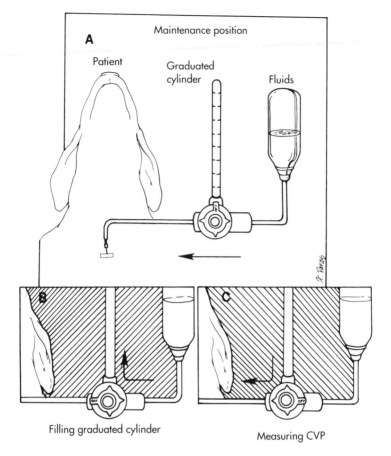

FIG. 17-6 Central venous pressure monitoring (*A*). A graduated cylinder at or below the level of the heart is filled with saline (*B*). The cylinder is then opened to the patient (*C*).

    E. Attach the fluid administration line to the other port of the three-way stopcock

    F. Suspend the graduated cylinder or pipette so that the three-way stopcock is below the animal's heart base. An imaginary line parallel to the floor is drawn between the animal's heart base and the cylinder. This marks the point of zero pressure on the cylinder

        1. The animal's heart base is marked by the sternum when the animal is in lateral recumbency

        2. The heart base is marked by the point of the shoulder when the animal is standing or in dorsal recumbency

    G. Let the fluid run through the system at the calculated flow (5 ml/lb/hr) until ready to record CVP

VIII. Use of Manometer (see Fig. 17-6)

    A. Turn the three-way stopcock so that the fluid line is open to the graduated cylinder

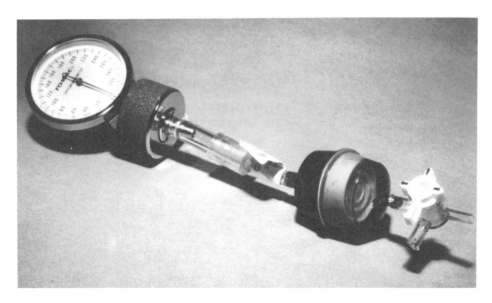

FIG. 17-7 A small blood filter attached to a three-way stopcock and then to a sphygmo-manometer is an inexpensive method of monitoring mean arterial blood pressure.

    B. When the cylinder has filled, turn the stopcock so that the cylinder is open to the patient

    C. The fluid column will fall to the level of the central venous pressure

    D. After the reading has been taken, open the patient line to the fluid, and administer fluids at the prescribed rate

ARTERIAL BLOOD PRESSURE

  I. The technique of invasive arterial pressure monitoring provides both an accurate quantitative value of the pulse pressure and a qualitative representation of the pulse waveform. This information provides knowledge of the hemodynamic state of the patient and the effects of various drugs and/or treatments. Blood pressure is not an indicator of cardiac output (see Fig. 17-7)

    A. Indications

      1. Detection of systemic arterial hypertension or hypotension

      2. Monitoring hemodynamic effects of drugs

      3. Verification of heightened or diminished pulse pressures

      4. Monitoring of arterial blood gases

  II. Physiological significance

    A. Blood pressure = lateral force per unit area of vascular wall

      1. Expressed clinically in millimeters of mercury (mm Hg)

      2. Pressure at the level of the right atrium is the zero reference level

    B. Blood pressure is needed to propel blood through high-resistance vascular beds

      1. Vascular beds of heart, brain, and kidney offer highest resistance

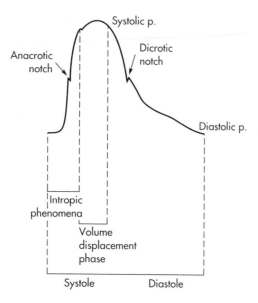

FIG. 17-8 Characteristics of the arterial pressure waveform.

    a. The mean pressure required to perfuse these organs is approximately 60 mm Hg
C. Systemic blood pressure oscillates about a mean pressure
    1. Maximum pressure = systolic
    2. Minimum pressure = diastolic
    3. Systolic/diastolic = pulse pressure
       a. Major determinant of palpable pulse strength
    4. Mean pressure: major determinant of perfusion pressure to most organs of the body
    5. Normal values (see Fig. 17-8)

systolic	110-160 mm Hg
diastolic	70-90 mm Hg
mean	80-110 mm Hg

D. The pulse waveform does not represent a fluid wave; rather, it is a pressure wave. The pressure pulse travels much faster through the arterial tree than the blood flow
    1. The pressure pulse reaches peripheral arterioles 200-300 msec after the onset of ventricular ejection
E. Components of the pressure pulse (see Fig. 17-8)
    1. Early systolic events: inotropic component
    2. Midsystolic events: volume displacement phase
    3. Events of late systole and diastole: runoff and reflection
F. Inotropic component: anacrotic rise or the steeply ascending limb of the pressure pulse
    1. Acceleration transient

a. The force caused when aortic valves open and the high energy state of intraventricular blood is communicated to the blood within the aorta, which is at zero velocity

2. Ejection pulse
   a. Continued upstroke resulting as stroke volume is ejected into aortic root
3. Steepness of the anacrotic rise is a qualitative indicator of myocardial contractility

G. Volume displacement phase: The abrupt phenomenon of the inotropic component is sustained by continuing ejection of stroke volume from the ventricle
   1. Pressure will continue to rise as long as flow into the vascular segment exceeds the volume of fluid leaving it
   2. Anacrotic notch is a discontinuity between the inotropic component and the sustained volume displacement curve
   3. Volume displacement phase may determine the maximum systolic pressure if stroke volume is large relative to peripheral runoff

H. Late systole and diastole: As the rate of runoff exceeds the volume input to the aorta, the pressure declines
   1. Dicrotic notch is a sharp deceleration of blood flow at closure of aortic valves
      a. Peripherally the dicrotic notch is an artifact of reflection
   2. Undulations on the diastolic decline are due to resonant waves in the great vessels and to reflections of energy from the periphery

I. There is an increase in pressure pulse amplitude with increasing distance from the aortic arch (see Fig. 17-9)
   1. Distensibility of peripheral arteries progressively decreases, resulting in an increased pulse wave
   2. The mean pressure is relatively unchanged along the arterial circulation

III. Primary factors affecting the arterial pressure
   A. Pulse pressure = cardiac output × total peripheral resistance
      1. Factors increasing stroke volume or cardiac output favor an increase in arterial pressure
      2. Factors increasing total peripheral resistance favor an increase in arterial pressure
   B. The inotropic component of the pulse pressure curve is modulated by three factors
      1. Preload—related to venous return
      2. Afterload—related to arterial pressure and peripheral resistance
      3. Heart rate
   C. Decreases in the inotropic component may reflect:
      1. Myocardial depression due to:
         a. Pathology
         b. Anesthesia
         c. Decreased β-adrenergic stimulation
      2. Decreased venous return

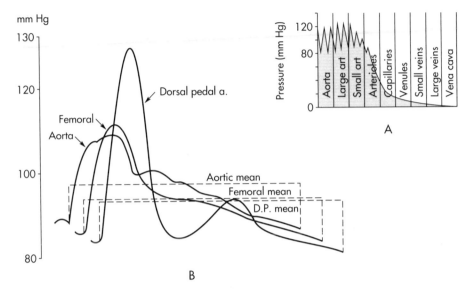

FIG. 17-9 Effects of distance from the aortic arch on the arterial blood pressure waveform.

     a. Relative or absolute hypovolemia
     b. Venodilatation
     c. Positive-pressure ventilation
   3. Decreased peripheral resistance
     a. Decreased sympathetic tone
     b. Anesthesia
     c. Endotoxin
 D. Volume displacement and the amplitude and duration of the pressure pulse reflect a balance between:
   1. Volume and rate of ejection fraction, which is related to venous return and contractility
     a. Small stroke volume yields narrow systolic peak and a precipitous downstroke
     b. Large stroke volume yields broad systolic peak with ramplike diastolic component
   2. Rate of runoff to the periphery, which is governed by changes in peripheral resistance
     a. Dicrotic notch will occur high on the pulse pressure curve with adequate stroke volume and low peripheral resistance
     b. Dicrotic notch will occur a few millimeters above the lowest diastolic value if the rate of runoff is rapid
 E. Late systole and diastole reflect the rate of runoff to the periphery and reflection from the periphery
   1. High peripheral resistance will diminish forward flow and increase reflection, creating a horizontal diastolic element
   2. Substantial volume displacement toward the periphery when vascular

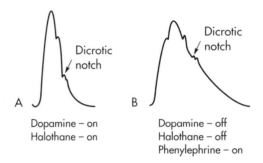

FIG. 17-10 Effects of peripheral artery vasodilation (A) and vasoconstriction (B) on the arterial blood pressure waveform.

resistance is low forms a diastolic tracing resembling an oblique but fairly steep ramp

F. Pulse pressure curves: examples recorded under anesthesia (see Fig. 17-10)

1. Myocardium initiates explosive systolic peak under the influence of a positive inotrope (see Fig. 17-10, A). Small stroke volume suggested by rapid downstroke in volume displacement phase

2. Discontinuation of halothane and dopamine (see Fig. 17-10, B): increased tone in venous capacitance vessels due to phenylephrine; decrease seen in anacrotic rise; broad volume displacement component. Dicrotic notch has moved upward on the descending limb of the systolic curve; this suggests a greater flow state

IV. Clinical value of arterial pressure monitoring

A. Depth of anesthesia

1. Anesthetic drugs, due to their effects on cardiac output and peripheral resistance, can markedly affect blood pressure

a. Light plane of anesthesia: Animal responds to painful stimulus by an increase in sympathetic tone

(1) Sudden elevation of blood pressure

b. Profound anesthetic depression: loss of homeostatic reflexes and impairment of myocardial function

(1) Decline in mean blood pressure, prolonged anacrotic rise, and decreased pulse pressure

B. Adequacy of fluid therapy

1. Narrow volume displacement phase may indicate need to volume-expand the patient

a. Marked discrepancy in the appearance of a pulse pressure curve before and after assisted ventilation is often an indicator of need for rapid IV fluid administration (see Fig. 17-11)

C. Maintenance of peripheral perfusion pressure

1. Prevention of tissue ischemia and subsequent metabolic acidosis relies on normal arterial oxygen values and mean blood pressure >60 mm Hg

a. If mean blood pressure <60 mm Hg, treatment may include:

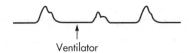

Ventilator

FIG. 17-11 Changes in arterial blood pressure waveform caused by assisted ventilation.

        (1) Rapid IV fluid administration
        (2) Decreased depth of anesthesia
        (3) Initiation of positive inotrope therapy if response to first two steps is poor
    b. Potential sequelae to inadequate tissue perfusion
        (1) Postoperative myositis—horse
        (2) Acute renal failure—all species
        (3) Cardiac arrhythmias—all species
        (4) Shock
  D. Assessment of ventilatory status
    1. Arterial blood gases, available through the arterial pressure line, are ideal for determining adequacy of ventilation. See Chapter 18: Acid-Base Balance and Blood Gases
V. Hazards of invasive arterial pressure monitoring
  A. Hematoma formation
  B. Air embolization
  C. Arterial thrombosis and occlusion (rare)
  D. Infection (rare)
  E. Formation of A-V fistula or aneurysm (rare)
VI. Equipment and procedure (see Chapter 14: Anesthetic Equipment and Maintenance
  A. Intra-arterial catheter with three-way stopcock
  B. Pressure sensing device
    1. Pressure transducer and oscilloscope
    2. Mercury manometer
    3. Aneroid gauge (see Fig. 17-7)
  C. Procedure
    1. Cannulate a peripheral artery aseptically with the arterial catheter
      a. Dog
        (1) Dorsal pedal artery
        (2) Femoral artery
      b. Ruminants
        (1) Caudal auricular artery
        (2) Coccygeal artery
        (3) Common digital artery
      c. Horse
        (1) Facial artery
        (2) Transverse facial artery
        (3) Great metatarsal artery

2. Flush the catheter with heparinized saline
   a. Always aspirate first to prevent air embolism
3. Attach the pressure transducer while stopcock is closed to the artery
4. Zero the pressure reading to atmospheric pressure with the transducer at about the level of the right atrium
5. Open the arterial line to the pressure transducer
   a. Pulse pressure curve should be displayed at this point
6. Reading pressures
   a. Systolic pressure: uppermost point of the pulse pressure curve
   b. Diastolic pressure: lowermost point of the pulse pressure curve
   c. Mean pressure
7. Upon removal of the arterial catheter, place manual pressure on the site of cannulation for 5 minutes to prevent hematoma formation

CHAPTER EIGHTEEN

Acid-Base Balance and Blood Gases

*"The management of a balance of power is a permanent undertaking,
not an exertion that has a foreseeable end."*

HENRY KISSINGER

OVERVIEW

The diagnosis of acid-base disorders is dependent on an interpretation of changes in blood pH, P_{CO_2}, and bicarbonate concentration. Very simply, changes in pH indicate whether an increase in hydrogen ions (acidosis) or a decrease in hydrogen ions (alkalosis) has occurred. The associated changes in carbon dioxide levels and bicarbonate help to determine the precise cause for the pH change. Evaluation of acid-base status of a patient provides information that can be used in the diagnosis of disease processes and the formulation of therapy. Electrolyte abnormalities are frequently associated with acid-base disorders, further emphasizing the importance of a basic understanding of pH, P_{CO_2} and bicarbonate regulation.

GENERAL CONSIDERATIONS

I. Many factors have an influence on a patient's acid-base balance
   A. Species
   B. Diet
   C. Physical status
   D. Temperature

II. Normal cellular metabolism continuously produces hydrogen ions, which are regulated and eliminated by the lungs, kidneys, and gastrointestinal system so as to maintain a pH of approximately 7.40
  A. The kidneys eliminate hydrogen ions by excreting fixed acids
  B. The lungs reduce plasma hydrogen ion concentration by eliminating carbon dioxide
III. Substances within the body referred to as buffers help to minimize changes in pH
IV. Determination of pH and blood gases are useful aids in determining patient status during anesthesia
  V. The absolute values of pH and blood gases must always be interpreted in relation to the patient's clinical history and physical status

FORMATION AND ELIMINATION OF ACIDS AND BASES IN ANIMALS

  I. The waste products of oral intake or metabolism are mostly acidic substances that release hydrogen ions
  A. Volatile acid: an acid that produces a gas
    1. $H_2CO_3 \rightarrow H_2O + CO_2$
  B. Nonvolatile, or fixed, acids: acids that cannot be converted to gas
    1. Lactate $+ H^+$
    2. Sulfate $+ H^+$
    3. Phosphate $+ H^+$
  II. The pathways for acid removal include the *kidney*, *lung* and *gastrointestinal tract*

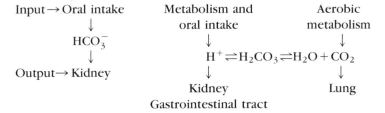

Note: This equation is called the carbonic acid equation or CO_2 hydration equation and is the basis for explaining acid-base kinetics in the body
  A. High-protein diets (cat, dog, pig, human)
    1. H^+ excess derived from oxidation of neutral sulfur in amino acids
    a. Methionine
    b. Cystine
    c. Cysteine
  B. Diets high in plant material and grain
    1. HCO_3^- excess from salts of:
    a. Fatty acids (acetate, proprionate)
    b. Citrate (fruits)
    c. Gluconates

Example:

$$H_2CO_3 \rightleftharpoons H^+ + HCO_3^-$$

$$\underset{\text{(sodium acetate)}}{H-\overset{\text{H}}{\underset{|}{C}}-\overset{\text{O}}{\overset{\|}{C}}-O-Na^+} + 2O_2 + H^+ \rightleftharpoons \underset{\text{Lung}}{2CO_2 + 2H_2O} + Na^+$$

Metabolizable salts of fatty acids yield HCO_3^- after metabolism

C. On the basis of primary dietary intake
  1. Herbivores: Alkaline urine or an excess base to excrete
  2. Carnivores: Acid urine or excess acid to excrete
D. Dietary and metabolic intake of acid or base equals the urinary and respiratory output, thereby maintaining the pH of the body fluids near 7.4

  1. $CO_2 + H_2O \overset{CA}{\rightleftharpoons} H_2CO_3 \rightleftharpoons H^+ + HCO_3^-$ (CA: carbonic anhydrase)

  2. $K_1 = \dfrac{[CO_2] + [H_2O]}{[H_2CO_3]}$

   $K_2 = \dfrac{[H^+] + [HCO_3^-]}{[H_2CO_3]}$

  3. $\dfrac{K_2}{K_1} = \dfrac{[H^+] + [HCO_3^-]}{[CO_2] + [H_2O]} = K_3$

  4. Given: $[CO_2] = \alpha \times P_{CO_2}$ ($\alpha = 0.0301$ — solubility coefficient)

  5. $\dfrac{K_3 \times \alpha P_{CO_2}}{[HCO_3^-]} = (H^+)$

   $-\log(H^+) = pH; -\log K_3 = pK$

   pK is that pH at which 50% of an acid or a base is in the ionized state. The pK of the acid (pK_a) H_2CO_3 is 6.1

  6. $-\log K_3 - \log \alpha P_{CO_2} + \log[HCO_3^-] = -\log[H^+]$

   $pH = pK_a + \log \dfrac{[HCO_3^-]}{\alpha P_{CO_2}}$: Henderson-Hasselbach equation

E. In the body: $pH = 7.4$, $pK_a = 6.1$, $P_{CO_2} = 40$ mm Hg

  1. $pH = pK_a + \log \dfrac{[HCO_3^-]}{\alpha P_{CO_2}}$

  2. $7.4 = 6.1 + \log[HCO_3^-] - \log \alpha P_{CO_2}$

3. $1.3 = \log [HCO_3^-] - \log \alpha P_{CO_2}$

4. Antilog $1.3 = \dfrac{[HCO_3^-]}{0.0301 \times 40}$ antilog $1.3 = 20$

$(HCO_3^-) = 20 \times 0.0301 \times 40 = 24$ mEq/L

ARTERIAL OXYGENATION TABLES[†]

I. Normal gas partial pressures (in mm Hg) during inspiration in ambient air, conducting airways, terminal alveoli (A), and arterial (a) and mixed venous (v) blood:

	Ambient air	Conducting airways	Terminal units	Arterial blood	Mixed venous blood
P_{O_2}	156	149	100	95	40
P_{CO_2}	0	0	40	40	46
P_{H_2O}	15*	47	47	47	47
P_{N_2}	589	564	573	573	573
P total	760	760	760	755	706

*P_{H_2O} varies according to humidity and has a proportionate effect on P_{O_2} and P_{N_2}

II. The inspired oxygen–arterial tension (FiO_2) relationship

FiO_2(%)	Predicted ideal Pa_{O_2} (mm Hg)
20	95-100
30	150
40	200
50	250
80	400
100	500

III. Causes of arterial hypoxia (a reduction in Pa_{O_2}) and their effect on alveolar-arterial (A-a) P_{O_2} differences ([A-a]O_2D)

Cause	Effect on Arterial P_{O_2}	Effect on (A-a) O_2D
Hypoventilation	Decreased	No change
Diffusion abnormality	No change or decreased*	No change or decreased*
Ventilation perfusion imbalance	Decreased	Increased
Right-to-left shunt	Decreased	Increased
Reduction to inspired P_{O_2}	Decreased	No change

*Effects of diffusion abnormalities are infrequently encountered at rest, but are more likely to be evident during exercise

[†]Taken from Murray JF: *The Normal Lung*, ed 2. Philadelphia, WB Saunders Co, 1986, pp 173, 174.

O_2 TRANSPORT

I. Dissolved

  A. Henry's law: Amount of O_2 dissolved is proportional to P_{O_2}. For each 1 mm Hg of P_{O_2}, there is 0.003 ml O_2/100 ml of plasma. Content = Solubility × Partial pressure

  B. Dissolved O_2 is not adequate to meet the animal's oxygen needs

II. Hemoglobin

  A. Conjugated protein of iron and porphyrin joined to the protein globin. Globin has two alpha and two beta chains made of differing amino acid sequences

    1. Hemoglobin A: adult

    2. Hemoglobin F: fetal

    3. Hemoglobin S: sickle (valine–glutamic acid)

  B. Hemoglobin A is transferred from a ferrous to a ferric ion by oxidation (methemoglobin), which is not useful in O_2 carriage

    1. Nitrites

    2. Sulfonamides

    3. Benzocaine

O_2 DISSOCIATION CURVE

I. $O_2 + Hb \rightarrow HbO_2$ (oxyhemoglobin)

  A. O_2 capacity is the amount of O_2 that can be combined with Hb Example: 1 g Hb can combine with 1.39 ml of O_2. If there are 15 g Hb, then $1.39 \times 15 = 20.8$ ml O_2/100 ml at 100% saturation

II. O_2 saturation

$$\frac{O_2 \text{ combined with Hb} \times 100}{O_2 \text{ capacity}}$$

III. O_2 content is the amount of O_2 present as dissolved O_2 and combined with Hb

Example: $P_{O_2} = 100$ 12 g Hb

       Sat = 96%

$$12 \times 1.39 \times 0.96 = 16.0$$
$$100 \times 0.003 = \underline{0.3}$$
$$16.3 \text{ ml } O_2/100 \text{ ml}$$

IV. O_2 dissociation curve shape

  A. Upper portion: P_{O_2} (partial pressure of oxygen) can fall slightly without affected O_2 loading of Hb

  B. Lower portion: Peripheral tissues can withdraw large amounts of O_2 with only small changes in P_{O_2}

    1. Reduced Hb: 5 g of reduced Hb can cause cyanosis (blue or purple discoloration)

V. Shifts in the O_2 dissociation curve are most commonly caused by changes in pH, P_{CO_2} (partial pressure of carbon dioxide), and temperature

    A. Increasing temperature and P_{CO_2} and decreasing pH shift the O_2 dissociation curve to the right

    B. 2,3-diphosphoglycerate (DPG) increases within the RBC occur in chronic hypoxia and shift the O_2 dissociation curve to the right

    C. Rightward shifts mean more unloading of O_2 at a given P_{O_2} in a tissue capillary. The normal P_{O_2} at 50% O_2 saturation is approximately 26 mm Hg

CARBON MONOXIDE

    I. $Hb + CO \rightarrow COHb$ (carboxyhemoglobin)

    II. CO has about 210 times the affinity for Hb than O_2

        A. Small amounts of CO can tie up large amounts of Hb, making it unavailable for O_2 carriage

        B. Results in a normal P_{O_2} but grossly reduced O_2 content

        C. Shifts the oxyhemoglobin curve to the left, thereby impairing O_2 unloading in tissues

CARBON DIOXIDE TRANSPORT

    I. Carried in blood

        A. As $[HCO_3^-]$

        B. Carbamino compounds

    II. Carried in plasma

        A. As $[HCO_3^-]$

    III. Carried in physical solution

NORMAL pH AND BLOOD GAS VALUES

    I. pH = 7.40; range 7.35-7.45

    II. Pa_{O_2} = 95 mm Hg; range 80-110 mm Hg

    III. Pv_{O_2} = 40 mm Hg; range 35-45 mm Hg

    IV. Pa_{CO_2} = 40 mm Hg; range 35-45 mm Hg

    V. Pv_{CO_2} = 45 mm Hg; range 40-48 mm Hg

    VI. HCO_3^- = 24 mEq/L; range 22-27 mEq/L

    VII. The Pa_{CO_2}-pH-HCO_3^- relationship

Pa_{CO_2} (mm Hg)	pH	HCO_3^- (mEq/L)
80	7.20	28
60	7.30	26
40	7.40	24
30	7.50	22
20	7.60	20

    VIII. Nomenclature

        A. Acidemia: pH < 7.35 (acid blood)

1. Metabolic acidosis: an abnormal physiologic process characterized by a primary gain of acid (H^+) or primary loss of base (HCO_3^-) from the extracellular fluid
2. Respiratory acidosis: an abnormal process in which there is a primary reduction in alveolar ventilation relative to CO_2 production ($Paco_2$ increase)

B. Alkalemia: pH > 7.45 (alkaline blood)
1. Metabolic alkalosis: an abnormal physiologic process characterized by a primary gain in base (HCO_3^-) or loss of acid (H^+) from the extracellular fluid
2. Respiratory alkalosis: an abnormal physiologic process in which there is a primary increase in alveolar ventilation relative to the rate of CO_2 production ($Paco_2$ decrease)

C. Compensation: An abnormal pH is returned toward normal by altering the component not *primarily* affected. For example, if the $Paco_2$ is elevated, the HCO_3^- should be elevated (retained) to compensate
1. If the Pco_2 or HCO_3^- values are outside normal limits, but the pH is within the normal range, then the patient is fully compensated
2. Because the process of compensation takes time to return the pH to within normal limits, a compensatory process implies a degree of chronicity

PRIMARY pH AND BLOOD GAS CLASSIFICATION

Classification	$Paco_2$	pH	HCO_3^-	BE
Acute ventilatory failure	↑	↓	N	N
Chronic ventilatory failure	↑	N	↑	↑
Acute alveolar hyperventilation	↓	↑	N	N
Chronic alveolar hyperventilation	↓	N	↓	↓
Uncompensated metabolic acidosis	N	↓	↓	↓
Compensated metabolic acidosis	↓	N	↓	↓
Uncompensated metabolic alkalosis	N	↑	↑	↑
Compensated metabolic alkalosis	↑	N	↑	↑

↓ = decreased; ↑ = increased; N = normal

I. Mixed respiratory and metabolic conditions can coexist. When this occurs, look at the individual values (pH, Pco_2, HCO_3^-) to determine the severity

RAPID QUALITATIVE INTERPRETATION OF pH AND BLOOD GASES

I. Determine pH: acidemia or alkalemia
A. The pH is the most important value in determining the animal's acid-base status. Match subsequent values to it
II. Determine Pco_2
A. Respiratory alkalosis: < 35 torr
B. Respiratory acidosis: > 50 torr
III. Determine HCO_3^-

A. Metabolic alkalosis: > 27 mEq/L

B. Metabolic acidosis: < 23 mEq/L

IV. Determine primary problem by matching either the P_{CO_2} or HCO_3^- or both with the pH. Determine if compensation exists

V. Make adjustments in HCO_3^-; for acute elevations or decreases in P_{CO_2}, as previously described

VI. Determine PaO_2

A. $PaO_2 < 80$ mm Hg—suspect hypoxemia

B. 5 g of reduced hemoglobin results in cyanosis

RULES OF THUMB

I. The HCO_3^- concentration rises about 1-2 mEq/L for each *acute* 10 mm Hg increase in $PaCO_2$ above 40. Maximum change in HCO_3^- is about 4 mEq/L

II. The HCO_3^- concentration falls 1-2 mEq/L for each *acute* 10 mm Hg fall in $PaCO_2$ below 40. Maximum change is about 6 mEq/L

III. *Acute* respiratory and nonrespiratory disorders can be distinguished by looking at the $PaCO_2$ and HCO_3^- values. HCO_3^- above 30 or below 15 mEq/L implies a nonrespiratory (metabolic) component

IV. During chronic elevation of the $PaCO_2$ (hypercapnea), each 10 mm Hg increase in $PaCO_2$ will cause a 4 mEq/L increase in HCO_3^- concentration

V. An *acute* 10 mm Hg increase in $PaCO_2$ results in a 0.05 unit decrease in pH. An *acute* 10 mm Hg decrease in $PaCO_2$ results in a 0.10 unit increase in pH

VI. Determining the predicted respiratory pH

A. Determine the difference between the measured $PaCO_2$ and 40 mm Hg, then move the decimal two places to the left

B. If the $PaCO_2$ is greater than 40, subtract half the difference from 7.40

C. If the $PaCO_2$ is less than 40, add the difference to 7.40

D. Examples

1. pH $= 7.01$; $PaCO_2 = 75$ ($PaCO_2 > 40$ mm Hg)

   $75 - 40 = 35$; $0.35 \times 0.5 > = 0.175$

   $7.40 - 0.18 = 7.22$

2. pH $= 7.43$; $PaCO_2 = 23$ ($PaCO_2 < 40$ mm Hg)

   $40 - 23 = 17$

   $7.40 + 0.17 = 7.57$

VII. Determining the metabolic component

A. A 10 mEq/L change in HCO_3^- concentration changes pH by 0.15 units. If the pH decimal is moved two places to the right, then a 10:15 or $2/3$ relationship exists

B. The absolute difference between the measured pH and the predicted respiratory pH is the metabolic component of the pH change. Moving the decimal point two places to the right and multiplying by $2/3$ will yield an estimate of the mEq/L variation of the buffer baseline (usually assumed as HCO_3^- concentration change)

VIII. Quantitative clinical determination of acid-base changes

A. Determine predicted respiratory pH

B. Estimate base excess or deficit
C. Examples
   1. pH = 7.02; $PaCO_2$ = 75
      Predicted respiratory pH:
      75 − 40 = 35; 0.35 × 0.5 = 0.175
      7.40 − 0.18 = 7.22
      Metabolic component:
      7.22 − 7.02 = 20 × 0.66 = 13.3 mEq/L, or 13.3 mEq/L base *deficit*
   2. pH = 7.64; $PaCO_2$ = 25
      Predicted respiratory pH:
      40 − 25 = 0.15
      7.40 + 0.15 = 7.55
      Metabolic component:
      7.64 − 7.55 = 9 × 0.66 = 6 mEq/L, or 6.0 mEq/L base *excess*

IX. Therapy
   A. Base deficits of less than 10 mEq/L are not routinely treated
   B. pH above 7.20 not routinely treated unless there is evidence of shock
   C. Since extracellular water is approximately 25-30% body weight, base deficits × body weight (kg) × 25% = Amount of HCO_3^- needed as replacement, or

$$\frac{\text{Base deficit} \times \text{wt (kg)}}{4} = \text{mEq } HCO_3^- \text{ required}$$

COMMON CAUSES OF ACID-BASE IMBALANCE

I. Respiratory acidosis
   A. Anesthesia or respiratory depressant drugs
   B. Obesity
   C. Brain damage
   D. Pulmonary disease
   E. Rib or thoracic disease or trauma

II. Respiratory alkalosis
   A. Anxiety, fear
   B. Fever
   C. Endotoxemia
   D. Pneumonia, pulmonary embolus
   E. Hypoxemia
   F. Left-to-right shunts
   G. Heart failure

III. Metabolic acidosis
   A. Renal disease (uremia)
   B. Chronic vomiting
   C. Diarrhea
   D. Severe exercise, hypoxia, ischemia, shock, trauma
   E. Diabetes

IV. Metabolic alkalosis
   A. Acute vomiting

    B. Hypokalemia

    C. Excessive use of diuretics

ACID-BASE AND ELECTROLYTE INTERRELATIONSHIPS

  I. Most CO_2 entering the blood passes into red blood cells, where:

    A. The majority of CO_2 enters into a reversible formation with HCO_3^-

$$CO_2 + H_2O \overset{CA}{\rightleftharpoons} H_2CO_3 \rightleftharpoons H^+ + HCO_3^-$$

    (CA = carbonic anhydrase)

      1. The HCO_3^- formed by this reaction diffuses out of RBCs. This movement sets up an electrostatic difference across the cell membrane, which is neutralized by the movement of Cl^- from plasma into the RBC (chloride shift)

 II. The location and absolute numbers of positively and negatively charged ions (strong ions) and their difference—strong ion difference [SID]—in combination with CO_2 production and the resultant P_{CO_2} determines pH ($[H^+]$) and $[HCO_3^-]$ changes in the body. The principal strong ions are Na^+, K^+, and Cl^-. SID = $[Na^+] + [K^+] - [Cl^-]$

 III. Changes in strong ions in various body fluids result in changes in SID, which provide the major mechanism for acid-base interactions

 IV. In order to maintain electrical neutrality, electrolyte shifts generally occur simultaneously with acid (H^+) or base (HCO_3^-) shifts. The most important electrolyte shift occurring with acid-base changes is K^+. For example, when HCO_3^- is added to the extracellular fluid, hydrogen ions (H^+) leave cells, causing K^+ to move intracellularly to maintain electrical equilibrium; therefore:

    A. Metabolic alkalosis—suspect hypokalemia

    B. Metabolic acidosis—suspect hyperkalemia

GLOSSARY

Acid: A substance that can donate hydrogen ion H^+

        Example: $H_2CO_3 \rightarrow H^+ + HCO_3^-$

Actual bicarbonate: The amount of bicarbonate (HCO_3^-), expressed in mEq/L of plasma

Base: A substance that can accept hydrogen ion H^+

        Examples: $OH^- + H^+ \rightarrow H_2O$

                       $HCO_3^- + H^+ \rightarrow H_2CO_3$

Base excess: The amount of base above or below the normal buffer base, in mEq/L, in blood. Positive value ($+$) reflect excess of base (or deficit of acid), and negative values reflect a deficit of base (or excess of acid)

Buffer: A mixture of substances in a solution that resists or reduces changes in hydrogen ion concentration (changes in pH)

Examples in whole blood:

	% buffering
Hemoglobin and oxyhemoglobin	35
Organic phosphate	3
Inorganic phosphate	2
Plasma proteins	7
Plasma bicarbonate	35
RBC bicarbonate	18
Total	100

Partial pressure: The pressure in mm Hg, an individual gas exerts on a column of mercury

Example—Gaseous components of air:

Gas	Fractional content (%)	Partial pressure (mm Hg)
Nitrogen (N_2)	78.084	593.44
Oxygen (O_2)	20.948	159.20
Argon (Ar)	0.934	7.10
Carbon dioxide (CO_2)	0.031	0.24
Others	0.003	0.02
Total	100.000	760.00 (atmospheric pressure)

pH: The negative log of the hydrogen ion (H^+) concentration. The pH is inversely proportional to the H^+ concentration

$$\text{Examples:} \quad (H^+) = 0.000001 = 1 \times 10^{-6} \quad pH = 6$$

$$(H^+) = 1 \times 10^{-7} \quad pH = 7$$

$$(H^+) = 1 \times 10^{-8} \quad pH = 8$$

Total CO_2 content: The amount of carbon dioxide gas extractable from plasma. Total CO_2 consists of:

HCO_3 (95% of the total CO_2 is HCO_3)
Carbonic acid ($H_2CO_3^-$)
Carbon dioxide

CHAPTER NINETEEN

Anesthetic Procedures and Techniques in Small Animals

"Come now let us reason together."

LYNDON BAINES JOHNSON

OVERVIEW

The anesthetic procedures and techniques developed for small animals are designed to produce a desirable end point safely, effectively, and economically. The use of a single drug to produce chemical restraint and anesthesia may be associated with specific side effects. Complete familiarity with a drug and its side effects offers the experienced anesthetist the advantages of knowing the drug's shortcomings and being prepared for those adverse responses that are likely to occur. The combination of several drugs, in reduced dosages, is used to provide chemical restraint and anesthesia while avoiding unwanted side effects and toxicity. Combination drug therapy offers the advantage of providing a more ideal anesthetic state, which includes hypnosis, analgesia, and muscle relaxation. Combination drug therapy, however, does require a more comprehensive knowledge of the pharmacology of the drugs and their interactions in order that all potential side effects may be anticipated.

GENERAL CONSIDERATIONS

I. A variety of anesthetic procedures and techniques can be used to safely produce chemical restraint and anesthesia in dogs and cats
II. The choice of anesthetic regimen is influenced by:
A. Breed

B. Health and physical condition
C. The purpose for chemical restraint and anesthesia
D. The familiarity of the personnel with the drugs being used
E. The amount of available assistance
III. Whenever possible, drugs that are reversible should be used
IV. Endotracheal intubation should always be performed in order to provide a patent airway
V. Careful monitoring is mandatory if adverse effects are to be averted
VI. Food and water should be withheld for approximately 12 hours prior to surgery, except in very small, very young, or diseased patients

PREANESTHETIC PERIOD

I. Review patient history
II. Perform physical examination
III. Review available laboratory data
IV. Formulate a specific anesthetic plan
    A. Decide if further preoperative tests are desired
    B. Choose drugs appropriate to case
V. Gather appropriate equipment and supplies
    A. Endotracheal tube
        1. Size determined by size of patient
        2. If using a cuffed tube, inject air into balloon and check for ability to hold volume
        3. Use a stylet for small-diameter, flimsy tubes (Fig. 19-1)
        4. A Cole catheter can be used in neonates, rodents, birds, and reptiles (Fig. 19-2)
    B. Laryngoscope
        1. Aids intubation by allowing close visual inspection and manipulation of tongue and laryngeal structures
        2. May be optional or required, depending on species anatomy and the physical size of the individual patient
    C. Anesthetic machine and breathing system
        1. Size and type of system determined by size of patient
            a. Patients less than approximately 400 pounds—small-animal anesthetic machine
                (1) Circle system for patients $\geq$ 15 pounds
                (2) Nonrebreathing system for patient $<$ 15 pounds
        2. Rebreathing bag approximately five times patient tidal volume
        3. Refill carbon dioxide–absorbent cannister if material is exhausted
        4. Evaluate system for possible malfunctions
            a. Fill vaporizer and check ease of operation
            b. Turn on flowmeters and check for free movement of indicator balls or slides
            c. Close pop-off valve and pressurize the system to 40 cm water using oxygen flush valve; check for leaks

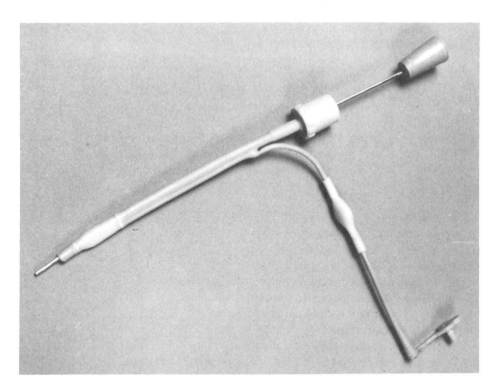

FIG. 19-1 A stylet can be used to stiffen small endotracheal tubes in order to facilitate tracheal intubation.

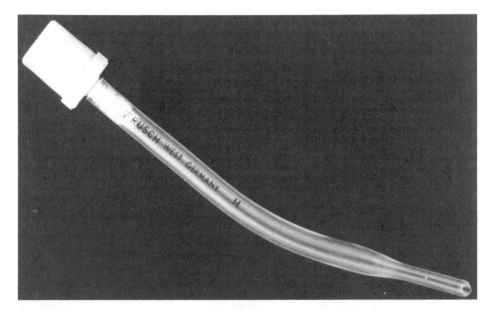

FIG. 19-2 A Cole catheter facilitates intubation of neonates, rodents, birds, and reptiles.

     5. Connect machine to waste gas scavenging system

  D. Fresh gases

     1. Oxygen

       a. Outside "house" supply

       b. Tanks mated to machine

         (1) Change oxygen tank if pressure gauge reads $\leq$500 psi

     2. Nitrous oxide

       a. Optional

       b. Change tanks mated to machine if pressure gauge reads $\leq$750 psi

  E. Intravenous administration supplies

     1. Catheter

     2. Appropriate IV fluids

     3. Administration set

  F. Drugs

     1. Calculate appropriate dosage volumes

     2. Withdraw drugs from vials into *labeled syringes*

  G. Ancillary supplies

     1. 4 $\times$ 4 inch gauze sponges

     2. Adhesive tape

     3. Roll gauze

     4. Esophageal stethoscope catheter and earpiece

PREMEDICATION

  I. Choice of drug determined by the patient's preoperative condition and any other special considerations pertinent to the procedure

  II. Drugs given IM or SQ should be administered 10-30 minutes prior to catherization and induction

 III. Drugs used as premedications

  A. Acepromazine 0.1 mg/lb IM, maximum total dose 4 mg

  B. Diazepam 0.1 mg/lb IV, maximum total dose 5 mg

  C. Innovar-Vet 1 cc/20-40 lb IM, 1 cc/40-80 lb IV

     1. Atropine 0.1 mg/lb IM or IV

     2. Glycopyrrolate 0.005 mg/lb IM or IV

  D. Anticholinergics

  E. Narcotics

     1. Morphine 0.2-0.3 mg/lb IM (dogs), 0.1 mg/lb IM (cats)

     2. Oxymorphone 0.05-0.15 mg/lb IM

     3. Meperidine 0.5-3 mg/lb IM

     4. Innovar-Vet 1 ml/30 lb IM (dogs), 1 ml/20 lbs IM (cats)

  F. Ketamine (cats) 3-5 mg/lb IM

  G. Xylazine 0.1-0.5 mg/lb IM

  H. Telazol 1-3 mg/lb IM

INDUCTION

  I. Intravenous

  A. Catheterize vein(s)

B. Start IV fluid administration immediately to ensure catheter patency
C. Lower fluid bag or bottle below patient's thorax with administration set valve completely open to allow blood to siphon back into catheter—this confirms placement within the vein
D. Inject induction agent(s) at appropriate rate(s), allowing time for patient equilibration before further increments are given
E. Specific IV induction drugs (see Chapter 8: Specific Intravenous Anesthetic Drugs
   1. Ultrashort-acting barbiturates
      a. Thiamylal 2-4%
      b. Thiopental 2-4%
      c. Methohexital 2%
   2. Pentobarbital
   3. Innovar-Vet
   4. Oxymorphone
   5. Etomidate
   6. Combinations
      a. Innovar-Vet 1 cc/40-60 lb IV plus pentobarbital 2-3 mg/lb IV
      b. Diazepam 0.1 mg/lb IV, thiamylal 2 mg/lb IV, lidocaine 2 mg/lb IV
         (1) Useful if animal is depressed
         (2) Stabilizes myocardium
         (3) Reduces thiobarbiturate dosage
      c. Diazepam-ketamine: simultaneous administration of diazepam (0.125 mg/lb IV) and ketamine (2.5 mg/lb IV)
         (1) Mix equal parts of diazepam (5 mg/ml in stock vial) and ketamine (100 mg/ml in stock vial) to yield a mixture that is 2.5 mg/ml diazepam and 50 mg/ml ketamine
         (2) Use 1 cc of mixture per 20 pounds
      d. Diazepam, narcotic, etomidate
         (1) Use etomidate at reduced dosage to produce hypnosis
II. Inhalant
   A. Face mask (Fig. 19-3)
      1. Be aware of potential for vomition and possible resultant aspiration
      2. Ensure adequate restraint during excitatory phase
   B. Induction box (Fig. 19-4)
      1. Cats, small dogs, rodents, birds, snakes
      2. Use high fresh gas flow rates
      3. Monitor patient closely for loss of righting reflex, then remove from box
      4. Atmospheric pollution with anesthetic gases is significant

ENDOTRACHEAL INTUBATION AND INITIATION OF INHALANT ANESTHESIA IN SMALL ANIMALS

I. Open patient's mouth, and manipulate tongue to side with endotracheal tube. Then grasp tongue with a gauze sponge, and retract tongue firmly between lower canine teeth to hold mandible open (see Fig. 19-5)

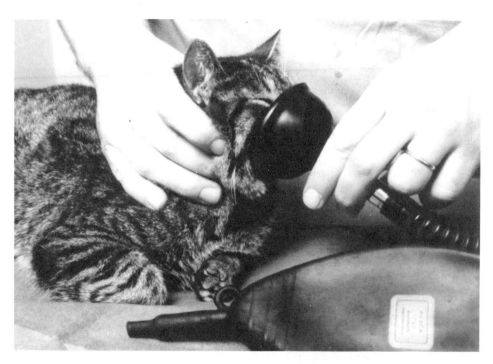

FIG. 19-3 A face mask is often used to induce cats and small dogs to anesthesia.

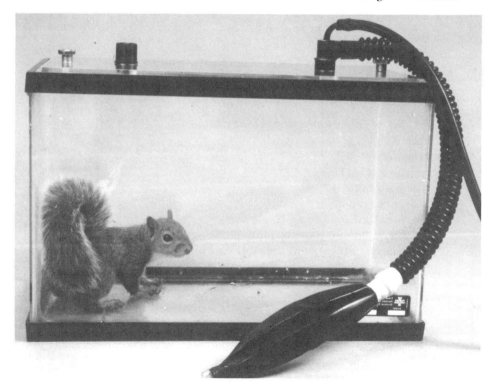

FIG. 19-4 An induction chamber is used to confine cats and small animals for induction to general anesthesia using an inhaled anesthetic.

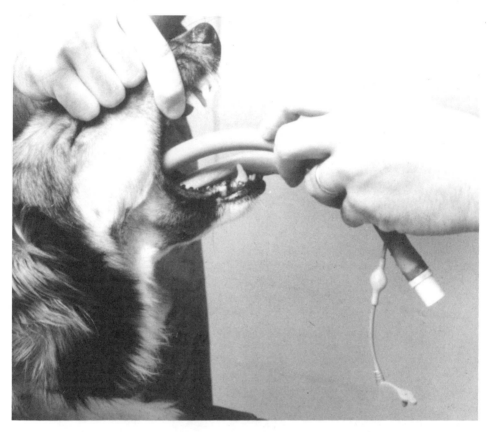

FIG. 19-5 Most dogs and cats are easily intubated without a laryngoscope.

II. Visualize larynx and insert endotracheal tube
  A. Direct
  B. Laryngoscope
  C. Potential difficulties
    1. Laryngospasm
      a. Patient too light
      b. Sensitized larynx
      c. 0.1 ml lidocaine sprayed into glottis reduces spasms
    2. Soft palate displacement prevents rostroventral movement of epiglottis
      a. Push soft palate dorsally with endotracheal tube to release epiglottis
  D. Turn on oxygen
  E. Connect breathing system to endotracheal tube, and secure tube to patient
    (see Fig. 19-6)
  F. Monitor respirations and pulse
    1. Pulses present—turn on vaporizer and nitrous oxide if desired
    2. Pulses absent—leave oxygen on and diagnose cause of absent or weak
      pulses; do not start inhalation agents
    3. Spontaneous ventilation—assist if required

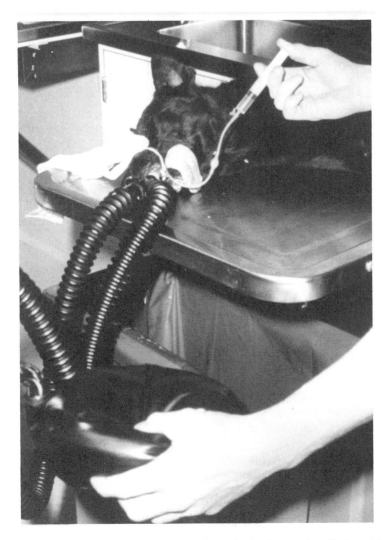

FIG. 19-6 Escape of gas from around the endotracheal tube can be eliminated by inflating the endotracheal tube cuff (right hand) until no gas escapes from the mouth during rebreathing bag compression (left hand) to 30 cm H_2O.

4. Apnea, dyspnea
   a. Patient's ventilatory drive may be depressed by anesthetic induction drugs; begin mechanical ventilation using the breathing system
   b. Endotracheal tube may be obstructed or kinked
   c. Bronchial intubation—withdraw tube into trachea
   d. Pneumothorax or pneumomediastinum
      (1) Relieve intrathoracic pressure by percutaneous needle insertion
      (2) Evaluate hemodynamic status

G. Set vaporizer to maintenance concentration at appropriate time determined by monitoring patient responses

MAINTENANCE OF ANESTHESIA

I. Monitoring (see Chapter 16: Patient Monitoring During Anesthesia)
II. Record concentrations and doses of anesthetic drugs given
   A. Readjust dosages according to response of patient and depth of anesthesia and analgesia needed
III. Continually check patency of airway through the endotracheal tube
   A. Blocked or kinked tube
   B. Overinflation of cuff
   C. Tube impinging at bifurcation of trachea
IV. Maintain endotracheal tube, head, and neck in a natural, slightly curved position to prevent kinking of the tube and maintain a patent airway. Position patient to avoid excessive flexion of neck, abduction of limbs, and pressure on thorax
V. Calculate intravenous fluids needed and adjust flow rate of drop. Record all fluids (total volumes), electrolytes, and other drugs administered
VI. Complete anesthetic record (Fig. 19-7)
   A. Start and end of anesthetic period
   B. Start and end of surgery period
   C. All major surgical events
   D. All changes in anesthetic status and technique
   E. All laboratory results during anesthesia, e.g., blood gases
VII. Nitrous oxide: Turn off before end of surgical period (usually 5-10 minutes before end). Methoxyflurane: Reduce concentration near end of surgery, and turn off 5-10 minutes before end
VIII. Halothane: Turn off at end of surgery or before, depending on depth of anesthesia
IX. Oxygen: Continue high flow rate (at least 3 L) into recovery period, until patient is swallowing. Empty rebreathing bag several times to dump anesthetic gases

POSTANESTHETIC RECOVERY

I. Deflate tube cuff and extubate when animal is swallowing
II. Administer oxygen as necessary (endotracheal tube, mask, oxygen cage)
III. Position animal in sternal recumbency with head extended
IV. Observe animal until it can maintain sternal recumbency
V. Maintain airway free of secretions (use postural drainage, sponges, suction tubes)
VI. Raise and maintain body temperature using towels and possibly covered heating pads
VII. Change animal's positions frequently, and stimulate by rubbing body, and flexing and extending limbs
VIII. Tranquilizers and analgesics may be needed if animal is distressed or in pain

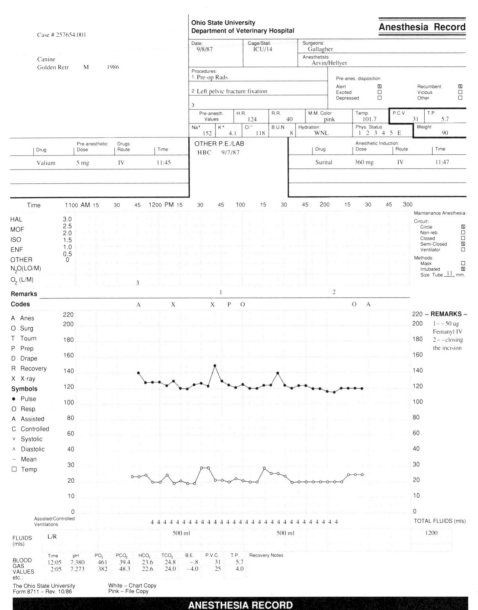

FIG. 19-7 Completed anesthesia record.

during recovery. Observe continuously for respiratory depression, especially if narcotic analgesics are given

IX. Maintain intravenous fluids as needed

X. Check periodically until patient is able to stand unsupported

XI. Use respiratory stimulants (e.g., doxapram HCl) only if needed

CHAPTER TWENTY

Anesthetic Procedures
And Techniques in Horses

"The little neglect may breed mischief . . . for want of a nail the shoe was lost;
for want of a shoe the horse was lost; and for want of a horse the rider was lost."
BENJAMIN FRANKLIN

OVERVIEW

The single most important rule in attempting to provide safe and effective anesthesia in horses is to be able to predict drug effects and drug actions. Patient temperament varies and has considerable influence upon drug dosages and anesthetic technique. Infusions of anesthetic drugs combined with physical restraint are frequently used to induce general anesthesia in the horse in order to prevent injury to the patient and attending personnel. The majority of anesthetic techniques are designed to produce rapid and safe induction to lateral recumbency and to maximize muscle relaxation and analgesia while maintaining normal cardiopulmonary status. Horses frequently require assistance in order to regain and maintain a standing position following general anesthesia.

GENERAL CONSIDERATIONS

I. Preparation of the equine surgical patient
   A. Food should be withheld for approximately 8-12 hours prior to surgery. Water should be withheld for at least 2 hours
   B. All shoes should be pulled, if this has not already been done. The surgical

site should be clipped and prepped prior to the induction to anesthesia (if possible)

C. The horse should be groomed and wiped with a moist cloth and have an intravenous catheter in place before the surgical area is entered

D. Each patient should receive a complete physical examination with emphasis on cardiopulmonary function

E. Each animal should be weighed, and the weight should be recorded in the anesthetic record

F. Each patient should be given a preanesthetic approximately 20-30 minutes prior to induction of anesthesia

G. Each patient should have its mouth rinsed with water before the surgical area is entered

H. The feet of all animals should be cleaned (bathed) before the surgical area is entered

II. All horses will develop acid-base disturbances, particularly respiratory acidosis with hypoxemia, the more prolonged the duration of anesthesia

III. Proper positioning and appropriate padding of the head, shoulder, and hip are paramount in order to minimize cardiopulmonary compromise and the development of neuropathies and myopathies

IV. Assisted or controlled ventilation is required in order to maintain normal arterial carbon dioxide concentrations during prolonged general anesthesia in the horse

V. Measurement of arterial blood pressure and its maintenance within normal levels will help to avoid postoperative complications, including myopathy

VI. All horses should be observed and, if possible, assisted to a standing position during the recovery period

PREANESTHETIC EVALUATION
(Neurologic, Cardiovascular, Pulmonary, and Hydration)

I. Physical evaluation
   A. Determine age, weight, sex
   B. Excitability of the animal
   C. ASA classification and disease, if any
   D. Concurrent or previous drug history
   E. Procedure to be performed
   F. Prepare anesthetic care plan

II. Laboratory evaluation
   A. Routine evaluation
      1. CBC (Hct, Hb)
      2. Total solids
   B. Suggested further evaluation
      1. Blood clotting mechanisms
      2. Serum electrolytes
      3. Serum chemistry

POPULAR PREANESTHETIC MEDICATIONS

I. Acepromazine (used to produce a calming effect)
  A. Dose: 10-30 mg/1,000 lb IM
        5-10 mg/1,000 lb IV
  B. Onset of tranquilization is within 10-20 minutes
  C. Duration of tranquilization lasts 2-3 hours
  D. Hypotensive effect may last for as long as 12 hours
II. Promazine
  A. Dose: 0.1-0.5 mg/lb IV
III. Xylazine (used to produce sedation, analgesia, and muscle relaxation)
  A. Dose: 0.7-1.0 mg/lb IM
        0.3-0.5 mg/lb IM
  B. Onset is within 2-3 minutes after IV and within 10-15 minutes after IM administration
  C. Duration is 30 minutes after IV and 60 minutes after IM administration
  D. First- and second-degree heart block may occur
IV. Chloral hydrate (used to produce sedation if the aforementioned drugs for premedication are ineffective)
  A. Dose: 10-50 mg/lb

GENERAL ANESTHETIC TECHNIQUES

I. Collect the necessary equipment
  A. Endotracheal tubes
    1. Choose the largest tube possible (30, 26, 20, or 15 mm)
      a. Most tube size designations are related to inside diameter
    2. Check the endotracheal tube cuff for leaks
    3. Use lubricating cream for endotracheal tube
    4. Use 25 and 60 cc syringe and three-way stopcock for inflating the cuff on the endotracheal tube
    5. Cotton mouth gag or speculum
  B. Intravenous catheter for intravenous anesthetic drug or fluid administration
  C. Pressure bag for administration of guaifenesin
  D. Chest rope for restraining front legs (see Fig. 20-1)
  E. Proper padding (see Fig. 20-1)
  F. Monitoring equipment (see Chapter 17: Hemodynamic Monitoring)
    1. ECG monitor
    2. Blood pressure recording device
    3. Pressure transducer
    4. Ultrasonic Doppler
    5. Oscillometric method
    6. Stethoscope
II. Before induction of general anesthesia
  A. The anesthetic machine should be examined to be sure the vaporizer has an adequate anesthetic level, and the circle system should be tested for leaks

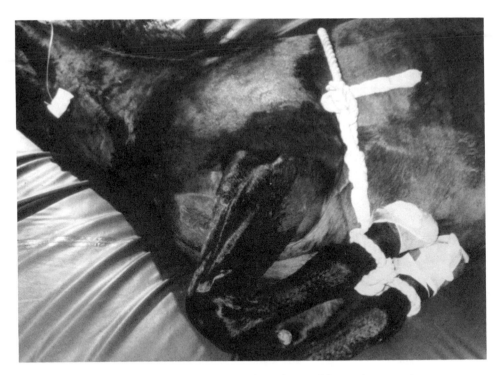

FIG. 20-1 Horses are usually positioned on large foam rubber pads or on air or water mattresses with their front legs restrained during general anesthesia.

   1. The system may be checked for leaks by occluding the Y piece that connects to the endotracheal tube, closing the pop-off valve, and flushing oxygen through the system. If pressure is maintained, the system is not leaking
   2. The circle system should be able to maintain a pressure of approximately 60 cm of water
 B. Check oxygen pressures in the tanks
   1. Oxygen = 2,500 psi
   2. Nitrous oxide = 750 psi (used in foals)
 C. Fresh carbon dioxide absorbent should be present in the cannister
 D. Describe flow rate
   1. Oxygen: 1 L/250 lb; minimum of 3 L/1,000 lb. High flow rates, 1 L/100 lb, are used during induction and recovery to denitrogenate and remove anesthetic vapors, respectively
   2. Nitrous oxide, if used, is added to the oxygen flow (e.g., 3 L oxygen and 3 L nitrous oxide = total flow 6 L)

ANESTHETIC INDUCTION AGENTS

I. Thiamylal sodium
 A. Dose:

        Without guaifenesin   3.0-5.0 mg/lb
        In combination with guaifenesin   1.5-2.0 mg/lb

  B. 4% solution—40 mg/ml
  C. Ultrashort-acting (5-10 minutes)
  D. Causes cardiovascular depression and may cause transient apnea (dose-dependent)

II. Guaifenesin
  A. Dose: 50 mg/lb to produce recumbency
            25 mg/lb to produce ataxia and relaxation
  B. 5% or 10% solution—50 or 100 mg/ml
  C. Administered before or with thiamylal sodium or ketamine
  D. Duration: 10-20 minutes
  E. Causes minimal analgesia and sedation
  F. Toxic signs include:
    1. Apneustic breathing pattern
    2. Muscle ridigity
    3. Hypotension

III. Ketamine
  A. Dose: 0.7-1.0 mg/lb IV
  B. 10% solution contains 100 mg/ml
  C. Administered in combination with, but after, xylazine and/or guaifenesin relaxation
  D. Short-acting (10-15 minutes)
  E. Causes apneustic breathing pattern

IV. Halothane
  A. 3-5% concentration of halothane and high oxygen flow can be used for induction for brief periods of time (e.g., 5 L by mask)

INDUCTION

  I. Induction (see Anesthetic induction agents)
    A. May be aided by prior placement of an intravenous catheter
    B. Tubing for an adult patient 500-1,000 pounds
      1. 240 polyethylene tubing or commercial catheter
      2. 10 gauge, 2-inch venapuncture needle
      3. 14 gauge disposable needle
      4. Three-way stopcock
      5. 12 cc syringe with heparinized saline solution

  II. Endotracheal intubation (Fig. 20-2)
    A. Practice makes perfect. Learn to intubate blindly
    B. If tube appears too small, choose a larger one
    C. Do not advance the tip of the endotracheal tube past the thoracic inlet
    D. Secure the tube with gauze, if necessary
    E. Nasal intubation can be performed in adults and foals (Fig. 20-3)
    F. Two *clean* endotracheal tubes and a speculum or mouth gag should be available for induction

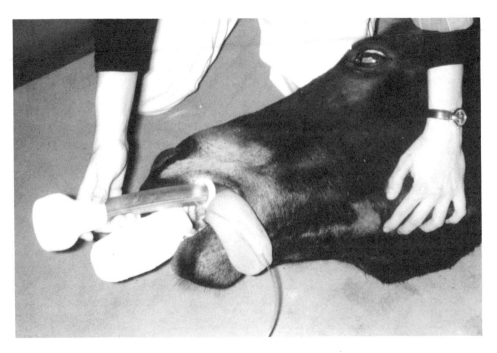

FIG. 20-2 Endotracheal intubation is performed blindly in the horse and foals.

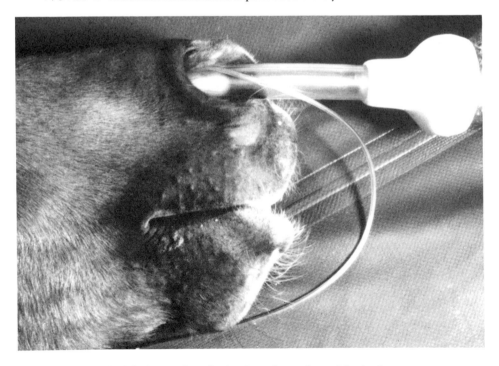

FIG. 20-3 Nasal intubation is easily performed in the horse.

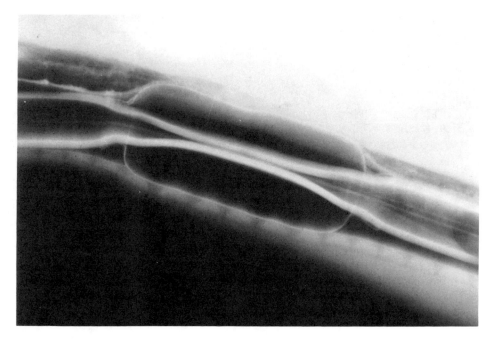

FIG. 20-4 Accidental overinflation of the endotracheal cuff can result in tube occlusion in the horse.

    G. Connect the endotracheal tube to the anesthetic system
        1. Circle system for large animals
            a. Rebreathing bag size should be at least five times the tidal volume
                (1) 30 L or 15 L bags are standard
    H. Inflate the endotracheal tube cuff, and check to see that it does not leak by squeezing the rebreathing bag, thereby expanding the animal's lungs
        1. 15-20 cm water or 10-15 mm Hg mercury pressure is sufficient
        2. Do not overinflate the cuff. Generally, 50-75 ml is adequate in a 1,000 pound patient (see Fig. 20-4)
III. Inhalation anesthesia
    A. Halothane: 1-3%
    B. Enflurane: 1-3%
    C. Isoflurane: 1-3%
IV. Monitoring (see Chapter 16: Patient Monitoring During Anesthesia, and Chapter 17: Hemodynamic Monitoring)
    A. Body temperature
        1. Generally increases in large animals during anesthesia
        2. May decrease in foals and during prolonged procedures
    B. Chart all anesthetic and surgical events and the animal's response
    C. A sample anesthesia record is illustrated (see Fig. 19-7)
    D. Monitor all vital signs (i.e., cardiovascular, respiratory) and the depth of anesthesia (unconsciousness, eye signs)

    V. Administration of fluids (see Chapter 24: Fluid Administration During Anesthesia)

   VI. Turn off anesthesia vaporizer and nitrous oxide before administering oxygen; this will minimize prolonged recovery and avoid diffusion hypoxia

  VII. Administer oxygen until the patient is swallowing, then extubate

     A. Use O_2 demand valve in recovery stall

 VIII. Postanesthetic recovery

     A. Oxygen is routinely administered via:

       1. O_2 humidifier

       2. O_2 demand valve

     B. Keep tranquilizer, ropes, and emergency drugs available in case of rough recoveries

       1. Make sure cuff on endotracheal tube is deflated

       2. Keep head and muzzle down to allow drainage

     C. Respiratory-assist devices

       1. North American Drager Ventilation

       2. Innovative Ventilator

CHAPTER TWENTY-ONE

Anesthetic Procedures and Techniques in Ruminants

"You've got to stop and eat the roses along the way."
ANONYMOUS

OVERVIEW

Physical restraint and local anesthetic techniques are frequently employed to provide immobility and analgesia to ruminants (cattle, sheep, and goats). Occasionally, however, general anesthesia is required and is produced using techniques similar to those for dogs, cats, or horses, depending on the size of the patient. Regurgitation of rumen contents and bloat (distention of the rumen) are potential hazards not encountered in normal dogs, cats, or horses. Close observation and monitoring of palpebral and ocular reflexes, eyeball position, and pupil size can be used to monitor the depth of anesthesia in ruminants. Recovery from anesthesia is generally quiet and uneventful and does not routinely require assistance.

GENERAL CONSIDERATIONS

I. Preparation of the ruminant surgical patient
  A. The most important factor in decreasing the risk of regurgitation is to decrease rumen pressure prior to anesthesia by:
    1. Withholding food for 24-36 hours in large ruminants
    2. Withholding water for 8-12 hours in large ruminants
    3. Withholding food for 12-24 hours in sheep and goats
      a. There is no need to withhold water before subjecting sheep and goats to general anesthesia
    4. Withholding food for 2-4 hours in calves, lambs, and young kids

      a. Calves, lambs, and young kids (less than 1 month of age) are essentially monogastric and are less prone to regurgitation during anesthesia

  B. The side effects of withholding food are minimal

    1. Mild metabolic alkalosis is observed in healthy animals

    2. Bradycardia is produced in adult cattle

  C. In the case of nonelective procedures, endotracheal and rumen tubes should be placed, when appropriate, to avoid bloat and aspiration of rumen contents

II. Due to the nature of cattle, most surgical techniques can be performed using local or regional anesthesia (see Chapter 5: Local anesthesia in cattle)

III. General anesthesia is required if local or regional anesthetic techniques are not adequate

  A. Light stages of anesthesia may predispose to stress

    1. Death may occur if painful procedures such as dehorning are attempted without adequate anesthesia

    2. Cardiac arrest may occur due to catecholamine-induced ventricular fibrillation or vagally induced asystole

IV. Preanesthetic evaluation is very similar to that of the horse

  A. Physical examination

  B. Basic laboratory tests

    1. CBC

    2. Liver enzymes

    3. Serum electrolytes

    4. BUN

V. The most frequently encountered problems associated with sedation and general anesthesia are

  A. Regurgitation

  B. Pulmonary aspiration

  C. Bloat

  D. Inadequate oxygenation

  E. Injury

  F. Respiratory depression and apnea

VI. Regurgitation is caused by a vagal effect on reticular contractions and parasympathetic effects on pharyngoesophageal and gastroesophageal sphincters

  A. Anesthetic drugs increase the risk of regurgitation by:

    1. Relaxing the pharyngoesophageal sphincter

    2. Relaxing the gastroesophageal sphincter

    3. Depressing the swallow reflex

  B. Recumbency also increases the risk of regurgitation

PREANESTHETIC MEDICATION

I. Preanesthetic drugs may be desired to calm an unruly bull or to decrease the dose of a more potent intravenous or inhalation anesthetic

II. Tranquilizers are not approved for use in food animals. Milk and meat drug residues must be taken into consideration

III. Popular preanesthetic medications
   A. Acepromazine (used to produce a calming effect)
      1. Dose: 20-40 mg/1,000 lb IM
             5-10 mg/1,000 lb IV
      2. Onset of tranquilization is within 10-20 minutes
      3. Duration of tranquilization is 2-4 hours
      4. Acepromazine (0.1-0.2 mg/kg IM) does not produce a great deal of useful sedation in goats
   B. Xylazine
      1. Must be dosed at one tenth the intravenous horse dose: 0.05 mg/lb IV or less
      2. It is recommended that only low-concentration xylazine (20 mg/ml) be used
      3. Moderate dose of 0.05-0.1 mg/lb IV generally induces recumbency and depresses or abolishes pharyngeal and laryngeal reflexes, thus allowing easy intubation and the use of inhalation anesthesia without barbiturates
      4. Side effects
         a. Cardiovascular depression
         b. Respiratory depression
         c. Rumen atony with bloat
         d. Hyperglycemia from decreased plasma insulin
         e. Diuresis
         f. Decreased hematocrit
         g. Abortion in late pregnancy
   C. Telazol
      1. Administered at 1 mg/lb IV or 1-3 mg/lb IM
      2. Prior administration of xylazine (0.1 mg/lb IM) decreases Telazol dosage by one half
      3. Ocular pharyngeal and laryngeal reflexes are depressed
      4. Compatible with inhalation anesthetics
      5. Side effects
         a. Respiratory depression
         b. Hypotension
   D. Atropine, glycopyrrolate
      1. The use of anticholinergic drugs (atropine, glycopyrrolate) preoperatively in ruminants is controversial
      2. Atropine sulfate 2 mg/100 lb IM or SQ may be useful in reducing bradycardia and hypotension during manipulation of viscera induced by vagal reflexes
      3. The duration of action of atropine in ruminants is short
      4. Anticholinergics increase the incidence of bloat due to a decrease in intestinal motility and an accumulation of gas from bacterial fermentation
      5. Anticholinergics increase the viscosity of the saliva (without decreasing the volume of saliva significantly)
      6. Saliva flow is controlled by having the head pointed downhill and an endotracheal tube with an inflatable cuff in place

ANESTHETIC INDUCTION

I. Barbiturates

    A. Thiopental sodium (Pentothal) and thiamylal sodium (Surital) are ultra-short-acting (10-15 minutes) barbiturates with predictable effects

        1. Doses of 3-5 mg/ml thiamylal or 5-7 mg/lb thiopental will achieve light surgical anesthesia within 12-15 seconds

        2. Less barbiturate is needed if the animal is premedicated or induced with guaifenesin

        3. Barbiturates should be used with caution in animals less than 3 months of age, as their ability to metabolize the drugs is inadequate

        4. Barbiturates rapidly cross the placental barrier and depress fetal respirations

    B. Pentobarbital (Nembutal, 30 mg/ml, 10 mg/lb IV) is infrequently recommended for induction of anesthesia prior to intubation and maintenance of anesthesia using an inhalation anesthetic

        1. Goats are very sensitive to the respiratory depression caused by pentobarbital

        2. Can produce significant cardiovascular depression

        3. Hemolysis and hematuria may be caused by the propylene glycol preservative in pentobarbital

        4. Anesthesia is produced within 5 minutes, with recovery in 30-60 minutes

II. Guaifenesin

    A. Dose: 50 mg/lb IV if used alone for recumbency

             25 mg/lb IV to effect

    B. 5% solution (50 mg/cc) with 5% dextrose

        1. More concentrated solutions may cause hemolysis

    C. Can be used in combination with xylazine, thiamylal, and/or ketamine

III. Xylazine-ketamine combination

    A. Dose: 0.04 mg/lb xylazine and 2 mg/lb ketamine

        1. Both drugs can be administered in the same syringe

        2. When given IV, immobilization occurs in less than 1 minute, providing anesthesia of 1-hour duration. Recovery occurs (standing) 2 hours or more after injection

        3. When given IM, induction time is 3-10 minutes; anesthesia and recovery time are increased

        4. Decreases heart rate, respiratory rate, and temperature; an apneustic respiratory pattern and salivation are seen in ruminants

IV. Xylazine-ketamine-guaifenesin combination

    A. Dose: 50 mg xylazine + 500 mg ketamine in 500 ml of 5% guaifenesin given to effect—approximately 1-2 ml/lb IV

        1. All three drugs are soluble in water

        2. Induction is gradual and generally uneventful but may require some physical restraint

        3. Anesthesia is adequate for periods of 30-90 minutes; respiration may need to be assisted

        4. Drug overdose causes apnea and hypotension

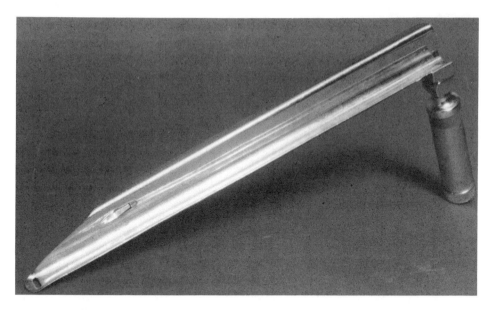

FIG.21-1 Endotracheal intubation in cattle, sheep, and goats can be facilitated with a long-blade laryngoscope.

V. Telazol
  A. 0.5-1.0 mg/lb IV; 1-3 mg/lb IM
    1. Produces excellent short-term (20-30 minutes) surgical anesthesia
    2. May produce respiratory depression
VI. Masking down with an inhalation agent
  A. Animals under 150 pounds can be induced using a mask induction technique with 3-4% halothane or 3% isoflurane, intubated and maintained on 1-2%
  B. Injury is prevented by casting the cow prior to induction or restraining it on a surgical table

ENDOTRACHEAL INTUBATION

  I. Intubation should immediately follow the induction of anesthesia
  II. Several techniques are useful
    A. A dental speculum or mouth gag can be placed
    B. Method 1: Insert an arm into the oral cavity of the adult cow, reflect the epiglottis forward manually, and guide the endotracheal tube into the larynx
    C. Method 2: Extend the patient's head and neck, and gently advance the tube into the trachea during inspiration
    D. Intubation may be facilitated by use of a laryngoscope and endoscopic light (Fig. 21-1)
    E. In small ruminants, a long, small-diameter wood or steel dowel may be placed into the trachea first and the endotracheal tube passed over it (Fig. 21-2)

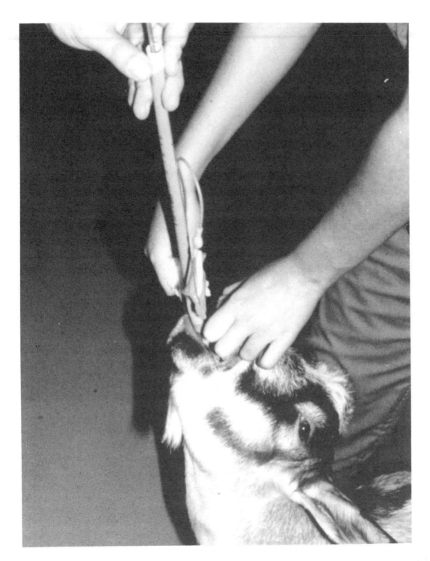

FIG. 21-2 A steel dowel can be placed in the trachea and the endotracheal tube slid over it to facilitate intubation in small ruminants.

   F. Whichever method is used, it should be done quickly to avoid regurgitation and aspiration of fluid
   G. A tracheostomy may be performed, if required

INHALATION ANESTHESIA

  I. Inhalation anesthetic drugs are an excellent means for producing anesthesia, particularly for prolonged operations on debilitated animals
 II. Induction is completed with 3-5% halothane or 2-4% isoflurane using 4-8 mg/lb/min O_2 flow rates

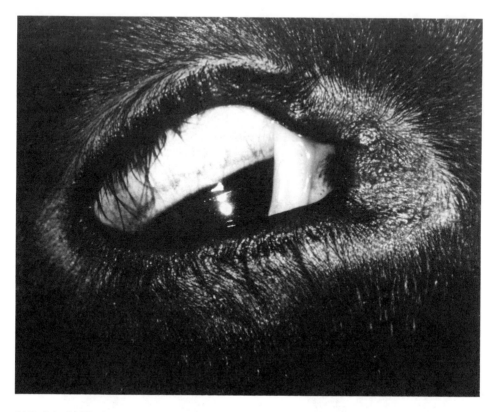

FIG. 21-3 The bovine eye rotates ventrally and medially during light planes of anesthesia.

III. Depending upon the individual, a surgical plane of anesthesia may be maintained at 0.5-2% halothane or 1-2% isoflurane

IV. A 50:50 mixture of nitrous oxide: oxygen may be used in small ruminants (preruminant)

V. Ruminants should be put on a mechanical ventilator to minimize respiratory acidosis, if surgical procedures last longer than 1 hour or blood carbon dioxide concentrations are greater than 60 mm Hg

MONITORING

I. The position of the eyeball provides a useful guide to anesthetic depth

A. Ocular reflexes are good indicators of anesthetic depth, as the corneal reflex should be active throughout anesthesia and the palpebral reflex is depressed by inhalation anesthesia

B. The eyeball is rotated medioventrally when the patient is in a light surgical plane of anesthesia (Fig. 21-3)

C. The iris and pupil are centered between the two lids when the patient is in a deep surgical plane of anesthesia or awake. Dilated pupils are a sign of anesthetic overdose when using inhalation anesthesia

    D. The auricular artery, located on the dorsal surface of the ear, can be cannulated to monitor arterial blood pressure

  II. See Chapter 16: Patient Monitoring During Anesthesia

III. Administration of fluids (see Chapter 24: Fluid Administration During Anesthesia)

RECOVERY

   I. The animal is allowed to breathe 100% oxygen for several minutes before being unhooked from the anesthetic machine

  II. The endotracheal tube should remain in place until the laryngeal reflex returns

III. If regurgitation occurs, the head should be positioned to allow drainage before pulling the endotracheal tube

 IV. The cuff should remain inflated while the endotracheal tube is being removed

  V. A stomach tube should be passed to decompress the rumen if the animal has bloated

 VI. Place a cow on its right side or, when possible, in sternal recumbency once the tube is pulled to avoid regurgitation and inhalation of the fluids

VII. Cattle generally recover needing little assistance following inhalation anesthesia

CHAPTER TWENTY-TWO

Anesthetic Procedures and Techniques in Pigs

"It is a bad plan that admits of no modification."

PUBLILIUS SYRUS

OVERVIEW

Pig anesthesia provides a unique and potentially challenging situation. There are few superficial veins that are easily accessible in pigs, other than those on the dorsal surface of the ear. These veins are frequently difficult to utilize because of identification and tagging procedures. Chemical restraining drugs can be administered intramuscularly. The pig is difficult to intubate because of its small oral cavity, dorsal displacement of the tongue, and the presence of a pharyngeal diverticulum. Respiratory depression and elevations of body temperature are frequently associated with chemical restraint and general anesthesia. Respiratory depression may be caused by the combined respiratory-depressant effects of the chemical restraining drugs chosen and the limited expansion of the chest wall due to abnormal body positioning and body fat. Elevation in body temperature is facilitated by the low ratio of body surface area to body mass, the relative absence of sweat glands, and inefficient thermoregulatory mechanisms. Hyperpyrexia and malignant hyperthermia have been reported in genetically predisposed pigs and can be triggered by a variety of intravenous and inhalation anesthetics. Physical restraint combined with sedatives, tranquilizers, and local anesthetic techniques are the usual methods used for simple surgical procedures in pigs. General anesthesia using inhalation anesthetics provides an excellent, stable state of anesthesia for prolonged or involved surgical procedures.

GENERAL CONSIDERATIONS

I. Surgical preparation of the pig
   A. Obtain a complete history, and do a complete physical examination, paying particular attention to the respiratory system

228

   B. Withhold food for 8-12 hours in adults, 2-4 hours in neonates
   C. Water need not be withheld
   D. If possible, use drugs that are potentially reversible, such as xylazine and narcotics
   E. Avoid stress by leaving the pig with other pigs until tranquilized, if possible

II. Respiratory depression is a frequent sequela to the administration of depressant drugs in pigs
   A. Use drugs that are potentially reversible, such as xylazine and narcotics
   B. Obtain an estimate of the size of the trachea prior to drug administration
      1. A pig's trachea is smaller than you may think
   C. Be prepared for respiratory emergencies
      1. Have a variety of endotracheal tube sizes available
      2. Be prepared to do a tracheotomy
         a. #10 blade and scalpel
         b. Hemostat
         c. Cuffed tracheostomy tube
         d. Respiratory stimulants, such as doxapram, may be necessary

III. Increases in body temperature are frequently associated with inhalation anesthesia in pigs
   A. The pig has a low body surface area relative to body mass
   B. The pig has relatively poor thermoregulatory mechanisms and relatively few sweat glands
   C. Depolarizing neuromuscular blocking agents and inhalation anesthetics can trigger malignant hyperthermia
      1. Several strains of pigs (Landrace, Poland China, and others) are genetically predisposed to malignant hyperthermia
      2. Dantrolene (1 mg/lb IV) is the only known truly effective therapy for malignant hyperthermia

IV. The preanesthetic evaluation should include:
   A. Physical examination
   B. Basic laboratory tests
      1. CBC

V. The most frequently encountered problems associated with sedation and general anesthesia are:
   A. Respiratory depression and apnea
   B. Increased body temperature
   C. Porcine stress syndrome

ANESTHETIC PROCEDURES

I. Lumbosacral epidural anesthesia is a commonly used local anesthetic technique in pigs (see Chapter 5: Local anesthesia in pigs)
   A. The major advantages are the minor systemic effects in debilitated animals and minimal effect of the fetuses during cesarean section
   B. Disadvantages include lack of anesthesia to the cranial half of the animal, necessitating physical restraint of the forelimbs

    C. A 3-5–inch, 18 gauge spinal needle is used, and 2% lidocaine hydrochloride solution is injected

    D. The dosage varies from 0.2 to 0.5 ml/10 lb, with the higher dosage providing anesthesia as far cranially as the paralumbar fossa

    E. Refer to Chapter 5 on local anesthesia

II. Intratesticular injection

    A. Large boars can be castrated by using restraint and the injection of 15-30 mg/kg of sodium pentobarbital into each testicle

    B. Anesthesia occurs in approximately 5 minutes

    D. The source of anesthetic is removed as soon as the testicles are removed; this should be done rapidly

III. Fentanyl-droperidol (Innovar-Vet) and ketamine combination

    A. IM Dosages

        1. < 200 pounds body weight:

	Innovar-Vet	1 ml/60-80 lb
	ketamine	3-5 mg/kg

        2. > 200 pounds body weight:

	Innovar-Vet	1 ml/100 lb
	ketamine	3-5 mg/lb

    B. Onset of analgesia is within 5-10 minutes and lasts for 30-45 minutes

    C. Supplemental doses of Telazol or ketamine (1-3 mg/lb) IM or sodium pentobarbital (1-3 mg/lb) IM may be given to prolong anesthesia

    D. Advantages

        1. Ease of administration

        2. Useful for longer procedures where some movement is allowable

        3. Reversibility of the depressant effects of fentanyl

    E. Disadvantages

        1. Pigs may develop muscle tremors and hyperpyrexia following ketamine administration

        2. Hyperthermia is occasionally observed

        3. Excitability, salivation, respiratory depression

        4. Atropine (0.02 mg/lb IM) may be necessary to prevent bradycardia caused by fentanyl

IV. Atropine-acepromazine-ketamine combination

    A. Dosage: 0.02 mg/lb atropine and 0.05-0.2 mg/lb acepromazine IM, followed in 30 minutes by 5 mg/lb IM ketamine

    B. Azaperone can be used as an alternative to acepromazine at dosages ranging from 0.2-1.0 mg/lb IM

    C. Useful for minor procedures, such as detusking or castration of large boars

    D. Advantages

        1. Ease of administration

        2. Some analgesia and muscle relaxation within 5 minutes and lasting 10-15 minutes

    E. Disadvantages

        1. Additional analgesia is required using a local lidocaine block

        2. 30-minute waiting period between administration of drugs

        3. Hypotension

V. Atropine-xylazine-ketamine combination

    A. Dosage: 0.02 mg/lb atropine and 0.1 mg/lb xylazine IM, followed in 10 minutes with 5 mg/lb IM ketamine

    B. Advantages

       1. Ease of administration

       2. Some analgesia and muscle relaxation within 5 minutes and lasting 10-15 minutes

    C. Disadvantages

       1. Xylazine has a short duration of action due to rapid metabolism

       2. Involuntary muscle movement during the anesthetic period

VI. Xylazine-ketamine-guaifenesin combination

    A. Dosage: 500 mg xylazine + 500 mg ketamine mixed in 500 ml 5% guaifenesin given to effect—approximately 1-2 ml/lb IV

    B. Advantages

       1. Gradual induction, stable hemodynamics, and good muscle relaxation

    C. Disadvantages

       1. Respiratory depression may require assisted ventilation

       2. Expensive

VII. Xylazine-Telazol

    A. Dosage: xylazine 0.1-0.5 mg/lb IM followed in 5 minutes by Telazol 1-3 mg/lb IM

    B. Advantages

       1. Ease of administration

       2. Good analgesia and muscle relaxation

       3. Minimal cardiovascular depression

    C. Disadvantages

       1. Occasional respiratory depression

       2. Light plane of anesthesia

       3. Short duration of action; therefore, may need to be supplemented

VIII. Atropine-acepromazine-thiamylal combination

    A. Dosage: 0.02 mg/lb atropine and 0.2 mg/lb acepromazine IM, followed in 10 minutes by 5 mg/lb thiamylal sodium (3-5% solution) administered into an ear vein

    B. Advantages

       1. Anesthesia immediate and lasts for 15-30 minutes

       2. Thiamylal can be redosed but produces respiratory-depressant and prolongs recovery time

    C. Disadvantages

       1. Difficulty of venapuncture

       2. Respiratory and cardiovascular depression

IX. Innovar-Vet–sodium pentobarbital combination

    A. Dosage: 1 ml/40-60 lb Innovar-Vet IV, followed in 10 minutes with 3 ml/lb IV sodium pentobarbital

    B. Advantages

       1. Excellent analgesia

       2. Good muscle relaxation

    C. Disadvantages

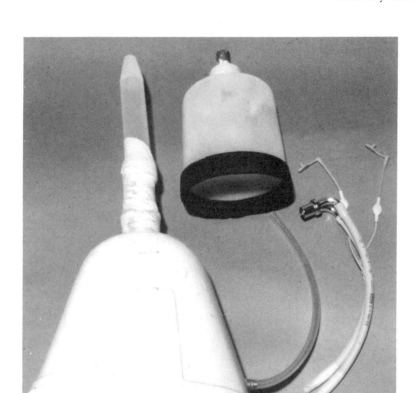

FIG. 22-1 Face masks and nasal endotracheal tubes can be used as an alternative to endotracheal intubation in pigs.

    1. Difficulty of venapuncture
    2. Respiratory depression
X. Inhalation anesthesia
    A. Inhalation agents, such as halothane, isoflurane, or methoxyflurane, can be administered:
        1. For induction (mask induction) to anesthesia
        2. For maintenance of anesthesia after the pig is induced with other drugs
    B. Delivery of inhalation drugs (see Fig. 22-1)
        1. Face mask
        2. Nasal tubes, which are made from human nasal tube adapters and small-animal endotracheal tubes (6-8 mm)
        3. Endotracheal intubation is preferred; long-bladder laryngoscope or long, rigid dowel rods can be used to pass the endotracheal tube

    C. Advantages
      1. Good control of anesthesia
      2. Excellent muscle relaxation
      3. Ease of administration
    D. Disadvantages
      1. Expensive equipment required
      2. Not generally suited for field conditions
      3. Halothane can induce hyperthermia in pigs

MONITORING

  I. Monitoring anesthetic depth in pigs is similar to that for other species (See Chapter 17: Hemodynamic Monitoring)
    A. The auricular artery, located on the dorsal surface of the ear, can be cannulated to monitor arterial blood pressure
  II. Signs of malignant hyperthermia include:
    A. Extreme muscle rigidity
    B. Increased temperature ($> 107°$ F)
    C. Tachycardia
    D. Tachypnea
    E. Metabolic acidosis
  III. Treatment of the hyperthermia in pigs
    A. Dantrolene 1.2 mg/lb per os
    B. Supportive treatment
      1. Bicarbonate
      2. Fluids
      3. Steroids
      4. Oxygen
      5. Body cooling

RECOVERY

  I. Oxygen and/or assisted ventilation if necessary
  II. Sternal positioning
  III. Well-ventilated, quiet environment
  IV. Periodic assessment of vital signs

CHAPTER TWENTY-THREE

Anesthetic Procedures and Techniques in Birds, Fish, Reptiles, Amphibians, Rodents, and Exotic Cats

"'The time has come,' the walrus said, 'to talk of many things.'"
LEWIS CARROLL

OVERVIEW

The domestication of a variety of exotic and wildlife species is increasing. Many of these species demonstrate idiosyncracies and widely varying sensitivities to drugs commonly used to produce chemical restraint and anesthesia. An overview of the important considerations and drugs used to produce chemical restraint and anesthesia follows. General textbooks on wildlife and exotic species should be consulted for a more detailed description of specific species' physiology and response to chemical restraining and anesthetic drugs.

BIRDS

I. Presurgical evaluation
  A. Complete physical examination
  B. Respiratory recovery time
    1. Time required for respirations to return to normal after the bird is captured and examined for 2 minutes
    2. Normal recovery time is 3-5 minutes
    3. A prolonged time may indicate an underlying respiratory problem
  C. Fecal parasite examination
  D. Fecal and choanal Gram's stain

E. PCV
  1. PCV < 25-30: Consider transfusion
     a. Loss of five drops of blood in small birds (e.g., canaries) is about 15% of total blood volume, potentially producing severe hypotension and cardiac arrest
  2. PCV > 55-60: Rehydrate with fluids
     a. Small birds may be given subcutaneous dextrose-saline injections
     b. Raptors may be given intravenous fluids 5 ml/kg/hr
F. Total protein (TP)
  1. TP < 3.0 g/dl: Consider plasma transfusion
G. Glucose
  1. Glucose < 200 mg/dl: Add 5% dextrose to fluids
H. Special tests
  1. Whole body radiographs
     a. Hepatomegaly is frequently seen with coagulopathies
  2. CBC and clotting time
  3. Culture and sensitivity of the cloaca and choana
  4. Serum profile
  5. Electrocardiogram
I. Systemic antibiotics
  1. Peak blood levels should be reached by the time of surgery
II. Preoperative preparation and precautions
  A. Fasting
    1. Small birds
       a. Need energy reserves in the gut to help them through the stress period
       b. Should not be fasted
    2. Medium-size birds
       a. Have high metabolic rate
       b. Should only be fasted for about 2 hours
    3. Large birds
       a. May regulate crop contents, resulting in aspiration
       b. Fast for 6-12 hours prior to anesthesia
  B. Avoid hypothermia
    1. Hypothermia depresses the respiratory control system, resulting in:
       a. Suppressed ventilation
       b. Possibly death
    2. Hypothermia may be diminished by
       a. Placing warm towels between birds and the stainless steel table
       b. Placing the bird on a circulating warm water blanket
  C. Consider having blood available for transfusion
    1. Use heparin as the anticoagulant
    2. Do not use EDTA, to avoid excessive binding of calcium
    3. Transfusion donors
       a. First choice is a bird of the same species
       b. Heterologous transfusions

(1) Are safe the first time

(2) Should not be repeated for at least 3 weeks

(3) Pigeon is the most common donor

D. Restrain to avoid trauma

  1. Secure wings to the back

  2. Tape legs together

  3. Use preanesthetic tranquilization

    a. Ketamine or Telazol

      (1) Parakeets: 1 mg/30 g IM

      (2) Small birds: 5 mg/kg IM

      (3) Pigeons: 25 mg/kg IM

    b. Droperidol: fentanyl citrate

      (1) Parakeets: 0.1 mg: 0.0002 mg IM

    c. Metomidate IM

      (1) Parakeets 5 mg/kg IM

    d. Phenothiazines are, for the most part, ineffective

E. Obtain precise body weight

  1. Gram scale

  2. Very important when calculating dosages of injectable drugs

III. Avian respiratory system and anesthetic consideration

A. Anatomy

  1. Upper respiratory tract

    a. External nares are situated at the dorsal base of the beak/bill

    b. Median choana is a slit on the roof of the pharynx through the center of soft palate, communicating with the nasal cavity

    c. Larynx is at the base of the tongue

      (1) Is easily visualized

      (2) Small stiff ring or slit

      (3) Is easily intubated

    d. Trachea

      (1) Calcified rings, usually complete

      (2) May be partially telescoped in some psittacines

      (3) May be serpentine in geese and swans

      (4) Lies to the left of the esophagus, as does the crop (when present)

    e. Syrinx—vocal organ

      (1) Cranial to trachea bifurcation

      (2) May be osseous in ducks and geese

      (3) Narrowest part in most birds

  2. Lower respiratory tract

    a. Bronchi cartilaginous semi-rings

      (1) Primary bronchus or mesobronchus enters lung craniomedially

      (2) Exits lung caudolaterally

    b. Secondary bronchi stem from primary bronchi

    c. Tertiary bronchi or parabronchi

      (1) Form dorsal and ventral parabronchial arcades

      (2) Visible on lung surface

       (3) Arcades from more distal parabronchi anastomose with proximal secondary bronchi

    d. Terminal part of mesobronchus

       (1) Connects directly with abdominal air sac

3. Lungs

    a. Small, relatively inelastic, and fixed in place by ribs 2-8

    b. Parabronchial arcades grossly seen on surface

    c. Each parabronchus gives rise to many microscopic air capillaries lying in close apposition to blood capillaries

    d. Air capillaries are respiratory exchange units

4. Diaphragm

    a. Incomplete, two membraneous parts

    b. Horizontal part—nonfunctional

    c. Oblique septum—may have some function

    d. Entering the abdomen = entering the thorax

5. Air sacs

    a. Cervical (paired)

    b. Cranial thoracic (paired)

    c. Caudal thoracic (paired)

    d. Caudal abdominal (paired)

    e. Clavicular (unpaired) with diverticula

    f. All but the cervical air sac have two or more communications with the lung

    g. All but the caudal thoracic air sac communicate with one or more pneumatic bones

    h. Entering pneumatic bones = entering the lung

    i. Air sac capacity is four to six times greater than the lung capacity

B. Physiology

1. Ventilation mechanics

    a. Both inspiration and expiration are dependent on active muscle contraction

    b. On inspiration, the sternal movement results in negative thoracoabdominal pressure, thereby drawing air into the caudalmost air sacs by a bellowslike action

    c. Expiration is a result of active compression of the thoracoabdominal air sacs

    d. Passive movement of the lungs by the ribs is essential to change the lung volume

       (1) If lungs are disconnected from ribs, bird will suffocate

2. Air flow

    a. Inspiration

       (1) Air enters mesobronchi, parabronchi, and air sacs

    b. Expiration

       (1) Air returns from air sacs through lungs

       (2) No stagnation period

    c. Air moves almost continually and unidirectionally

    3. Air sac function
      a. Air reservoirs for bellows ventilation
        (1) Up to six times the lung volume
      b. Surfaces for evaporating, cooling
        (1) Increase in temperature = increase in respiratory rate
        (2) Decrease in temperature = decrease in respiratory rate
      c. Surfaces for limited gas exchange
    4. Anesthetic considerations
      a. Positioning and restraint
        (1) Bird must be able to freely move sternum
      b. Abdominal surgery
        (1) Positive-pressure ventilation is required since diaphragm is incomplete
      c. Tidal volume
        (1) Is usually larger than in mammals of comparable size
        (2) 15 ml/kg (0.015 ml/g)
      d. Anesthetic gas concentrations
        (1) Fast induction
        (2) Fast recovery
        (3) Induction and recovery are more rapid than in mammals since gas exchange occurs during both inspiration and expiration
      e. Air sac rupture is possible with overinflation
      f. Cannulation of the clavicular air sac is possible
        (1) To administer volatile anesthetics
        (2) To provide ventilation

IV. Contraindications to anesthesia
  A. Shock
  B. Ascites
  C. Severe anemia
  D. Respiratory distress
  E. Fluid-filled crop
  F. Severe emaciation
  G. Dehydration
  H. Acidosis

V. Choice of anesthetic (listed in order of decreasing safety)
  A. Isoflurane
  B. Telazol IM
  C. Ketamine and xylazine IV
  D. Ketamine and xylazine IM
  E. Halothane
  F. Methoxyflurane

VI. Parenteral agents
  A. These agents are contraindicated in kidney disease, which is often manifested by anuria
  B. Use a minimal dose (one eighth to one quarter of the calculated dose)

C. Repeat the minimal dose until the desired plane of anesthesia is reached
D. When determining the dose, consider the following
   1. Species of the bird
   2. Age
   3. Weight
   4. Amount of body fat
   5. Condition of bird
   6. Procedure
E. Intramuscular administration
   1. Administer in pectoralis muscle
   2. Avoid the large vessels near the sternum
   3. Avoid the leg muscles
      a. Possibility of nerve damage
      b. First-pass effect due to the renal portal system
F. Intraperitoneal administration
   1. Should be avoided due to variability in absorption rates

VII. Ketamine-xylazine combination
A. The most common parenteral drug combination
B. Drug concentrations
   1. Ketamine 100 mg/ml (see Tables 23-1, 23-2)
   2. Xylazine 20 mg/ml (see Table 23-3)
      a. Xylazine is drawn up first
      b. Maximum doses in milliliters/bird
   3. Ketamine IM dosage for 45 minutes—minor surgical procedures
      a. Birds > 250 g: 10 mg/kg
      b. Birds < 250 g: 30 mg/kg
   4. Ketamine IV dosage
      a. Use an initial injection of one eighth to one quarter of calculated IM dose
      b. Repeat injection in 5-10 minutes if a deeper plane of anesthesia is required
C. Anesthetic effects
   1. Good muscle relaxation
   2. Good analgesia
   3. Relatively smooth recovery
   4. Xylazine eliminates many of the problems associated with the use of ketamine alone

VIII. Telazol
A. Alternative to xylazine-ketamine
B. 1:1 mixture of tiletamine-zolazepam
C. Dose is highly variable, ranging from 4.0 to 25.0 mg/kg IM
   1. Larger birds require lower dosages
      a. Mallard: 5-10 mg/kg IM
      b. Parakeet: 15-20 mg/kg IM

IX. Inhalation agent

TABLE 23 - 1

DOSAGES OF CHEMICAL RESTRAINING DRUGS NECESSARY TO PRODUCE SEDATION IN VARIOUS EXOTIC ANIMALS

Species	Ketamine	Fentanyl-droperidol (Innovar-Vet)	Pentobarbital	Xylazine	Chloral hydrate–pentobarbital (Equithesin)
Primates	10-20 mg/lb IM	0.01 ml/lb IM	1-2 mg/lb IM	0.5 mg/lb IM	
Skunk	5 mg/lb IM	0.05 ml/lb IM	3-5 mg/lb IM	1 mg/lb IM	
Raccoon	5 mg/lb IM	0.05 ml/lb IM	3-5 mg/lb IM	1 mg/lb IM	
Ferret	5 mg/lb IM	0.05 ml/lb IM	3-5 mg/lb IM	1 mg/lb IM	
Rabbit	10 mg/lb IM	0.08 ml/lb IM	2-3 mg/lb IM	1-2 mg/lb IM	
Guinea pig	10 mg/lb IM	0.02 ml/lb IM	0.01 mg/g IP	3 mg/lb IM	
Rat	10 mg/lb IM	0.05 ml/lb IM	0.01 mg/g IP	3 mg/lb IM	
Mouse	10 mg/lb IM	0.005 ml/lb IM	0.01 mg/g IP	3 mg/lb IM	
Gerbil, hamster	10 mg/lb IM		0.01 mg/g IP		
Birds:					
Parakeet	0.05-0.1 mg/g IM		0.1-0.3 mg/g IM	5-25 mg/lb IM produces apathy	0.5 ml/lb IM produces sedation in most birds (1.0 ml/lb IM produces anesthesia)
Parrot	0.05-0.1 mg/g IM				
Pigeon	0.01-0.05 mg/g IM				
Chicken	0.01-0.03 mg/g IM				
Duck	0.01-0.03 mg/g IM				
Snake	10-25 mg/lb IM		5-10 mg/lb IP		
			3-4 mg/lb IM		
Lizard	10-25 mg/lb IM		3-4 mg/lb IM		
Turtle	25-50 mg/lb IM		3-5 mg/lb IM		

DOSAGES OF CHEMICAL RESTRAINING DRUGS NECESSARY TO PRODUCE ANESTHESIA IN VARIOUS EXOTIC SPECIES

Species	Ketamine	Fentanyl-droperidol (Innovar-Vet)	Pentobarbital	Xylazine	Telazol
Primates	5-10 mg/lb IM	0.04 ml/lb IM	9-13 mg/lb IV —	0.5-1.0 mg/lb IM	2-15 mg/lb IM
Exotic cats	5-20mg/lb IM	0.05 ml/lb IM			5-15 mg/lb IM
Skunk	15 mg/lb IM	0.1 mg/lb IM	15-20 mg/lb IP		5-15 mg/lb IM
Raccoon	15 mg/lb IM	0.1 ml/lb IM	15-20 mg/lb IP		
Ferret	15 mg/lb IM	0.1 ml/lb IM	15-20 mg/lb IP		5-15 mg/lb IM
Rabbit	20 mg/lb IM	0.1 ml/lb IM	8-10 mg/lb IM		10-20 mg/lb IM
Guinea pig	20 mg/lb IM	0.06 ml/lb IM	0.03-0.05 mg/g IP		20-30 mg/lb IM
Rat	20 mg/lb IM	0.09 ml/lb IM	0.03-0.05 mg/g IP		10-20 mg/lb IM
Mouse	20 mg/lb IM	0.001 ml/lb IM	0.03-0.05 mg/g IP		
Gerbil, hamster	20 mg/lb IM		0.03-0.05 mg/g IP		20-30 mg/lb IM
Squirrel					2-10 mg/lb IM
Birds:					
Parakeet	0.1-0.2 mg/g IM		0.3-0.5 mg/g IM produces anesthesia of 30 minutes duration	50-75 mg/lb IM produces sleep of 15-30 minutes duration	10-20 ml/lb IM
Parrot	0.1-0.2 mg/g IM				15-30 mg/lb IM
Pigeon	0.02-0.1 mg/g IM				
Chicken	0.02-0.05 mg/g IM				
Duck	0.02-0.05 mg/g IM				
Snake	25-50 mg/lb IM (1-3 day recovery)		10-15 mg/lb IP,IM		5-20 mg/lb IM
Lizard	25-50 mg/lb IM		10-15 mg/lb IP,IM		5-15 mg/lb IM
Turtle	25-50 mg/lb IM		6-10 mg/lb IP,IM		2-10 mg/lb IM

TABLE 23-3

MAXIMUM DOSES OF XYLAZINE FOR USE WITH BIRDS

Species	IM	IV
Budgerigar	0.01	0.005
Cockatiel	0.02	0.010
Amazon	0.05	0.025
Cockatoo	0.15	0.06
Raptors:		
Kestrel, saw-whet owl	0.03	
Goshawk	0.05	
Great grey owl	0.10	
Bald eagle	0.15	
Gyrfalcon	0.15	
Turkey vulture	0.15	

A. Delivery
 1. Mask
 2. Endotracheal tube
    a. Pediatric tube
    b. Urinary catheter
    c. Feeding tube
    d. Polyethylene tubing
 3. Trocar placed into air sac
B. Precautions
 1. Eliminate as much dead space as possible since the tidal volumes are small
 2. Do not kink tubes
C. Isoflurane
 1. Inhalation agent of choice
 2. Advantages
    a. Lack of toxic preservatives
    b. Minimal effect on liver function
    c. Minimal effect on kidney function
    d. Respiratory depression is partially antagonized by surgical stimulation
 3. Clinical concentrations
    a. Induction: 3-5% with 2-3 L oxygen flow
    b. Maintenance is species-dependent, ranging from 0.5 to 3% with O_2 flow from 0.5 to 2.0 L/min
D. Halothane
 1. Next safest inhalation agent
 2. Disadvantages
    a. Contraindicated during systemic disease
    b. Sensitization of the heart to arrythmias

TABLE 23-4

LEVELS OF NARCOSIS AND ANESTHESIA IN BIRDS

Type	Light	Medium	Deep
Narcosis	Sedate Lethargic Eyelids droop	Feathers ruffled Head hangs down Arousable, does not resist handling	Rapid, regular respirations Deep respiration No response to sound
Anesthesia	Palpebral and corneal reflexes present. Lack of voluntary movement No response to postural changes or vibration	Palpebral reflex absent Corneal reflex sluggish Slow, deep, regular respirations (best level for surgery)	All reflexes absent Too deep, emergency pending

     c. Brief interval between apnea and cardiac arrest, making precise monitoring extremely important

  3. Clinical concentrations

     a. Induction: 3-4%

     b. Maintenance: 1.5-2%, 0.5% with nitrous oxide

  E. Methoxyflurane

    1. Concerns

     a. Highly metabolized by the body, leading to a high potential for organ toxicity (e.g., liver toxicity)

     b. Prolonged, sluggish recoveries

  F. Ether

    1. Safe anesthetic in proper doses

    2. Flammability limits use

X. Monitoring during anesthesia

  A. One person should devote full attention to monitoring and have no other assigned duties

  B. Parameters to be monitored

    1. Respiratory rate and depth

    2. Heart rate (ECG and auscultation)

    3. Cloacal temperature

    4. Level of narcosis and anesthesia (Table 23-4)

XI. Anesthetic emergencies

  A. Clinical signs

    1. Heart rate < 120 beats/min

    2. Respirations < 25/min in large birds

             < 35/min in small birds

3. Loss of all reflexes
  B. Treatment
    1. Turn off the anesthetic, and flush the system
    2. Administer 100% oxygen
    3. Begin CPR with digital pressure on the ventral carina 60 times/min
    4. Administer doxapram 5-10 mg/kg IV or IM
    5. IV fluids
    6. Administer epinephrine for cardiac arrest (5-10 μg/kg)
XII. Recovery from anesthesia
  A. Provide 85-90° F environment
  B. Wrap the bird in a newspaper or large towel
    1. Discourage thrashing or excitement
  C. Recovery time
    1. From isoflurane, 10 min
    2. From halothane, 20 min
    3. From average doses of ketamine/xylazine, 45 minutes to 3 hours
  D. Water, food, toys, and perches should be removed from the cage until the bird is recovered

FISH

  I. Indications
    A. Tagging
    B. Fin clipping
    C. Measuring and stripping eggs
    D. Stripping milt (milk of fish)
    E. Transporting
      1. From rearing to fattening units
      2. To new streams or lakes
      3. To laboratories
        a. To decrease stress
        b. To prevent injury by jumping out of the tank
        c. To allow more fish to be maintained in a smaller volume of water
    F. Physical examination
    G. Surgical procedures
      1. Enucleation
      2. Removal of skin growths
      3. Removal of skin parasites
      4. Clipping fins to mark fish
    H. Handling dangerous fish
      1. Piranhas
      2. Electric eels
      3. Lionfish
      4. Stingrays
    I. Intensification of color by dispersing chromatophores
  II. Restraint is limited because of:
    A. Shape of fish

TABLE 23-5

STAGES OF ANESTHESIA IN FISH

Stage O	Excitement, fright, finning, and increased opercular movement
Stage I	
Phase 1	Fright, change in color
Phase 2	Visual response absent
Stage II	
Phase 1	Loss of balance, distress; color darkens
Phase 2	Complete loss of equilibrium and swimming movements; may be upside down
Stage III	Respirations very slow; no response to stimuli; opercula spread
Stage IV	Medullary collapse; respiratory and cardiac functions cease

   B. Mucolaginous covering
   C. Muscular activity
 III. Monitoring of anesthesia
   A. Behavioral patterns are similar to those of mammals (see Table 23-5)
   B. Factors affecting stages of anesthesia
     1. Size and species of fish
     2. Dose or concentration of anesthetic agent
     3. Quality of water
 IV. Anesthetic procedures
   A. Immersing in a bath containing anesthetic drugs is the most common
   B. Parenteral injections require preanesthesia by bath
     1. Intramuscular
     2. Intravenous
     3. Intraperitoneal
     4. Intracranial
   C. Stunning (hitting the fish over the head) is poor anesthetic practice
  V. Anesthetic agents (Table 23-6)

TABLE 23-6

DOSAGES OF CHEMICAL RESTRAINING AGENTS FOR FISH

Method/drug	Dose	Approximate duration of action
Carbonated H_2O	1:1	5-10 min
Diethyl ether	10-15 ml/L H_2O	15 min
Chloral hydrate	0.8-1.0 gm/L H_2O	15 min
MS-222 (Finquel)	50-100 mg/L H_2O	15 min

Notes: 1. Activity is related to H_2O temperature.
    2. Fast for 24 hours prior to procedure.
    3. Remove fish from anesthetic containing H_2O shortly after all movement stops.
    4. Use boiled aquarium H_2O as diluent.

A. Carbon dioxide (CO_2)
   1. Produces anesthesia at 200 ppm in water
      a. Induction time: 1-2 minutes
      b. Recovery time: 5-10 minutes
   2. Methods of making CO_2 solutions
      a. Club soda and water (1:1 ratio)
      b. Two or three Alka-Seltzer tablets added to 12 oz (360 ml) water
      c. Balanced solution of dissolved sodium bicarbonate and diluted sulfuric acid
         (1) Any of the three solutions can be neutralized with sodium carbonate if the fish becomes hypoxic
B. Chloral hydrate
   1. Sedation is produced at 0.8-0.9 g per liter of water
   2. Induction time: 8-10 minutes (slow)
      Recovery time: 20-30 minutes
C. Diethyl ether
   1. 10-15 ml per liter of water
   2. Induction time: 2-3 minutes
   3. Disadvantages
      a. Highly volatile
      b. Highly flammable
      c. Highly irritative at larger doses (e.g., 40-50 ml/L)
D. Tricaine methanesulfonate (Finquel, MS-222)
   1. Most widely used fish anesthetic
   2. Sedative dose: 25-35 mg per liter of water
      a. Transport fish in moss and chipped ice
      b. Mortality is approximately 10% after 4 hours of anesthesia
   3. Anesthetic dose: 50-100 mg per liter of water
      a. Induction time: 1-3 minutes
      b. Maintenance: provides excellent anesthesia for up to 4 hours
      c. Recovery: 3-15 minutes
   4. Precautions
      a. MS-222 is an acid and can be neutralized before fish are added
      b. Neutralization decreases induction and recovery time
      c. Side effects
         (1) Toxic when used in salt water
         (2) Toxic when used in sunlight
         (3) Major disadvantage is its cost
E. Urethane
   1. Wide margin of safety between effective and lethal doses
   2. Anesthetic dose: 5-40 mg per liter of water
      a. Induction time: 2-3 minutes
      b. Recovery time: 10-15 minutes
   3. Urethane was once a popular choice for fish anesthesia
      a. It has been proven to be a carcinogenic and leukopenic agent in man
         (1) Neither of these effects has been documented in fish

F. Alternative anesthetic agents
  1. Halothane
    a. 40 ppm per liter of water
    b. 1-3 minutes of induction
    c. Good maintenance
    d. 3-15 minutes of recovery
  2. Benzocaine
    a. 25-100 mg per liter of water
    b. 1-3 minutes of induction
    c. Excellent maintenance
    d. 3-15 minutes of recovery
  3. Saffan
    a. 24 mg/kg
    b. 1-5 minutes of induction
    c. Excellent maintenance
  4. Quinaldine (Kodak)
VI. Treatment of anesthetic overdose
  A. Place fish in pure water
  B. Increase water flow over the gills to enhance oxygen exchange and anesthetic elimination
    1. If respiratory movements do not spontaneously return in 1-2 minutes
      a. Pull fish back and forth through the water
      b. Put fish under stream of running water
  C. Thoracic massage may be attempted

ANESTHESIA IN REPTILES AND AMPHIBIANS

I. Indications
  A. Surgery
  B. Immobilization
    1. Diagnostic procedures
    2. Therapeutic
  C. Sedation for shipping
II. Forms of anesthesia
  A. Topical or local anesthesia
  B. Hypothermia
  C. Electroanesthesia
  D. Immersion in solutions with anesthetic
  E. Injectable anesthetics
  F. Inhalation
III. Topical or local anesthetics
  A. Require physical restraint for administration
  B. Effective anesthesia for small species
    1. Lidocaine, 1-2% with or without epinephrine
IV. Hypothermia
  A. Refrigeration at 5° C up to 2 hours
  B. Immersion in ice water

   1. Use a shallow tray of ice water

   2. Best supplemented with a local anesthetic

  C. Not unusually recommended, due to secondary tissue damage and questionable analgesia

V. Electroanesthesia

  A. Technique

   1. Bitemporal electrodes

   2. Low- and high-frequency sine waves

    a. As the interval between pulses decreases (cycle per second) and current (mA) increases, induction becomes rapid

  B. Respiratory arrest nearly always occurs

   1. Animal must be ventilated

  C. Recovery is immediate on cessation of current

VI. Immersion in a solution containing anesthetic agent

  A. Immerse until desired level of sedation is achieved

  B. Tricaine methanesulfonate (Finquel, MS-222) is used

   1. Induction time: 5 minutes

   2. Recovery time: 15-30 minutes

   3. 0.1-0.5% is the anesthetic of choice for amphibians

VII. Injectable anesthetics (see Tables 23-1, 23-2)

  A. Absorption and excretion of anesthetic drugs are directly affected by environmental temperature

   1. Ectothermic or poikilothermic animals don't want environments too cold or too hot

   2. Ideal environmental temperature is 75-90° F

   3. Ideal humidity is 40-60%

  B. Route of administration

   1. Intravenous

    a. Turtles

     (1) Inject into ventral abdominal vein after drilling through plastron

    b. Crocodilians

     (1) Caudal vein

     (2) In hemocanal in ventral spinous processes of the coccygeal vertebrae

    c. Snakes

     (1) Large central abdominal vein

     (2) Buccal vein

   2. Intraperitoneal

    a. Snakes

     (1) In midsection of pleuroperitoneal cavity, anterior to cloaca (10% of body length), off to one side of midline

    b. Crocodilians

     (1) In mesogastric area

   3. Intramuscular

    a. Snakes

        (1) In longitudinal musculature along the dorsum

        (2) Inject small volumes

        (3) At multiple sites

    b. Crocodilians

        (1) In base of the tail

  4. Intracardiac

    a. Difficult technique

    b. Turtles

        (1) For rapid induction

        (2) A long needle is introduced between the neck and forelimb

    c. Alligator

        (1) A needle is introduced on the ventral side caudal to the sternum at the level of the sixth row of scales caudal to the pectoral girdle

        (2) The needle is moved in dorsocranial direction

C. Preferred injectable anesthetics

  1. Ketamine has been used effectively in:

    a. Snakes

    b. Lizards

    c. Small crocodilians

    d. Turtles

        (1) Doses of intramuscular ketamine

           (a) 44 mg/kg is adequate for sedation and minor surgery

           (b) 66-88 mg/kg is necessary for major surgery in most turtle species

           (c) >132 mg/kg requires support with positive respiratory pressure

    e. Ketamine or Telazol appear to be the most satisfactory injectable anesthetics in reptiles

    f. Fatalities in reptiles have been observed

        (1) Prolonged recovery times of up to 6 days

        (2) Permanent aggressivity of many reptiles, particularly snakes, after recovery from ketamine anesthesia

  2. Telazol

    a. Useful in a wide variety of reptiles

        (1) Turtles: 5-10 mg/kg IM

        (2) Snakes: 50-100 mg/kg IM

        (3) Iguana: 10-25 mg/kg IM

    b. Response is similar to ketamine, although there is better relaxation

  3. Saffan

    a. Active Ingredient: alphaxalone (9 mg) and alphadolone acetate (3 mg)/ml, 12 mg total steroid/ml

    b. Dose: 9-18 mg total steroid/kg IM

    c. Effects

        (1) No given effect (if given s.c.) to deep anesthesia (if given in epaxial musculature)

    d. Surgical anesthesia
      (1) Induction time: 25-40 minutes
      (2) Duration: 15-35 minutes
    e. Advantages
      (1) No local reaction at injection site
      (2) Minimal discomfort
      (3) No alteration in behavior
  4. Etorphine HCl (M99)
    a. Intraperitoneal injection may reduce induction time as much as 50% compared with IM injection
    b. Snakes
      (1) Dose (mg) per 7-9 inches of body weight
        (a) 1 mg for snakes < 4 feet long
        (b) 0.5 mg for snakes > 4 feet long
      (2) Induction time: 10-30 minutes
      (3) Duration of anesthesia: 3 hours
    c. Turtles
      (1) 0.25-1.25 mg/kg
      (2) Duration of anesthesia: 45-100 minutes
    d. Crocodilians
      (1) 0.05-2.0 mg total dose
      (2) Anesthesia time: 60 minutes
      (3) Subcutaneous injection of etorphine in alligators is ineffective
  5. Other injectable drugs (IP, IV, or IC) that provide 6-7 hours of anesthesia or restraint in reptiles are:
    a. Phencyclidine 2.5-5 mg/kg
    b. Telazol 35 mg/kg
    c. Succinylcholine 0.06-1.0 mg/kg IM
VIII. Inhalation agents
  A. Indications
    1. Painful surgical procedures
    2. Prolonged procedures
  B. Techniques
    1. Cotton ball soaked with the volatile anesthetic agent is placed in a box or bag with the patient
    2. Anesthetic machine is attached to the chamber until the patient loses its righting reflex
    3. Face mask
    4. Intubation
      a. The glottis in snakes is easily seen cranially to the floor of the mouth, making intubation easy
      b. The trachea in snakes is mobile, allowing ventilation during ingestion of food
      c. The right lung is responsible for ventilation
      d. Air sacs extend caudally from the right lung

C. Peculiarities in reptiles
1. Can maintain apnea for long periods (e.g., up to $4^{1/2}$ hours in iguanas)
2. Can convert to anaerobic metabolism (e.g., some species of turtles)
3. Low concentrations of volatile agents are required in certain species of snakes
   a. Consult available literature
   b. Use personal experience
4. Oxygen flow rate should be twice the animal's minute volume
   a. 300-500 ml/min in reptiles < 5 kg
   b. A nonrebreathing system is best for maintenance of anesthesia
D. Specific inhalation agents
1. Ether
   a. Induction time: 20-60 minutes
   b. Recovery time: up to 10 hours (e.g., in turtles)
   c. Is explosive (electrocautery is precluded)
2. Methoxyflurane
   a. Induction time: 8-25 minutes (e.g., snakes)
   b. Recovery time is variable
3. Halothane
   a. Induction time (at 3 vol%): 1-30 minutes
   b. Maintenance at 1.5%
      (1) An increased concentration ($> 1.5\%$) is required in poisonous snakes
   c. Recovery time is variable and prolonged
      (1) Up to 7 hours
4. Isoflurane
   a. Induction time (at 3 vol%): 1-15 minutes
   b. Maintenance at 1.5%
   c. Recovery time: up to 3 hours
5. Nitrous oxide
   a. Can be added to anesthetic-O_2 mixtures at 40-72%
6. Chloroform
   a. Used in rattlesnakes prior to removing their venom sacs
IX. Recovery
A. Reptiles and amphibians recovering from any type of anesthesia should be kept in an atmosphere that is:
1. Warm ($85°$ F)
2. Draft-free
3. Oxygen-enriched
B. Warm water baths may be helpful if precautions against drowning are taken

RODENTS

I. Pocket pets
A. Rabbit
B. Guinea pig

    C. Gerbil

    D. Hamster

    E. Ferret

    F. Rat

II. Blood sampling

    A. Cutting a nail bed (guinea pig)

    B. Incising the tail vein (other rodents)

    C. Puncture of the ear vein (rabbit)

III. Injection sites

    A. Intravenous

      1. Dorsal vein of penis (guinea pig, rat)

      2. Saphenous vein (by venous cutdown)

      3. Tail vein (rat and mouse)

        a. Pull tail through piece of cardboard

        b. Tail may be warmed to dilate vein

      4. Lateral tarsal vein (rat)

      5. Sublingual vein (rat under anesthesia)

      6. Ear vein (rabbit)

    B. Intramuscular

      1. Biceps, semitendinosus, semimembranosus

    C. Intraperitoneal

      1. Given off the midline with the animal's foreparts down

IV. Preoperative considerations

    A. Responses to anesthetic drugs are highly variable

    B. Factors affecting responses to anesthesia

      1. Age

      2. Sex

      3. Weight

        a. Cecum of rabbit or guinea pig may be filled with ingestion (causing an inaccurate body weight measurement)

      4. Percentage body fat

      5. Strain and genetic background

      6. General health and nutrition

      7. Time of day

        a. Anesthesia may be prolonged during the afternoon in the nocturnal species since hepatic metabolism is at its lowest point

      8. Type of bedding

        a. Cedar and pine beddings induce hepatic enzymes and therefore decrease anesthetic time

V. Premedication (see Table 23-1)

    A. Atropine

      1. To decrease respiratory tract secretions

      2. To decrease vagal tone

        a. 0.05 mg/kg s.c.

        b. 15 mg/100 g body weight for rats and rabbits since they have serum atropinase

TABLE 23-7

PHYSIOLOGIC DATA IN POCKET PETS

Species	Heart rate	Respiratory rate	Body weight (g)	Tidal volume (ml/kg)
Rabbit	130-330	30-60	2000-6000	4-6
Guinea pig	230-280	40-100	700-1200	2.3-5.3
Gerbil	320-360	80-90	70-100	—
Hamster	250-500	40-130	85-150	0.4-1.4
Mouse	325-780	90-160	20-40	0.09-0.23
Ferret	220-240	30-40	680-1360	—
Rat	250-450	70-115	250-520	0.6-2.0

   B. Acepromazine
      1. 1-2 mg/kg IM
      2. Used with caution in gerbils as it lowers the seizure threshold
         a. 50% of gerbils exhibit spontaneous epileptiform seizures
   C. Chlorpromazine
      1. 3-5 mg/kg IV
      2. 3-35 mg/kg IM
         a. May cause myositis
         b. Prolongs barbiturate anesthesia
      3. Same precaution as observed with acepromazine when used in gerbils
VI. Anesthesia (see Table 23-2)
   A. Induction
      1. Chamber
      2. Face mask
      3. Nose cone
      4. Injection
   B. Controlling the depth of anesthesia
      1. Taking off or putting on the nose cone or mask
   C. Monitoring
      1. Respiratory rate (see Table 23-7)
      2. Heart rate (ECG) (see Table 23-7)
      3. Mucous membrane color
      4. Loss of reflexes
         a. Tail jerk
         b. Toe pinch
         c. Corneal
         d. Pedal
            (1) This reflex in guinea pigs may give a false impression of waking up when more anesthesia may kill the animal
   D. Intubation
      1. Is difficult but possible with practice
         a. Small mouth

b. Large teeth
c. Large tongue, hiding larynx
d. Small glottis
   (1) Smaller in diameter than the trachea
   (2) Angled anteriorly so that glottis is not seen
2. Size of tubes
   a. 2 mm for guinea pigs
   b. 1-4.5 mm for other rodents
3. Technique for intubation
   a. After mask induction
   b. Upper incisors should be fixed to keep the trachea straight
   c. Tracheal tube
      (1) Made from polyethylene tubing
      (2) Metal stylet; may be made from a paper clip
   d. Laryngoscope must be inserted to the side of the incisors
   e. The tongue must be pulled ventrally and kept on the midline
   f. The tube tip is placed on the epiglottis to see the glottis
   g. The tube is placed blindly during inspiration when the vocal folds abduct
   h. Some rodents cough when the tube is correctly placed
4. Complications from manipulating the laryngoscope
   a. Pharyngeal edema
   b. Pharyngeal bleeding
E. Gas flow rates
   1. 300 ml/min for induction chamber
   2. 200 ml/min for face mask
   3. 20-100 ml/min for surgical plane of intubated rodents
F. Inhalation agents
   1. Ether
      a. Advantages
         (1) Cheap, therefore the most frequently used anesthetic in laboratory rats
         (2) Easy to use
         (3) Dose is not related to body weight
         (4) Good muscle relaxation
      b. Disadvantages
         (1) Flammable
         (2) Explosive
         (3) May cause excessive salivation
         (4) May cause pulmonary irritation, predisposing to respiratory infection
         (5) May inhibit hypothalamic function
         (6) May affect the liver
   2. Methoxyflurane
   3. Halothane

4. Isoflurane
5. Nitrous oxide and oxygen (1:1 ratio) at 100 ml/min
   a. Induction: May be used with any of the inhalation agents
   b. Maintenance: May be used with any of the inhalation agents
G. Hypnosis for minor procedures in rabbits (e.g., radiography)

VII. Rabbit (and related lagomorphs)
A. Injectables
   1. There is considerable variability to injectable anesthetics
   2. Ketamine, 50-55 mg/kg IM is used for restraint and can be used with:
      a. 15 mg promazine
      b. 2 mg acepromazine
      c. 2-5 mg/kg xylazine, in addition to above combination
         (1) Provides improved surgical anesthesia for 10-20 minutes
         (2) No movement in response to surgical stimuli
   3. Innovar-Vet, 0.13-0.22 mg/kg IM for premedication or light neurolep-
      tanalgesia
   4. Telazol 5-10 mg/kg IM

VIII. Guinea pig
A. Preparation
   1. Should be fasted for 6-12 hours
      a. To prevent vomiting
      b. To prevent dose miscalculation
B. Anesthetics
   1. Ketamine, 20-40 mg/kg IM
      a. With acepromazine, 2 mg/kg
      b. With xylazine, 5 mg/kg
         (1) Reduces heart rate, cardiac output, and mean arterial blood
             pressure for $2^1/2$ hours
   2. Ketaset Plus (Bristol) 125 mg/kg IM
      a. Ingredients
         (1) Ketamine (100 mg/kg)
         (2) Promazine (7.5 mg/ml)
         (3) Aminopentamide (0.0625 mg/ml)
      b. Pharmacologic effects
         (1) Somatic analgesia
         (2) Muscle relaxation
         (3) Decreased salivation
         (4) Coughing and swallowing are retained but suppressed
   3. Sodium pentobarbital (1% solution)
      a. May be injected at 28-35 mg/kg IM to provide surgical anesthesia
         for $1/2$-$1^1/2$ hours
      b. With chlorpromazine 25 mg/kg IM, anesthesia is prolonged to $2^1/2$
         hours

IX. Gerbil
A. Pentobarbital, 6% solution

    1. 0.01 ml per 10 g s.c. at the scruff of the neck or IP to induce surgical anesthesia for 30-45 minutes

    2. Ceiling dose: 6 mg

    3. Hypothermia is a major concern

  B. Ketamine

    1. 44 mg/kg IM

    2. Used as an induction agent for methoxyflurane (0.5 ml in a nose cone)

  C. Diazepam

    1. 10 mg/kg IP; can be substituted for ketamine

      a. Is of particular value since epilepsy is apparently hereditary in gerbils

  D. Telazol

    1. 15-20 mg/kg IM can be used as an alternative to ketamine

X. Hamsters

  A. Is probably the most popular pocket pet

  B. Surgical procedures

    1. Drain absess

    2. Remove neoplasms

    3. Repair hernia

  C. Popular anesthetics

    1. Pentobarbital, 6% solution IP just lateral to the umbilicus

      a. 0.01 ml/10 g of body weight

      b. Induction of anesthesia: 5 minutes

      c. Duration of anesthesia: 30 minutes

  D. Other injectable combinations

    1. Ketamine, 80 mg/kg and xylazine, 5 mg/kg IM

    2. Innovar-Vet, 0.15 ml/100 g IM

      a. Induction of anesthesia: 6 minutes

      b. Duration of anesthesia: 60 minutes

    3. Telazol 15-20 mg/kg IM

XI. Mouse

  A. Is the smallest of the pocket pets

  B. Hypothermia is a concern

  C. Popular anesthetics

    1. Pentobarbital, 6% solution, IP at 90 mg/kg

      a. Males and thin mice are more sensitive to the drug

  D. Other injectable combinations

    1. Ketamine, 50 mg/kg and xylazine, 50 mg/kg IM

      a. Induction time: 5 minutes

      b. Duration of anesthesia: 60-100 minutes

    2. Innovar-Vet (diluted in saline)

      a. Dose: 0.02 ml per 100 g

      b. Duration of anesthesia: 30-60 minutes

    3. Telazol

      a. 20-30 mg/kg IM

XII. Ferret
  A. Indications for anesthesia
    1. Neutering
    2. Descenting
  B. Intramuscular drug combinations
    1. Ketamine, 26 mg/kg and acepromazine, 1.1 mg/kg
    2. Ketamine, 25 mg/kg and xylazine, 2 mg/kg
      a. Surgical anesthesia: 30 minutes
        (1) Ketamine alone at 20-30 mg/kg is useful for restraint
        (2) Ketamine even at 60 mg/kg IM may be inadequate for surgical anesthesia
    3. Telazol 20-30 mg/kg IM
XIII. Rat
  A. Injectables
    1. Pentobarbital
      a. Dose: 10-20 mg/kg IP in young rats
             30-50 mg/kg IP in older rats
      b. LD_{50} is 60 mg/kg
        (1) Young rats, females, albinos, and cold rats are more susceptible
        (2) Males, rats on low-calorie diets, and rats on cedar bedding are less susceptible
      c. Induction time: 5-20 minutes
         Duration of surgical anesthesia: $1/4$-1 hour
      d. Side effects
        (1) Poor analgesia
        (2) Decreased blood pressure
        (3) Decreased cerebral blood flow
        (4) Respiratory depression
      e. Peculiarity: Rats cannot vomit, so there is no need to worry about aspiration of stomach contents
    2. Ketamine
      a. Does not work well in rats
      b. Can accelerate stress-induced ulcers
  B. Other injectable combinations
    1. Fentanyl-droperidol (Innovar-Vet), 0.2 ml/kg IM
      a. Neuroleptanalgesia for $1/2$-1 hour
    2. Fentanyl (0.315 mg)–fluanisone (10 mg) per ml solution (Hypnorm), 0.3 ml/kg IM
      a. Neuroleptanalgesia for $1/2$-$3/4$ hour
      b. Side effects
        (1) Bradycardia
        (2) Prolonged recovery
        (3) Poor muscle relaxation
    3. Neuroleptanalgesia in combination with diazepam 2.5 ml/kg induces increased tolerance to postoperative pain

4. Midazolam (1.25 mg/ml)–fluanisone (2.5 mg/ml)–fentanyl (0.79 mg/ml)
   a. Mixture can be given IP
   b. Two parts water: one part Hypnorm: one part midazolam induces neuroleptanalgesia for 2 hours
   c. Naloxone, 0.1 mg/kg IP or IV may be used to reverse the respiratory depression
5. Telazol 20-30 mg/kg IM

EXOTIC CATS

I. Prerestraint considerations
  A. Patient data
    1. Species
    2. Physical condition
      a. Depressed
      b. Age
      c. Sex
      d. Gestation, lactation
      e. Excitability
        (1) High catecholamine release may override effects
        (2) Running during capture causes acidosis
    3. Accurate body weight may be difficult to obtain
  B. Types of restraint
    1. Physical (manual)—animals less than 35 pounds
    2. Snare
    3. Net
    4. Shield
    5. Squeeze cage
    6. Chemical
      a. Allows restraint for limited period of time
      b. Safer for handler
      c. Less stressful for patient
II. Delivery methods for chemical restraint
  A. Oral
    1. Difficult administration (confinement necessary)
    2. Some drugs not absorbed through digestive tract (mucous membranes)
  B. Hand-held syringe
    1. Animal must be confined and restrained
    2. Wait for animal to present suitable muscle area to side of cage
    3. Use large-gauge needle for faster injection
    4. Preferable to use locking hub on needle
  C. Pole syringe
    1. Allows injection from distance
    2. Must maintain contact with animal until all drug is injected
  D. Syringe or dart for long-range projection
    1. Blowgun

a. Advantages
(1) Silent projection
(2) Less trauma on impact
(3) No parts requiring maintenance
(4) Inexpensive
b. Disadvantage
(1) Limited range of fire (15 meters)
E. Firearms
1. Short-range pistol (CO_2-powered); range 15 meters
2. Long-range rifle (CO_2-powered); range 35 meters
3. Extra-long-range rifle (percussion cap–powered); maximum range 80 meters
a. Advantage
(1) Extended range
b. Disadvantage
(1) Noisy
(2) Patient trauma at injection site
III. Problems associated with various restraint methods
A. Equipment failure
1. Needle breaks on impact
2. Not enough breath to work blowgun
3. Plugs in end of needle; side injection eliminates this
4. Faulty CO_2 cartridges in dart guns, making propelling charge insufficient
B. Operator failure
1. Inaccurate impact
a. Needle must be perpendicular to skin
b. Weak propelling charge—needle doesn't penetrate skin
2. Excessive impact force—syringe blown through leg
3. Drug leaks out at injection site because needle hole is too large
4. Needle too small
a. Dart falls out before all drug is injected
b. Syringe bounces out because of force of injection
C. Patient complications
1. Infection develops at injection site
2. Injury during fall
3. Only partial sedation
4. Adverse drug reactions
IV. Chemical restraint (see Tables 23-1, 23-2)
A. Utility of agent based on:
1. Drugs that can be given by IM injection
2. Drugs with high therapeutic index (effective dose/lethal dose range)
3. Short induction period desirable (10-20 minutes)
4. Effective dose (volume) small enough for use in darts
5. Reversibility

CHAPTER TWENTY-FOUR

Fluid Administration During Anesthesia

"One can drink too much, but one never drinks enough."
GOTTHOLD EPHRAIM LESSING

OVERVIEW

Fluid and blood replacement therapy are vital adjuncts to any anesthetic plan. Their use is extremely important during prolonged surgical and anesthetic procedures when hemorrhage is excessive or if the patient is debilitated or shocky. Almost all drugs used to produce chemical restraint and anesthesia decrease the force of cardiac contraction and relax blood vessels, thereby increasing vascular volume. The net effect of these actions can lead to a decrease in cardiac output (blood flow) and arterial blood pressure. The routine administration of maintenance fluids during anesthesia is indicated in order to replace insensible losses during prolonged surgical anesthetic procedures, maintain an adequate and effective circulating blood volume, and maintain near-normal cardiac output. Blood loss must be replaced with at least two to three times the amount of isotonic fluids, since most fluids do not contain protein and will distribute throughout the extracellular fluid space, which is approximately three times the vascular volume. When blood loss is excessive, it should be replaced with blood on a one-to-one basis.

GENERAL CONSIDERATIONS

I. Anesthesia, surgery, and many of the diseases for which surgical intervention is required interfere with water, electrolyte, and acid-base balance and decrease the effective circulating blood volume

A. Diseases producing changes in fluid, electrolyte, and acid-base balance (see Table 24-1)
B. Imbalances due to anesthesia
   1. Most inhalation and intravenous anesthetic agents:
      a. Depress myocardial contractility; cardiac output is decreased and metabolic acidosis may ensue
      b. Induce generalized vasodilatation; relative hypovolemia and hypotension may result
      c. Depress minute ventilation; respiratory acidosis may occur
   2. The sympathoadrenal response to hypercapnia and decreased effective circulating blood volume is usually depressed under general anesthesia
C. Imbalances due to surgical procedure
   1. Blood loss
   2. Drying of exposed tissues
   3. Removal of effusions
II. Fluid losses leading to a decrease in effective circulating blood volume usually cause the development of metabolic acidosis
III. Blood loss can be replaced with fluids, providing the hematocrit remains above 20%
IV. Fluid administration to young or small patients should be supplemented with a source of calories (dextrose) and monitored very closely in order to prevent overhydration
V. The administration of large quantities of room-temperature fluids can produce hypothermia
   A. Warm fluids should be administered cautiously with close hemodynamic monitoring in order to prevent the development of hypotension and shock
VI. Fluid administration
   A. Fluid administration sets deliver 10 drops/ml (regular) or 60 drops/ml (mini-drip)
   B. Larger-diameter needles or intravenous catheters offer less resistance to fluid flow and increase the rate of fluid administration
   C. Occasionally, fluids are administered at extremely rapid rates using electrical fluid pumps
   D. Infusion pumps facilitate accurate volumes of fluid delivery (Fig. 24-1)

NORMAL BODY WATER DISTRIBUTION

I. Total body water represents 55-75% (use 60%) of body weight
   A. Primarily dependent on age and body fat
II. Extracellular water constitutes 23-33% (use 30%) of body weight; percentage is greater in very young animals
III. Plasma water constitutes approximately 5% of body weight
IV. Blood volume constitutes 8-10% of body weight, depending on the hematocrit
   A. Blood volume equals plasma water plus red blood cell volume
V. Interstitial water constitutes 15-25% of body weight
VI. Extracellular water equals plasma water plus interstitial water
VII. Intracellular water constitutes 35-45% of body weight

TABLE 24 - 1

COMMON DISEASES AND ASSOCIATED ELECTROLYTE ABNORMALITIES

Disease syndrome	Water	Na$^+$	K$^+$	Ca^{++}	Mg^{++}	HPO$_4^-$	Cl$^-$	HCO$_3^-$
Gastric loss, vomiting	Loss	→	→		→		→	–↑
Pancreatic or intestinal fluid loss	Loss	→→	→		→		→→	→
Diarrhea	Loss		→	→	→		→	→
Starvation	Loss	→	→		→			
Acute hemorrhagic pancreatitis	Loss	–↓	–↓	→	→		→	→
Malabsorption syndrome	Loss			→	→	→		
Acute renal failure (oliguric)	Excess	–↑↓	←	→	→	←	–↑↓	→
Renal tubular dysfunction	Loss	→	–↓					→
Chronic renal disease	Loss	–↓	–↓	–↓	→	–↑	–↓	→
Diabetes insipidus	Loss	←					←	

Burns	Loss	
Primary aldosteronism	Excess	
Stress, surgery, including ADH	Excess	
Hypoadrenocortisolism (Addison's)	Loss	
Hypopituitarism	Excess	
Hyperadrenocortisolism (Cushing's)	Excess	
Excess citrated blood		
Hyperparathyroidism		
Excess lactation (milk fever)		
Acidosis (metabolic)		
Alkalosis (metabolic)		

↑ = increased serum concentration
↓ = decreased serum concentration
— = normal serum concentration

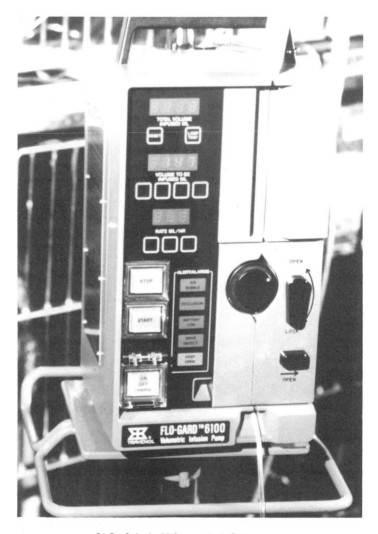

FIG.24-1 Volumetric infusion pump.

ELECTROLYTE DISTRIBUTION

I. Extracellular water contains large quantities of sodium and chloride ions

II. Intracellular water contains large quantities of potassium ions

III. Normal electrolyte composition of serum (Table 24-2)

PRINCIPLES OF FLUID ADMINISTRATION

I. Whenever possible, dehydration and electrolyte and acid-base imbalances should be corrected prior to anesthesia

II. Do not attempt to replace chronic fluid losses acutely

    A. Severe dilution of plasma proteins, blood cells, and electrolytes may be detrimental

TABLE 24-2

NORMAL ELECTROLYTE COMPOSITION OF SERUM

	Na^+	K^+	Ca^{++}	Mg^{++}	HPO_4^-	Cl^-	HCO_3^-
Dog	145-155	4.0-5.4	9.8-12.8	1.8-2.4	2.5-7.3	104-117	18-25
Cat	150-170	3.7-6.0	9.1-12.3	—	2.8-8.7	111-128	18-22
Horse	137-143	3.2-4.5	11.6-13.4	2.2-2.8	1.5-5.1	98-105	23-31
Cow	137-148	3.1-5.1	8.9-11.6	2.2-3.4	4.5-8.2	84-102	23-31

III. When intravenous fluids must be given rapidly (e.g., for shock) special care must be given to renal and cardiac functions
  A. Renal function
    1. Improve or reestablish GFR (renal perfusion) before anesthesia
    2. When hydration has been restored, administer mannitol at 0.5-1 g/lb over 30 minutes
    3. Monitor urine output
  B. Cardiac function
    1. CVP should be monitored if right-sided or biventricular heart failure is suspected (see Chapter 17: Hemodynamic Monitoring)
    2. If possible, pulmonary capillary wedge pressures should be monitored in cases of left-sided heart failure
    3. Careful attention must be given to thoracic auscultation
      a. If the total protein drops below 4 g/dl from fluid administration, there is increased likelihood of pulmonary edema

FLUID ADMINISTRATION DURING ANESTHESIA

  I. Fluids administered during anesthesia are usually polyionic isotonic crystalloid solutions (see Table 24-3)
  II. Rates of administration depending on fluid loss during surgery
   Small animals   5-10 ml/lb/hr
   Large animals   3-5 ml/lb/hr
    A. This rate may be surpassed if significant hypotension develops
    B. Special care must be taken not to produce pulmonary edema
  III. Blood loss should be estimated and 3 ml of crystalloid solution administered for each milliliter of blood loss (unless blood transfusion is indicated) over and above the basic fluid rate provided during anesthesia
  IV. Maximum rate of fluids that can be administered safely in cases of shock therapy is 40 ml/lb/hr

POSTOPERATIVE MAINTENANCE FLUID THERAPY

  I. When continued IV fluid therapy is necessary postoperatively, the normal fluid rates are:
    A. 20-30 ml/lb/24 hr (mature animal)
    B. 30-45 ml/lb/24 hr (young animal)

TABLE 24 - 3

COMPOSITION OF COMMONLY USED FLUIDS

	Tonicity	pH	Calorific value	Na$^+$	K$^+$	Ca^{++}	Mg^{++}	Cl$^-$	Lactate	HCO$_3^-$
Normal saline (0.9% NaCl)	Isotonic	5.0	0	155	0	0	0	155	0	0
2.5% dextrose (0.45% NaCl)	Isotonic	4.5	85	77	0	0	0	77	0	0
5% dextrose	Isotonic	4.0	170	0	0	0	0	0	0	0
Ringer's	Isotonic		0	147	4	5	0	156	0	0
Lactated Ringer's	Isotonic	6.5	9	130	4	3	3	109	28	0
Eltrad			0	140	10	5	3	103	55	0
Mannitol 10% or 20%	Hypertonic		0	0	0	0	0	0	0	0
Whole blood	Isotonic	6.5	150	144	5.3	10	0	103	0	23
THAM*	Hypertonic		0	0	0	0	0	0	0	300

*Contraindicated in anuria and uremia

Notes: Potassium chloride: 20 or 40 mEq/ampule; 50 g/1 gal = isotonic
Sodium bicarbonate: 84 g = 1000 mEq; 50 g/1 gal = isotonic

CLINICAL ASSESSMENT OF HYDRATION

	Minimal (4%)	Moderate (6-8%)	Severe (10-12%)
Skin resiliency	Pliable	Leathery	Absolutely no pliability
Skin tenting	Twist disappears immediately and tent persists up to 2 seconds	Twist disappears immediately and tent persists 3 seconds or more	Twist as well as tent persists indefinitely
Eye	Bright Slightly sunken	Duller than normal Obviously sunken	Cornea dry Deeply sunken, 2-4 mm space between eyeball and bony orbit
Mouth	Moist, warm	Sticky to dry, warm	Dry, cyanotic, warm to cold

I. Calculation of replacement fluid volume in animal suffering from dehydration
   A. Body weight (kg) × % dehydration (expressed as decimal quantity) = fluid deficit (L) (e.g., 20 kg (dog) × 10% dehydration = 2 L fluid deficit)
      1. When administering replacement fluids, periodic reassessment is indicated to determine response to volumes administered
   B. Replacement fluids can be administered over a 4-6–hour period or added to the maintenance fluid volume and administered over a 24-hour period

BLOOD TRANSFUSION—MAJOR BLOOD GROUPS

I. Dog
   A. Eight specific antigens have been identified on the dog erythrocyte
      1. DEA_1, DEA_2, and DEA_7 have the greatest potential to induce hemolytic antibody production in recipients
         a. Dogs negative for these RBC antigens are desirable as donors
      2. Transfusion reactions related to the remaining blood group antigens are considered clinically insignificant
      3. Dogs should be heartworm-negative
II. Cat
   A. Three antigens have been identified on the cat erythrocyte
      1. Transfusion reactions are rare in the cat, so blood typing is rarely performed
      2. Decreased survival time for infused RBCs may develop after multiple transfusions
III. Horse
   A. At least nine specific blood group antigens have been identified in the horse
      1. Whenever possible, compatibility testing should be done in horses prior to transfusion
         a. Blood typing

   b. Major and minor antigen agglutination
   c. Lysis cross-matching test
  2. In situations where compatibility cannot be tested, a healthy male horse that has never had a transfusion is the most suitable donor

IV. Cow
 A. 11 antigenic blood groups recognized
V. Swine
 A. 15 antigenic blood groups recognized
VI. Sheep
 A. Eight antigenic blood groups recognized

INDICATIONS FOR BLOOD TRANSFUSION

 I. Restoration of oxygen carrying capacity
  A. Anemia
   1. PCV < 20%, Hb < 5 g/dl in a normally hydrated patient that is being prepared for surgery
   2. A nonsurgical chronic anemic patient may not require transfusion until PCV < 15 in dogs or PCV < 10 in cats
  B. Massive hemorrhage
   1. 30-40% of total blood volume loss is considered moderate hemorrhage that may still be adequately treated by appropriate amounts of crystalloid infusion
   2. If more than 50% of the total blood volume is lost, whole blood is necessary for replacement
 II. Restoration of blood volume
 III. Coagulation factor replacement
  A. Poor viability of platelets and coagulation factors in stored blood
  B. Choose fresh blood (storage < 12 hours) when treating coagulopathies

COLLECTING AND STORING BLOOD FOR TRANSFUSION

 I. Obtain blood from jugular vein or cardiac puncture
 II. Anticoagulant solutions used
  A. ACD (acid citrate dextrose)
  B. CPD (citrate phosphate dextrose) maintains higher pH, ATP, and 2,3 DPG content during storage
  C. Heparin
   1. Heparin activates platelet aggregation and inhibits thrombin formation by inhibiting factor IX activation
   2. Blood collected with heparin as the anticoagulant should not be transfused if stored 48 hours
 III. Plastic containers are recommended for blood collection. They are less likely to activate platelet and coagulation factors
 IV. Suggested guidelines for blood storage
  A. Maintain between 1° and 6° C

1. ACD anticoagulant: 21 days
2. CPD anticoagulant: 28 days
3. Feline blood: 30 days

B. 70-75% of red blood cells are viable at the end of storage times listed above

MODIFICATIONS OF STORED BLOOD

I. RBCs become less deformable as the fluidity of cytosol decreases due to:
   A. Hypertonicity of anticoagulant solution
   B. Decreasing erythrocyte ATP content

II. Decreased erythrocyte 2,3-DPG content
   A. Shift of oxygen dissociation curve to the left
      1. Decreased oxygen release at the tissue level
   B. 2,3-DPG content in RBCs is restored within hours of transfusion

III. Decreased pH (pH < 6.5 after 3 weeks of storage)
   A. Citrate anticoagulants are converted to bicarbonate within minutes by the liver
      1. Unless inadequate liver blood flow or altered liver metabolism is suspected, bicarbonate therapy with blood transfusion is not necessary

IV. Decreased platelet numbers
   A. Functional platelets nonexistent after 2-3 days of storage

V. Increased ammonia content
   A. May be detrimental in patient with impaired hepatic function

VI. Increased plasma potassium concentration
   A. Occurs due to progressive hemolysis during storage

VII. Metabolic transformations in stored blood are largely reversed during the first 24 hours following transfusion

BLOOD ADMINISTRATION

I. Blood administration sets
   A. Must contain a filter to remove aggregated debris
      1. Micropore filter with pore size 20 to 40 μm
      2. Cloth filter of administration set with 170 μm pore
   B. Tubing must be flushed prior to introducing blood
      1. Reduces resistance to blood flow
      2. Isotonic saline is fluid of choice
      3. Lactated Ringer's or other calcium-containing solutions may recalcify blood and trigger coagulation
      4. Dextrose solutions may cause agglutination and/or hemolysis

II. Sites of blood administration
   A. Peripheral or jugular vein is recommended
   B. Intraperitoneal administration
      1. Slow administration
      2. Poor recovery of RBCs into system; approximately 40% of blood is absorbed in 24 hours

    C. Medullary cavity of femur or humerus
      1. Adequate for neonatal small animals
      2. Use 20 gauge needle or bone marrow aspiration needle
      3. 95% of blood will be absorbed in 5 minutes

III. Rewarm stored blood in order to decrease viscosity and prevent hypothermia in recipient
    A. Immerse transfusion tubing in water bath maintained at a temperature below 40° C
      1. Autoagglutination will occur at higher temperatures

IV. Volume of blood to be administered
    A. General rule: 1 ml whose blood/lb raises the PCV by 1% (assuming a donor PCV of 40%)
    B. Amount of donor blood needed (ml) =

$$\text{recipient blood volume} \times \frac{\text{desired PCV} - \text{actual patient PCV}}{\text{PCV of anticoagulated donor blood}}$$

      1. Total blood volume is estimated at 40 ml/lb (30 ml/lb in the cat)

V. Rate of blood administration depends upon the clinical circumstance
    A. Rapid administration in the face of massive hemorrhage
    B. In other cases:
      1. Transfuse slowly at 0.1 ml/lb during the first 30 minutes, and observe for adverse reactions
      2. Afterward the rule of thumb is 5 ml/lb/hr until the desired PCV is achieved
      3. As with any fluid administration, monitor for signs of fluid overload (CVP, thoracic auscultation)

ADVERSE EFFECTS OF TRANSFUSION—IMMUNE MEDIATED

  I. Hypersensitivity nonhemolytic reactions
    A. Activation of kallikrein-kinin system or IgE
    B. Release of biogenic amines
    C. Clinical signs are muscle tremor, pyrexia, hypotension, tachycardia, and urticaria

  II. Hemolytic reactions
    A. Hemolysis results from:
      1. Recipient antibodies interacting with incompatible antigen of donor
      2. Antibodies of a previously sensitized donor interacting with recipient antigen
    B. Immediate transfusion reactions are unlikely during a first transfusion
    C. Clinical signs usually develop within an hour posttransfusion and include hypotension, pyrexia, muscle tremor, emesis, convulsions, hemoglobinemia/uria, bilirubinemia/uria
    D. Shock, renal failure, and DIC may ensue
    E. Delayed transfusion reactions for up to 2 weeks posttransfusion

1. The recipient mounts an immune response to incompatible erythrocytes
2. Clinical signs include pyrexia, anorexia, jaundice, and bilirubinuria
F. Hemolysis in the newborn resulting from previous sensitization of the mother (neonatal isoerythrolysis) can be avoided by preventing colostrum absorption
   1. Withhold mother's milk from neonate for first 48 hours of life

NONIMMUNOLOGIC ADVERSE TRANSFUSION REACTIONS

I. Sepsis
   A. Improper collection, storage, or handling may result in bacterial contamination and overgrowth
II. Transmission of infectious or parasitic diseases
III. Circulatory overload
IV. Citrate toxicity
   A. Rarely seen due to rapid metabolism of citrate by the liver
      1. More likely in animal with liver dysfunction or excessively rapid blood administration
   B. Excessive circulating citrate causes chelation of serum ionized calcium

PLASMA TRANSFUSION

I. Indications
   A. Hypoproteinemia: Total protein < 4 g/dl

   Albumin < 1.5 g/dl
   B. Failure of passive transfer
      1. Inadequate colostral antibody absorption
   C. Thrombocytopenia ⎱ *Note*: Use fresh plasma
   D. Coagulopathies ⎰
II. Plasma can be stored in a conventional freezer for up to 1 year

CHAPTER TWENTY-FIVE

Respiratory Emergency

*"Each person is born to one possession which outvalues all his others —
his last breath."*

MARK TWAIN

OVERVIEW

Respiratory depression is by far the most common complication associated with chemical restraint and anesthesia. All too frequently, respiratory depression can lead to a respiratory emergency by causing apnea and hypoxemia. Hypoventilation cannot always be determined by visual inspection but can be assessed by arterial blood gases. Although potentially devastating, respiratory depression if recognized early is easily treated by establishing a patent airway and providing adequate inflation of the lungs to ensure appropriate gas exchange.

GENERAL CONSIDERATIONS

I. Definition: Respiratory emergency is the inability to maintain adequate ventilation and normal blood gas values
II. Common causes
   A. The causes are diverse and may vary between animal species
   B. Major causes
      1. Hypoventilation due to drug-induced respiratory depression
      2. Airway obstruction
      3. Parenchymal pulmonary disease
      4. Pleural cavity disease
      5. Iatrogenic

       a. Laryngeal spasm with intubation of cats

       b. Small or plugged endotracheal tube

III. Patient age and size determine respiratory frequency, rate of lung inflation, inflation pressure, and volume delivered in the use of assisted or controlled ventilation. Generally speaking, large adult patients require slower inflation rates, lower frequencies of inflation, and larger inflation pressure and volumes

    A. Pulmonary lesions leading to pneumothorax must be corrected immediately in order to ensure adequate lung expansion

IV. A total lack of respiratory effort or increased respiratory frequency and the use of the accessory muscles of respiration, particularly the abdomen, are signs of a respiratory emergency

V. Support of ventilation should be continued until the patient can maintain consciousness, normal mucous membrane color, and normal blood gases

CLINICAL SIGNS

  I. Apnea or dyspnea

 II. Respiratory rate, depth, and effort are generally increased in animals with respiratory disease

III. Stridor or strenuous breathing are sounds associated with airway obstruction

 IV. Cyanosis; may be absent in severely anemic animals

  V. Abnormal upper airway and lung sounds (wheezes, crackles)

 VI. Deformities of head, neck, and thorax

VII. Abnormal positions

    A. Extension of the head and neck

    B. Abduction of the forelimbs

    C. Sternal recumbency

HYPOVENTILATION

  I. Treat primary cause

 II. Control or assist breathing when necessary

III. Use respiratory stimulants when necessary

    A. Doxapram 0.05-0.2 mg/lb IV; repeat if necessary

AIRWAY OBSTRUCTION

 I. Partial airway obstructions are frequently associated with respiratory disease and endotracheal intubation

II. Anatomical conformations that predispose dogs to airway collapse

    A. Stenotic nares

       1. Brachycephalic breeds

    B. Elongated soft palate

       1. Brachycephalic breeds

       2. Beagle and cocker spaniel

       3. Horses

      C. Collapsing arytenoid cartilages
        1. Congenital in Bouvier, bull terrier, Siberian husky
        2. Acquired in giant-breed dogs (e.g., St. Bernard)
      D. Everting laryngeal ventricles
        1. Brachycephalic breeds
        2. English bulldog
        3. May be associated with hypothyroidism
      E. Collapsing trachea
        1. Middle-aged to older obese toy-breed dogs
        2. Especially miniature poodle, Yorkshire terrier, Chihuahua
      F. Laryngeal paralysis
        1. Congenital, especially in Bouvier, bull terrier, Siberian husky
        2. Acquired in giant-breed dogs, especially St. Bernard
        3. Postsurgically in horses
      G. Hypoplasia of the trachea
        1. Congenital in brachycephalic breeds
        2. English bulldog
III. Other causes of airway obstruction
      A. Endotracheal or tracheotomy tubes
      B. Nasal disease (e.g., tumor, fungal)
      C. Chronic obstructive pulmonary disease
      D. Other species
        1. Cat—asthma
          a. Stage I (asymptomatic)
          b. Stage V (severe distress)
        2. Horse—gutteral pouch infections, ethmoidal hematoma, tumors
        3. Sheep—nasal parasites
        4. Pig—atrophic rhinitis
IV. Clinical signs
      A. Noisy striduous or strenuous breathing
        1. Loudest at larynx and pharynx during upper airway obstruction
        2. Low-pitched honking sound during tracheal collapse
      B. History of exercise intolerance, cyanosis, and collapse
      C. Choking, retching, and vomiting
      D. Severely distressed animals may paw or claw at the face and throat
V. Diagnosis
      A. History of facial injuries, epistaxis, or wounds to the neck
      B. The presence of stenotic nares, foreign bodies or tumors, and soft tissue swelling
      C. Radiography
        1. Survey
        2. Contrast
        3. Fluoroscopy
      D. Bronchoscopy to confirm presence or absence of lower airway obstruction
      E. Electromyography to confirm denervation of laryngeal muscles

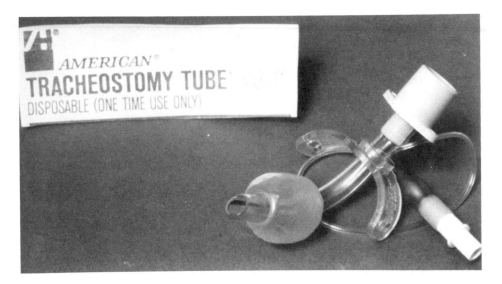

FIG. 25-1 Tracheotomy tubes are available in different sizes and are cuffed or uncuffed. Cuffed tubes are preferred.

VI. Treatment

  A. Avoid stress

  B. Establish patent airway

    1. Intubate

    2. Remove oral, nasal, or tracheal foreign material or blood using forceps, suction, and postural drainage

    3. Perform tracheotomy if necessary to bypass obstruction (see Fig. 25-1)

    4. Apply local anesthetic creams (5% lidocaine) to prevent laryngospasm

  C. If apneic, institute artificial ventilation with air or, preferably, oxygen

    1. Mouth-to-mouth

    2. Mouth-to-nose

    3. Nasal tube intubation, with oxygen administration

    4. Face mask and oxygen

    5. Deliver oxygen to endotracheal or tracheotomy tube

  D. Control breathing rate if apneic; assist ventilation if breathing

    1. Rate: 6-15/min

    2. Inspiratory time: 1-3 seconds, depending on size of patient

    3. Maintain proper inspiratory:expiratory ratio of 1:2, 1:3, or 1:4

    4. Inflate lungs to 15-20 cm water if chest is closed (up to 30-50 cm water in large animals)

    5. Inflate lungs to 20-30 cm water if chest is open or atelectasis of lungs has occurred (up to 50 cm water in large animals)

    6. Tidal volume

      a. Approximately 5 ml/lb

      b. 10 ml/lb if mechanical ventilator is used

    E. Discontinue all anesthetic agents, including nitrous oxide

    F. Supportive care

       1. Intravenous fluid therapy

       2. Bronchodilators

       3. Respiratory stimulants when necessary

       4. Sedation

       5. Antibiotics

       6. Corticosteroids

       7. Maintain normal body temperature

    G. Treat coexisting problems

       1. Prepare for surgery

          a. Removal of foreign bodies or tumors

          b. Repair fractures and wounds of the respiratory system

          c. Chest drainage

          d. Correct anatomical defects when necessary

    H. Care of tracheotomy tube

       1. Suction every 2 hours using aseptic technique

       2. Nebulization with saline or acetylcysteine diluted with saline

       3. Maintain normal hydration

       4. Monitor body temperature

       5. Take periodic chest radiographs

PARENCHYMAL EXCHANGE DISEASES

  I. Classification

    A. Life-threatening pneumonias

       1. Acute fulminating bronchopneumonia

       2. Smoke inhalation

       3. Aspiration pneumonia

    B. Pulmonary contusion

    C. Pulmonary edema

    D. Cat asthma

  II. Diagnosis

    A. Physical signs, including lethargy

    B. Radiographs of the chest

    C. Laboratory tests

       1. CBC

       2. Transtracheal aspirate

       3. Bronchoscopy

       4. Blood gas determination

  III. Treatment

    A. Removal of aspirated material

    B. Maintaining the patency and function of the airways

    C. Positive end-expiratory pressure (PEEP) ventilation

    D. Treating infection

    E. Enhancing removal of secretions (acetylcysteine, guaifenesin)

    F. Supportive care

1. Oxygen administration ($\geq 40\%$) via:
   a. Face mask
   b. Pediatric incubator
   c. Oxygen cage
   d. Tracheotomy and positive-pressure ventilation, if laryngeal spasm or airway obstruction with secretions persist
2. Humidification of the air by nebulization with normal saline improves removal of secretions
3. Normal body hydration must be maintained with fluids IV or SQ to prevent drying and thickening of secretions
4. Periodic coupage (percussion of the chest)
5. Physiotherapy with deep breathing aids removal of secretions, increases lymphatic drainage of the lungs, and activates surfactant
6. The use of diuretics, corticosteroids, and antiprostaglandins in pneumonia is controversial
7. Bronchodilators are helpful in reversing bronchial spasm and constriction
8. Pneumonias with viscous secretions may require expectorants (guaifenesin)
9. Antibiotic usage should be based on culture and sensitivity results
10. Analgesics may be used for extreme pain and apprehension in selected patients
11. Medical therapy of pulmonary edema includes:
    a. Decreasing the work load of the heart by cage rest, administering oxygen, sedation, and digitalization
    b. Improving ventilation by endotracheal suctioning
    c. Nebulization with 40% ethyl alcohol
    d. Eliminating excessive fluids by use of diuretics and vasodilators

PLEURAL CAVITY DISEASE

I. Definition: Pleural cavity disease includes problems that decrease the functional capacity of the lungs due to occupation of space in the pleural cavity and damage to the integrity of the thoracic wall

II. Classification
   A. Pneumothorax
      1. Open
      2. Closed
      3. Spontaneous
      4. Tension
   B. Pleural effusion
      1. Chylothorax
      2. Pyothorax
      3. Hydrothorax
      4. Hemothorax
      5. Neoplastic effusion
      6. Infectious, inflammatory effusion

    C. Diaphragmatic hernia

    D. Flail chest

III. Causes

    A. Spontaneous pneumothorax: accumulation of free air in the pleural cavity

    B. Tension pneumothorax: Air accumulates in pleural space during inspiration and is not expelled during expiration

       1. Trauma is the most common cause of pneumothorax resulting in pleural or parenchymal lacerations or tracheobronchial ruptures

          a. Diaphragmatic hernias

            (1) Displacement of the lungs with abdominal viscera

          b. Flail chest: proximal and distal fractures of several consecutive ribs

            (1) Chest wall is drawn inward with expiration and blown outward with expiration (paradoxical movement)

            (2) Lung contusion and hemopneumothorax may be present, precipitating acute respiratory distress

       2. Other causes

          a. Penetrating injuries from bite wounds and projectiles

          b. Rupture of congenital bullous emphysematous or granulomatous lung lesions (blebs or bullae)

          c. Rupture of parasitic cysts (Paragonimus); neoplasia

          d. Hardware disease in cattle

          e. Pleuritis

          f. Iatrogenic

            (1) Intrathoracic surgical procedures

            (2) Cardiopulmonary resuscitation

            (3) Overzealous intermittent positive-pressure ventilation

          g. Rarely, following pneumomediastinum from trauma to trachea or esophagus

    C. Pleural effusion: abnormal fluid accumulation within the pleural cavity

       1. Hemothorax

          a. Rupture of cardiac and intrathoracic blood vessels from trauma

          b. Clotting disorders

          c. Bleeding neoplasms (e.g., hemangiosarcoma)

          d. Lung lobe torsion

          e. Pleuritis

       2. Chylothorax

          a. Rupture of the thoracic duct

          b. Idiopathic lymphatic obstruction

       3. Hydrothorax

          a. Hypoproteinemia

          b. Heart failure and cardiomyopathy

       4. Pyothorax

          a. Penetrating wounds of thorax or esophagus

          b. Migrating foreign bodies

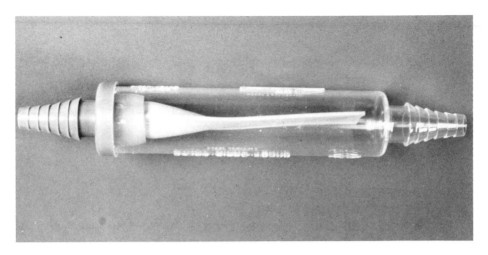

FIG. 25-2 A unidirectional valve (Heimlich valve) is used to aid in evacuating air from the chest.

  c. Spread of pulmonary infection and pleuritis
  d. Organisms: *E. coli, Staphylococcus, β-streptococcus, Pasteurella, Nocardia*
IV. Diagnosis
 A. Thoracic radiography
 B. Thoracentesis
V. Treatment
 A. Establish a patent airway
 B. Oxygen therapy
 C. Shock therapy
 D. Thoracic examination
  1. Auscultation
  2. Percussion
  3. Bandage penetrating wounds, flail segments
 E. Assess status of animal
 F. Tube thoracostomy
  1. Indications
   a. Acute severe pneumothorax
   b. Tension pneumothorax
   c. Pneumothorax associated with rib fractures, emphysema, or hemothorax
   d. In situations where repeated needle evacuations are necessary
   e. Post-thoracotomy
  2. Methods of drainage
   a. Intermittent aspiration using a syringe and three-way stopcock
   b. Unidirectional flutter (Heimlich) valves (Fig. 25-2)

      c. Intermittent connection of the chest tube to a suction pump (10-15 cm water negative pressure)

      d. Connection of chest tube to underwater seal units

        (1) One-bottle system

        (2) Two-bottle system

        (3) Three-bottle system

   3. Complications

      a. Chest tube attaches to underwater seal and requires constant monitoring

      b. Accumulation of fibrin and blood

      c. Displacement of tube

      d. Kinking of tube

      e. Subcutaneous emphysema

      f. Lung tissue entrapment and infarction after vigorous suction

      g. Infection

IATROGENIC CAUSES OF RESPIRATORY EMERGENCIES

I. Inadequate evaluation of the patient

II. Faulty anesthetic techniques

   A. Anesthetic overdose (e.g., barbiturates)

   B. Excessive dead space in anesthetic equipment

   C. Lack of delivery of oxygen

      1. Nitrous oxide on; oxygen off

      2. Oxygen supply depleted

      3. Anesthetic system not connected properly

      4. Endotracheal tube too small

      5. Overdistended endotracheal tube cuff

        a. Stenosis of trachea in horses

        b. Postsurgical stenosis of trachea

      6. Inappropriately placed endotracheal tube

        a. In esophagus

        b. In pharynx

        c. At or caudal to bifurcation of trachea

   D. Kinked or obstructed anesthetic delivery hoses and tubes

   E. Overdistention of lungs during mechanical ventilation

   F. Neuromuscular paralysis of diaphragm and intercostal muscles without ventilatory support

III. Restrictive bandages

IV. Inadequate monitoring of the patient

   A. Abnormal patterns of respiration

      1. Eupnea: normal rate and rhythm

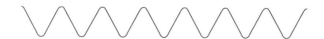

2. Tachypnea: increased respiratory rate

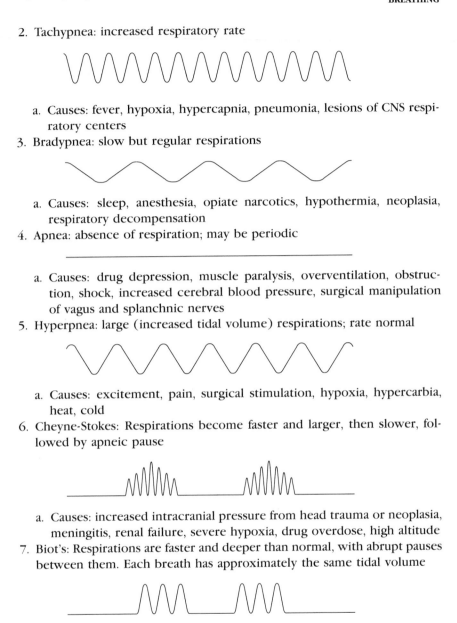

    a. Causes: fever, hypoxia, hypercapnia, pneumonia, lesions of CNS respiratory centers

3. Bradypnea: slow but regular respirations

    a. Causes: sleep, anesthesia, opiate narcotics, hypothermia, neoplasia, respiratory decompensation

4. Apnea: absence of respiration; may be periodic

    a. Causes: drug depression, muscle paralysis, overventilation, obstruction, shock, increased cerebral blood pressure, surgical manipulation of vagus and splanchnic nerves

5. Hyperpnea: large (increased tidal volume) respirations; rate normal

    a. Causes: excitement, pain, surgical stimulation, hypoxia, hypercarbia, heat, cold

6. Cheyne-Stokes: Respirations become faster and larger, then slower, followed by apneic pause

    a. Causes: increased intracranial pressure from head trauma or neoplasia, meningitis, renal failure, severe hypoxia, drug overdose, high altitude

7. Biot's: Respirations are faster and deeper than normal, with abrupt pauses between them. Each breath has approximately the same tidal volume

    a. Causes: anesthesia in normal athletic horses and greyhounds, spinal meningitis, drugs that cause generalized CNS depression

8. Kussmaul's: regular and deeper respirations without pauses. Patient's breathing usually sounds labored, with breaths that resemble sighs

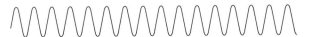

    a. Causes: renal failure or metabolic acidosis, diabetic ketoacidosis

  9. Apneustic: prolonged gasping inspiration, followed by extremely short, inefficient expirations

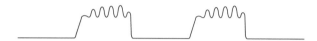

    a. Causes: high doses of drugs (e.g., ketamine in cats and horses, guaifenesin in horses), lesions in the pons and thalamus

OTHER CAUSES OF PULMONARY INSUFFICIENCY

  I. Ventilation-perfusion inequalities
    A. Decreased cardiac output
    B. Atelectasis
    C. Gravitational effects
    D. Severe abdominal distention (e.g., obesity, neoplasia)
    E. Airway obstruction
    F. Hypoventilation
  II. Increased venous admixture (shunts)
    A. Pulmonary arterial-venous shunts
    B. Bronchial vessel shunts
    C. Atelectasis (physiologic shunt)
    D. Pulmonary neoplasia

RESPIRATORY ARREST

  I. Cessation of breathing from any of the previously discussed causes
  II. Correction must be made immediately (within 3-5 minutes)
 III. Treatment
    A. Establish a patent airway
      1. Remove obstruction, foreign material
      2. Intubate
      3. Consider tracheostomy
    B. Provide artificial ventilation
      1. Room air delivered via Ambu bag
      2. 100% oxygen delivered via anesthetic system
      3. Refer to Chapter 15: Ventilation and Mechanical Assist Devices
    C. Proceed with CPR (see Chapter 26: Cardiac Emergency and Shock)
    D. Interestingly, an acupuncture resuscitative technique has been used successfully in an emergency situation
      1. 25-28 gauge hypodermic needle, 25-50 mm long
      2. Insertion 10-20 mm into the nasal septum at point VG 26, along the midline of the nasolabial cleft at the left of the lower canthi of the nostril
      3. The needle is twirled strongly and moved up and down
      4. The technique can be used as adjunct but not a replacement for conventional techniques

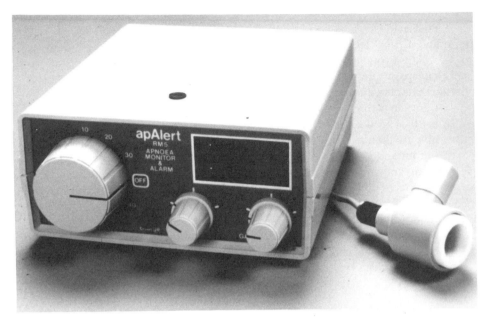

FIG. 25-3 A modified temperature device can be attached to the endotracheal tube to monitor respiratory rate.

PREVENTION OF RESPIRATORY EMERGENCIES

   I. Proper preanesthetic evaluation
      A. Clinical signs
      B. Auscultation
      C. Radiography
      D. Blood gas analysis
  II. Use of proper anesthetic equipment
 III. Adequate inspection of anesthetic equipment
  IV. Proper administration of preanesthetic and anesthetic agents
   V. Careful monitoring during anesthesia (see Fig. 25-3)
  VI. Be cognizant of possible problem

USE OF ANALEPTICS, BICARBONATE, BRONCHODILATOR DRUGS; OTHER DRUGS

   I. Doxapram hydrochloride (1-2 ml/lb, small animals; 0.1-0.3 mg/lb, large animals, IV)
      A. Centrally acting respiratory stimulant; increases tidal volume and, in larger doses, respiratory rate. Causes small elevations in arterial blood pressure and heart rate, and may cause arousal from anesthetic depression
  II. Sodium bicarbonate (0.5-2 mEq/lb)
      A. To correct metabolic acidosis, which may occur in severe hypoxia, hypercapnea, or complete respiratory and cardiac arrest. Excessive administration

may produce hypokalemic metabolic alkalosis or paradoxical cerebrospinal fluid acidosis

III. Aminophylline (up to 2 mg/lb IV slowly over 30 minutes, 1-2 mg/lb IM)

    A. Dilates bronchial smooth muscle and may be useful in asthmatics and bronchospasm; Inotropic action on heart

IV. Nikethamide (2-4 mg/lb IV slowly)

    A. Centrally acting respiratory stimulant due to stimulation of chemoreceptors in the carotid and aortic bodies; excessive doses cause convulsions. The myocardium may be depressed, but large doses may slightly increase cardiac output and coronary flow. Short duration of effect (10-15 minutes)

V. Narcotic antagonists (naloxone, nalorphine, levallorphan)

    A. Nalline (nalorphine), 1 mg/5 lb, acts by competitively displacing narcotic analgesics from opiate and nonopiate receptors

VI. Other specific antagonists

    A. Neostigmine, edrophonium: reversal of nondepolarizing neuromuscular blocking drugs (see Chapter 11: Neuromuscular Blocking Drugs)

    B. α_2 antagonists (yohimbine, tolazoline): reversal of xylazine (see Chapter 3: Drugs Used for Preanesthetic Medication)

CHAPTER TWENTY-SIX

Cardiac Emergency and Shock

"It is by presence of mind in untried emergencies
that the native metal of a man is tested."

JAMES RUSSELL LOWELL

OVERVIEW

Bradycardia, hypotension, and decreased peripheral perfusion leading to shock can occur following the administration of chemical restraining drugs and anesthetics. The possibility of these emergencies increases in severely debilitated or traumatized patients. A variety of physical and pharmacologic approaches to patients with poor cardiovascular function have been developed in order to prevent further deterioration of the circulation or return abnormal hemodynamics to normal. Since it is difficult to perform external/internal cardiac massage in animals in excess of 500 pounds, it is imperative that a working knowledge of the various pharmacologic approaches to cardiopulmonary resuscitation be understood. Generally, most therapeutic approaches to acute cardiovascular crises must be followed by continued care and close patient monitoring.

GENERAL CONSIDERATIONS

I. Definition: Cardiac emergency is any acute or chronic condition involving the heart that results in the inability to maintain an adequate cardiac output
II. Common causes

A. Respiratory failure (hypoxia)
   1. Hypoventilation
   2. Low inspired P_{O_2}
   3. Ventilation-perfusion abnormality
   4. Shunt
   5. Diffusion abnormality
B. Acid-base imbalance
   1. Respiratory acidosis
   2. Metabolic acidosis leading to myocardial depression
   3. Respiratory alkalosis
   4. Metabolic alkalosis leading to myocardial irritability
   5. Mixed metabolic and respiratory alkalosis or acidosis
C. Electrolyte imbalance
   1. Hypokalemia (tachycardia)
   2. Hyperkalemia (bradycardia)
   3. Hypocalcemia (hypocontractility, hypotension)
D. Autonomic imbalance
   1. Increased sympathetic tone
      a. Increased myocardial automaticity and irritability
   2. Increased parasympathetic tone
      a. Predisposition to bradycardia and various forms of heart block; pre-disposition to atrial arrhythmias, including atrial fibrillation
E. Hypothermia
F. Air embolism
G. Toxicity
   1. Myocardial depressant factors produced by ischemic organs (i.e., pancreas)
   2. Any hypersensitivity or overdose
      a. Hypotensive crisis secondary to phenothiazine administration
         (1) Most commonly observed after IV drug administration
         (2) Can occur in any species, but reported to occur most frequently in horses
         (3) Treatment includes fluids, steroids, and occasionally vasopressors
H. Excessive or inappropriate drug administration
   1. Administration of catecholamines during inhalation anesthesia with halothane (ventricular arrhythmias, tachycardia)
   2. Accidental intraarterial drug administration, for example, accidental intracarotid administration of preanesthetic drugs (phenothiazines, xylazine) in horses and cattle. Treatment should include adequate padding, anticonvulsants (diazepam), fluids, and steroids
I. Cardiac disease and/or arrhythmias (see Table 26-1)
   1. Bradycardia
      a. Increased parasympathetic tone
      b. Hypothermia

TABLE 26 - 1

DISTINGUISHING CHARACTERISTICS OF SEVERAL TYPES OF CARDIAC FAILURE OR ARREST

Cause	Peripheral pulse	Auscultation of heart sounds	Electrocardiogram	Visual observation
Ventricular tachycardia	Rapid, irregular Pulse deficit	Muffled; may be of variable intensity	Wide QRST complexes; absence of PQRS relationship	Disorganized, rapidy beating heart
Ventricular fibrillation	None	None	Absence of QRST complexes; fibrillation waves	Fine to coarse rippling of the ventricular myocardium
Bradycardia	Slow; may be irregular	Slow	Infrequent or irregular PQRST complexes; juctional or ventricular escape complexes	Infrequent coordinated ventricular contractions
Ventricular asystole	None	None	Absence of QRST complexes; straight-line ECG	No cardiac movement
Electro-mechanical dissociation	None	None	Normal PQRST complexes	Feeble or absent cardiac contractions

    c. Hyperkalemia

    d. Specific drug medication (narcotics, xylazine)

    e. Drug overdosage

  2. Tachycardia

    a. Increased sympathetic tone

      (1) Pain

      (2) Excitement, stress

      (3) Hypotension

      (4) Hypoxia

      (5) Hypokalemia

    b. Specific drug administration (catecholamines, atropine, ketamine)

  3. Atrial or ventricular arrhythmias

    a. Associated with ischemia, hypoxia, hypotension, hypercarbia, metabolic acidosis or alkalosis, hypothermia, hypotension, surgical manipulation, anesthetic agents being used, cardiac catheterization, etc.

  4. Ventricular fibrillation

    a. Most likely to occur during induction and recovery from anesthesia due to instability of autonomic reflexes and endogenous release of catecholamines

    b. May be associated with too rapid an infusion of thiobarbiturates or high initial concentrations of inhalation anesthetics

    c. May follow severe hypercarbia, hypoxia, hypovolemia, or acidosis

  5. Ventricular asystole

    a. Usually associated with drug (anesthetic) overdose

    b. Seen in shock or in toxic animals that must be anesthetized

  6. Electromechanical dissociation

    a. Hypoxia and ischemia

    b. Drug overdose

  7. Cardiovascular collapse

    a. Cardiac failure that is unresponsive to therapy

    b. Seen primarily in those patients that have chronic heart disease or are extremely toxic

INDICATIONS OF POOR CARDIAC FUNCTION

    I. Cyanosis (not seen in anemic patients)

   II. Poor perfusion

     A. Prolonged refill time (>2 seconds)

  III. Irregular or absent pulse or heart sounds

   IV. Signs of shock (see Shock)

    V. Cardiac arrhythmias

   VI. Abnormal breathing pattern or apnea

  VII. Dilated pupils

 VIII. Depression or loss of consciousness

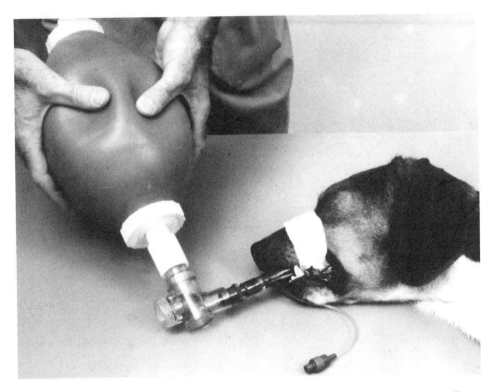

FIG. 26-1 A self-inflating Ambu bag can be used to assist or control breathing in small animals.

EQUIPMENT

I. Should be readily accessible in the event of collapse
    A. Cuffed endotracheal tubes
        1. Small
        2. Medium
        3. Large
    B. Lighted laryngoscope with small, medium, and large tongue blades
    C. Ambu bag, demand valve, or anesthetic machine (Fig. 26-1 and 26-2)
    D. Tongue depressors
    E. Syringes
        1. Five 3 cc
        2. Five 5 cc
        3. Five 12 cc
        4. Five 30 cc
    F. Three-way valve
    G. One roll 1-inch adhesive tape
    H. One roll 2-inch gauze
    I. Pack of sterile 4 × 4–inch gauze pads

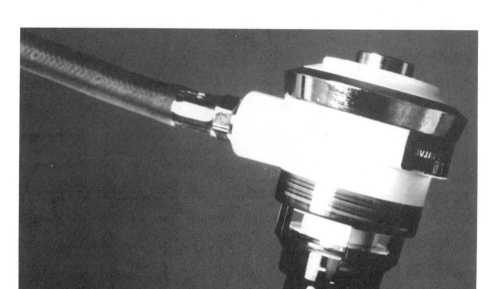

FIG. 26-2 A demand valve connected to an oxygen hose can be attached to an endotracheal tube for assisting or controlling breathing in small or large animals.

   J. One roll elastic bandage
  K. Blood administration set
   L. Needles
      1. Five 20 gauge
      2. Five 18 gauge
      3. Two 16 gauge
  M. Butterfly administration needles
      1. Two 21 gauge
      2. Two 19 gauge
  N. IV fluid administration set
  O. Sterile emergency surgery pack
      1. Scalpel handle
      2. Blades: Two #10, two #15
      3. Two small hemostats
      4. Thumb forceps
      5. One pair Metzenbaum scissors

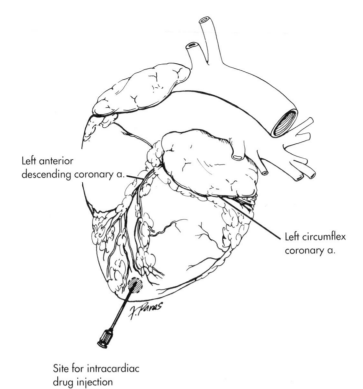

Left anterior
descending coronary a.

Left circumflex
coronary a.

Site for intracardiac
drug injection

FIG. 26-3 Site for injection of drugs into the left ventricle of the heart.

6. One pair curved forceps
7. Several packages of suture of preference swaged to needles
8. Needle holders
9. One set medium-sized rib retractors
P. Intravenous catheters: one 16 gauge, one 18 gauge
Q. Chest tube: Heimlich valve

TREATMENT

See Tables 26-2 to 26-4 and Figs. 26-3 and 26-4
   I. Airway
  II. Breathing
 III. Circulation
  IV. Drugs
   V. Electrocardiogram
  VI. Defibrillation

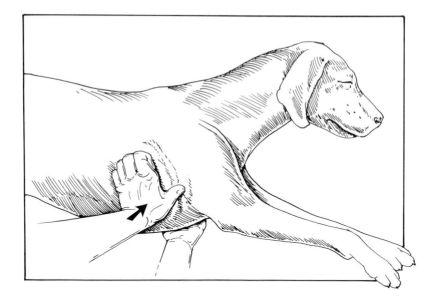

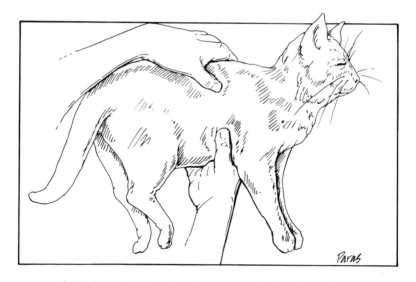

FIG. 26-4 External cardiac massage in the dog and cat.

TABLE 26-2

TREATMENT OF CARDIOPULMONARY ARREST

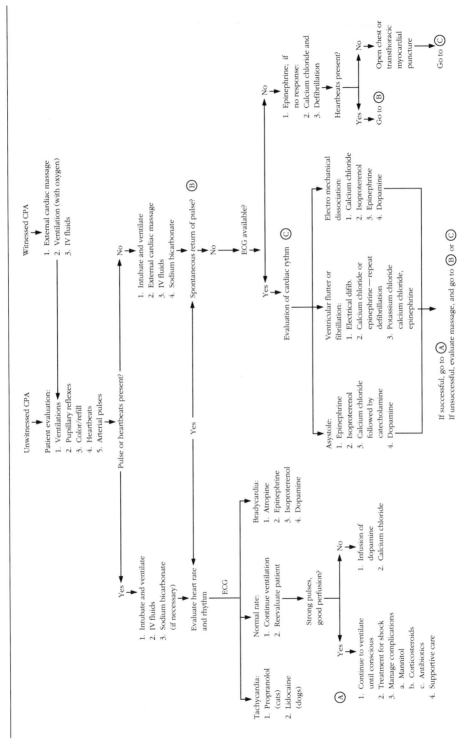

TABLE 26-3

TREATMENTS FOR VENTRICULAR FIBRILLATION

I. Direct-current defibrillators
  A. 0.5-2.0 watt-seconds (ws)/kg internal
  B. 5-10 ws/kg external
    1. Small patient (<7 kg)
      a. 5-15 ws internal
      b. 50-100 ws external
    2. Large patient (>10 kg)
      a. 20-80 ws internal
      b. 100-400 ws external
II. Alternating-current defibrillators
  A. Small patient
    1. 30-50 V internal
    2. 50-100 V external
  B. Large patient
    1. 50-100 V internal
    2. 150-250 V external
III. Chemical defibrillation
  A. 1 mg potassium chloride and 6 mg acetylcholine/kg followed by 1 ml/10 kg of 10% calcium chloride
IV. Unresponsive ventricular fibrillation
  A. Evaluate ventilation
  B. Evaluate chest or cardiac compression
  C. Repeat epinephrine and calcium chloride administration (see Table 26-4)
  D. Repeat sodium bicarbonate administration
  E. Administer lidocaine
  F. Repeat electrical defibrillation

SHOCK

I. Definition: Shock is an acute disease syndrome characterized by impairment of the cardiovascular system and a decreased effective circulating blood volume. The key factor in shock is derangement of the microcirculation, resulting in *inadequately oxygenated and perfused tissues*
II. Etiology (Table 26-5 on page 300)
  A. Hypovolemic
  B. Cardiogenic
  C. Distributive
  D. Obstructive
III. Pathophysiology
  A. Decreased effective circulating blood volume (see Table 26-6 on page 301)
    1. Endotoxins
      a. Endotoxin-induced extravasation of fluids (third-space loss)

Text continues on p. 300.

TABLE 26-4

ESSENTIAL DRUGS USED IN THE MANAGEMENT OF CARDIOPULMONARY ARREST

Generic name	Trade name	Beneficial effects (recommended use)	Adverse or side effects	Dose and route of administration
Vasoactive and cardiostimulatory agents				
Epinephrine HCl	Adrenaline	Positive inotrope. Initiates heartbeats; increases heart rate and cardiac output. Initially increases, then decreases mean arterial blood pressure and coronary blood flow	Intense vasoconstriction of renal and splanchnic vasculature; causes decreased perfusion of these tissues; increases myocardial oxygen consumption and cardiac work. Arrhythmogenic	6-10 μg/kg IC 20-30 μg/kg/IV 0.1-0.2 ml/20 kg, small animals 1-3 ml/450 kg, large animals
Isoproterenol HCl	Isuprel	Positive inotrope. Initiates heartbeats; increases heart rate and cardiac output	Lowers mean arterial pressure, requiring concurrent blood volume exanpsion; may decrease coronary perfusion; increases myocardial work load and oxygen consumption. Arrhythmogenic	1-6μg/kg IC 2-10 μg/kg/IV Use low range for bradyarrhythmias
Dopamine HCl	Inotropin	Positive inotrope. Increases heart rate, cardiac output, and mean arterial blood pressure; improves blood flow to coronary, renal, and mesenteric circulation	May produce severe tachycardia if given rapidly. Arrhythmogenic. Vasoconstriction at higher doses	To effect, add 5.0 mg to 250 cc 5% dextrose; drip slowly at rate of 2-10 μg/kg/min
Dobutamine HCl	Dobutrex	Positive inotrope. Less chronotropic and vasopressor effect than dopamine	Tachyarrhythmias, vasoconstriction, and arrhythmias at higher dosages	To effect, 2-15 μg/kg/min
Ephedrine sulphate	Ephedrine	Vasopressor	Tachycardia, hypertension	5-10 μg/kg

Continued

ESSENTIAL DRUGS USED IN THE MANAGEMENT OF CARDIOPULMONARY ARREST

Generic name	Trade name	Beneficial effects (recommended use)	Adverse or side effects	Dose and route of administration
Drugs used specifically to increase contractility				
Calcium chloride		Positive inotrope	May cause asystole	0.05-0.10 ml/kg of the 10% solution IV, IC
Digoxin	Lanoxin	Positive inotrope. Increases vagal tone. Used only in cases of CPA caused by congestive heart failure	Arrhythmogenic. Increases oxygen consumption; causes vasoconstriction when given IV	0.02-0.04 mg/kg IV; given in 4 divided doses; dosed every hour to effect; monitor ECG
Drugs used to combat acidosis				
Sodium bicarbonate		Buffers acidosis; allows more effective defibrillation	Excessive administration may produce alkalosis, hyperosmolarity, paradoxial cerebrospinal fluid acidosis	1-2 mEq/kg, IV, to effect
Drugs used to treat acute cardiac arrhythmias				
Atropine sulfate		Parasympatholytic effects; may correct supraventricular bradycardia or a slow ventricular rhythm by stimulating supraventricular pacemakers	May cause excessive tachycardia; increases myocardial oxygen consumption; lowers ventricular fibrillatory threshold. May predispose to sympathetic-induced arrhythmias	10-40 μg/kg IV

Glycopyrrolate	Robinul-V	Parasympatholytic (anticholinergic); may correct supraventricular bradycardia	May cause excessive tachycardia	0.005-0.01 mg/kg IV
Propranolol HCl	Inderal	β-adrenergic blocker; antiarrhythmic; may correct supraventricular and ventricular tachycardia	Decreases contractility, an important adverse effect; may increase airway resistance	1.0 mg diluted in 1 cc saline; this dilution is given as 0.05-0.1 cc boluses IV to effect
Lidocaine	Xylocaine	Ventricular antiarrhythmic	Dosage must be considerably decreased when used in cats	2-6 mg/kg IV
Bretylium tolysolate	Bretylol	Ventricular antifibrillatory drug	Of questionable value for treatment of ventricular fibrillation in dogs	?
Acetylcholine KCl cocktail		Chemical defibrillator	Parasympathomimetic side effects	6 mg/kg ACh + 1 mEq/kg KCl, IC
Drugs used to stimulate ventilation				
Doxapram HCl	Dopram	Direct action on centers in the medulla	Respiratory alkalosis, hyperkalemia	1-4 mg/kg IV
Methetharimide	Mikedimide	Competitive effect against barbiturate-induced respiratory depression	Overdose causes convulsions	0.4-0.8 mg/kg IV (can repeat this)

Continued

TABLE 26 - 4—cont'd

ESSENTIAL DRUGS USED IN THE MANAGEMENT OF CARDIOPULMONARY ARREST

Generic name	Trade name	Beneficial effects (recommended use)	Adverse or side effects	Dose and route of administration
Drugs used to combat cerebral edema				
Oxygen		Prevents vasodilation	May cause pulmonary edema with prolonged administration; may suppress ventilatory drive	2-4 L/min
Mannitol	20% Osmitrol	Osmotic diuretic; reduces cerebral edema (See Shock)	May volume-overload the circulatory system, causing edema	1-2 mg/kg IV
Dexamethasone	Azium			
Drugs used to combat acute pulmonary edema				
Furosemide	Lasix	Potent loop diuretic promoting loss of Na^+, Cl^- and H_2O	May cause dehydration or lead to hypokalemic metabolic alkalosis if used excessively	1-2 mg/kg IV 2-4 mg/kg IM
Steroids				
Prednisolone sodium succinate	Solu-Delta-Cortef	Stabilizes lysosomal membranes; induces vasodilation; regulates fluid and electrolyte homeostasis		30 mg/kg IV

Drug	Trade name	Action	Notes	Dosage
Dexamethasone	Azium	Increases cardiac output	May increase edema in cats with congestive heart failure; fluid administration rate generally should not exceed 90 ml/kg/min; administer at high rates initially to improve venous return	8 mg/kg IV
Isotonic IV fluids Lactated Ringer's 0.9% saline		Expand the blood volume; hypotension; increase tissue perfusion		20-80 ml/kg/hr to effect

Specific drug antagonists

Drug	Trade name	Action	Notes	Dosage
Nalorphine	Nalline	Narcotic antagonist	Narcotic-like effects at increased dosages	0.4 mg/kg
Levallorphan	Lorfan	Narcotic antagonist	Narcotic-like effects at increased dosages	1 mg followed by 0.5 mg if necessary
Naloxone	Narcan	Narcotic antagonist	None	50 µg/kg
Neostigmine	Prostigmine Stiglyn	Cholinesterase inhibitor; used to reverse nondepolarizing neuromuscular blocking agents	Cholinergic effects; a parasympatholytic must be given prior to drug administration, e.g., atropine, glycopyrrolate	0.02 mg/kg
Pyridostigmine	Regonol	Cholinesterase inhibitor; used to reverse nondepolarizing neuromuscular blocking agents	Cholinergic effects; a parasympatholytic must be given prior to drug administration, e.g., atropine, glycopyrrolate	0.1 mg/kg

TABLE 26-5

CAUSES OF SHOCK

Category	Cause
Hypovolemic shock	
Exogenous	1. Blood loss caused by hemorrhage
	2. Plasma loss caused by thermal or chemical burns and inflammation
	3. Fluid and electrolyte loss caused by dehydration, vomiting, diarrhea, renal disease, severe exercise, heat stress, or excessive diuresis
Endogenous	1. Extravasation of fluids, plasma, or blood into a body cavity or tissues (third-space losses) caused by trauma, endotoxins, hypoproteinemia, anaphylaxis, or burns
Cardiogenic shock	1. Myocardial mechanical problems caused by regurgitant or obstructive defects
	2. Myopathic defects caused by inheritable traits, chemicals, or toxins
	3. Cardiac arrhythmias
Distributive shock	
High-resistance	1. Distribution of blood volume and flow to vital organs caused by endotoxins, anesthetic drug overdose, CNS trauma, anaphylaxis
Low-resistance	1. Distribution of blood away from vital organs caused by severe infections, abscesses, or arteriovenous fistulas
Obstructive shock	1. Obstruction to blood flow through the heart (pericardial tamponade, neoplasia, embolism), aorta (embolism, aneurysm), vena cava (gastric bloat, heartworm, neoplasia), lungs (embolism, heartworm, positive-pressure ventilation)

    b. Release of vasoactive substances (histamine, catecholamines, serotonin, bradykinins)

    c. Generalized vasoconstriction (occurs early in septic shock)

    d. Capillary damage with loss of volume

    e. Selective capillary dilatation

    f. Relative hypovolemia

    g. The opening of arteriovenous shunts may result in blood flow bypassing capillary beds regardless of cardiac output

  2. Traumatic, hemorrhagic (see Table 26-6)

    a. Blood loss

      (1) 20% blood loss: mild signs of shock

      (2) 40% blood loss: obvious signs of shock

      (3) Acute fall of PCV below 20 results in greater than 50% mortality

    b. Release of catecholamines

COMPENSATORY AND CORRECTIVE RESPONSES TO A DECREASE IN THE EFFECTIVE CIRCULATING BLOOD VOLUME

Causes of shock
|
Decreased effective circulating blood volume
|
Increased sympathoadrenal response

Arteriolar constriction
|
Increased vascular resistance
|
Increased blood pressure

Venular constriction
|
Increased venous return

Increased cardiac output

Increased cardiac contractility

Increased heart rate

Increased renin secretion
|
Angiotensin II formation
|
Aldosterone secretion
|
Salt (Na$^+$) and H$_2$O resorption

Antidiuretic hormone release
|
Increased H$_2$O resorption

Compensatory acute changes

Corrective chronic changes

  c. Vasoconstriction
  d. Hypovolemia
 3. Septic, traumatic, hemorrhagic, or cardiogenic shock, if uncorrected, eventually will lead to:
  a. Ischemic anoxia due to:
   (1) Decreased circulatory volume
   (2) Decreased venous return
   (3) Reduced cardiac output
   (4) Increased total peripheral resistance
   (5) Decreased tissue perfusion
   (6) Increased catecholamines
   (7) Further vasoconstriction
  b. Stagnant anoxia due to:
   (1) Anoxia
   (2) Stagnation
   (3) Acidosis
   (4) Microthrombosis
   (5) Ateriovenous shunting (admixture); bacteria-tissue interaction and/or atelectasis in the lung may contribute to shunting
   (6) Tissue injury
  c. Time
   (1) Ischemic anoxia to stagnant anoxia may take hours to occur in hemorrhagic shock; occurs in seconds or minutes in septic shock
  d. The ultimate outcome is cell damage and death
B. Cellular events
 1. Reduced oxygen and nutrient supply
 2. Anaerobic metabolism occurs
 3. Decreased ATP and energy
 4. Increased membrane permeability
 5. Influx of sodium and water
 6. Efflux of potassium
 7. Cellular edema
 8. Mitochondrial damage (swelling)
 9. Intracellular acidosis
 10. Lysosomal membrane rupture
 11. Extracellular lytic enzymes
 12. Extracellular acidemia
 13. Cell damage and death

CLINICAL AND LABORATORY FEATURES

 I. Shock may be divided into early (reversible) and late (irreversible) stages (See Table 26-7)
 II. Laboratory findings: The laboratory data in shock vary greatly and depend, in many instances, on the cause of the shock syndrome and the stage of shock
 A. Packed cell volume

TABLE 26-7

STAGES OF SHOCK

Characteristic	Early stage	Late stage
Cardiovascular		
Heart rate	Moderately increased	Markedly increased
Heart rhythm	Regular, rapid	Regular or irregular
Pulse pressure	Normal	Reduced (weak, thready pulse)
Capillary refill time	Minimally prolonged	Markedly prolonged (>3 sec)
Mucous membrane color	Pale pink (injected in septic shock)	White (red or blue in septic shock)
CVP	Minimally reduced	Markedly reduced (<1 cm H_2O)
Arterial blood pressure	Normal or decreased (elevated in septic shock)	Decreased (mean pressure <60 mm Hg)
ECG	Normal, tachycardia	Normal, arrhythmic, ST segment deviation
Respiratory		
Respiratory rate	Increased	Rapid, shallow breathing
Pattern of respiration	Regular	Normal, intermittent dyspnea
Auscultation	Normal, increased tracheal sounds	Increased bronchovesicular sounds, crackles
Tidal volume	Increased	Decreased
Arterial oxygen tension	Normal	Normal or decreased
Arterial carbon dioxide	Decreased	Normal, decreased, or increased
Central nervous system		
Level of consciousness	Alert, anxious, minimally depressed	Depressed, semiconscious, coma
Laboratory evaluation		
Packed cell volume	Normal or increased	Normal or decreased
Total protein	Normal or increased	Decreased
Blood lactate	Normal	Increased
Serum K^+	Normal or decreased	Increased
BUN and creatinine	Normal	Normal or increased
Urine volume and Na^+	Decreased	Markedly decreased
White blood cell count	Increased (left shift)	Decreased (left shift)

1. In hemorrhagic shock
   a. Below normal in hypovolemic and progressive phases of oligemic shock. Plasma volume increased as interstitial fluid moves into vascular system during the first 30 minutes after hemorrhage (0.25 ml/kg/min). In many species (particularly the horse), the spleen serves as a blood reservoir and buffers the effects of acute blood loss on PCV. Because of the ability of splenic contraction to restore blood volume, hemorrhage must be severe before PCV decreases
   b. In traumatic burn, endotoxic shock, colic
      (1) Packed cell volume increased, hemoconcentration
2. Blood glucose elevated; epinephrine release
3. Blood serum protein concentration may be normal or increased early and is generally reduced during later stages of shock
4. The platelet count is usually decreased
5. The blood urea nitrogen and creatinine are elevated, and creatinine clearance is reduced
6. The urinalysis generally shows no specific abnormalities
7. Electrolyte patterns vary considerably, but there is a tendency to a low serum sodium and low serum chloride
8. The serum potassium may be high, low, or normal
9. The plasma bicarbonate is usually low, and blood lactate is elevated
10. Respiratory alkalosis occurs early in shock and is manifested by a low Pa_{CO_2} and elevated arterial pH
11. Hypoxia and metabolic acidosis develops as shock progresses with Pa_{CO_2} values below 70 mm of mercury (normal: 75-100 mm Hg)
12. Blood cultures should reveal the causative pathogens, but bacteremia is often intermittent, and the blood cultures are often negative

B. The lung in shock: Respiratory failure is the most frequent cause of death in patients with shock, particularly after the hemodynamic alterations have been corrected. This syndrome is characterized by pulmonary congestion, hemorrhage, atelectasis, edema, and the formation of capillary thrombi. Pulmonary surfactant decreases, and pulmonary compliance becomes progressively compromised

THERAPY (Table 26-8)

I. Support of respiration: In many patients with shock, arterial Po_2 is markedly depressed. Oxygen may be administered nasally or by mask. Endotracheal intubation and the use of a positive-pressure respirator may be helpful in achieving proper ventilation

II. Volume replacement: With the CVP or pulmonary wedge pressure as a guide, blood volume should be replaced with appropriate fluids. Oliguria in the presence of hypotension is not a contraindication of continued vigorous fluid therapy

III. In addition to fluids, inotropes, antiarrhythmics, antibiotics, and glucocorticosteroids may be indicated. Small volumes (3-4 mg/kg) of hypertonic saline (7%)

THERAPEUTIC MANAGEMENT OF PROBLEMS ASSOCIATED WITH SHOCK

Problem	Treatment	Trade name	Dosage	Side effects or contraindications
Hypovolemia				
Fluid loss	Crystalloid	Lactated Ringer's	50-100 ml/kg/hr IV	Hypervolemia, pulmonary edema, hypoproteinemia
Plasma loss	Colloid expander	Gentran 40 (Travenol)	20-40 ml/kg IV	Hypervolemia, pulmonary edema, allergic reactions
Blood loss	Whole blood	—	10-40 ml/kg IV	Hypervolemia, allergic reactions
Hypotension	Correct hypovolemia first			
	Calcium chloride	—	1 ml 10% sol./10 kg IV	
	Phenylephrine	Neo-Synephrine (Winthrop)	10-50 μg/kg IV	
	Epinephrine	Adrenaline (Parke-Davis)	3-5 μg/kg, IV	Hypertension, tachycardia, arrhythmias
	Dopamine	Intropin (Arnar-Stone)	3-10 μg/kg/min IV	
	Dobutamine	Dobutrex (Lilly)	3-10 μg/kg/min IV	
Cardiac arrhythmias				
Bradycardia	Atropine	—	0.01-0.02 mg/kg IV	Tachycardia
	Glycopyrrolate	Robinul (Robins)	0.005-0.01 mg/kg IV	Tachycardia
Tachycardia	Digoxin	Lanoxin (Burroughs-Wellcome)	0.01-0.02 mg/kg IV slowly	Bradycardia, cardiac arrhythmias
	Propranolol	Inderal (Ayerst)	0.05-0.01 mg/kg IV	Bradycardia, cardiac failure
Atrial arrhythmias	Quinidine	Quinidine gluconate (Lilly)	4-8 mg/kg/10 min IV	Hypotension
Ventricular arrhythmias	Lidocaine	Xylocaine (Astra)	2-4 mg/kg IV	CNS excitement
	Procainamide	Pronestyl (Squibb)	4-8 mg/kg/5 min IV	Hypotension

Continued

305

THERAPEUTIC MANAGEMENT OF PROBLEMS ASSOCIATED WITH SHOCK

Problem	Treatment	Trade name	Dosage	Side effects or contraindications
Acute heart failure	Calcium chloride		1 ml 10% sol./10 kg IV	
	Epinephrine	Adrenaline (Parke-Davis)	3-5 µg/kg IV	Hypertension, tachycardia, cardiac arrhythmias
	Dopamine	Intropin (Arnar-Stone)	3-10 µg/kg/min IV	
	Dobutamine	Dobutrex (Lilly)	3-10 µg/kg/min IV	
Respiratory failure				
Hypoxia	O$_2$, nasal catheter; oxygen cage		2-4 L/min	Decreased venous return, respiratory alkalosis
	Ventilation			
Hypercarbia	Doxapram	Dopram V (Robins)	1.0-2.0 mg/kg	CNS excitement
	Ventilation		V$_T$ = 14 ml/kg	Decreased venous return, resp. alkalosis
Dyspnea	Tracheostomy			
	Chest tubes	Heimlich valve		
	Ventilation		V$_T$ = 14 mg/kg	Decreased venous return, respiratory alkalosis
Sepsis	Surgery			
	Gentamicin	Gentocin (Schering)	4 mg/kg qid IM	Muscle weakness, renal toxicity
	Kanamycin	Kantrim (Bristol)	10 mg/kg qid IM	Muscle weakness, renal toxicity
	Ampicillin	Omipen (Wyeth)	10 mg/kg qid IM	
Metabolic acidosis	Sodium lactate*		Bicarbonate dose = Base deficit × 0.3 × wt(kg)	Metabolic alkalosis, hyperosmolarity, CSF acidosis, hyperkalemia
	Sodium acetate*		or 0.5 mEq/kg/10 min IV to effect	hypocalcemia
	Sodium bicaronate			

Condition	Treatment	Agent	Dose	Complications
Hyperkalemia	Sodium bicarbonate		0.5-1.0 mg/kg IV	As above
	0.9% NaCl solution		10-40 ml/kg/hr IV	Hypervolemia, hypoproteinemia
	Calcium gluconate		0.5 ml/kg of 10% sol. IV	Tachycardia
	Hyperventilation		V_T = 14 ml/kg	Decreased venous return, respiratory alkalosis
Hypoglycemia	50% dextrose		1-2 ml/kg IV 0.5-1.0 g/kg/hr 10% glucose	Hyperosmolarity
Renal ischemic	Fluids	Lactated Ringer's	10-40 ml/kg/hr IV	Hypervolemia, hypoproteinemia, pulmonary edema
	Mannitol (20%)	Osmitrol (Travenol)	0.5-2.0 mg/kg IV	Hyperosmolality
	Furosemide	Lasix (National)	1.0-2.0 mg/kg IM, IV	Decreased cardiac output
Hypothermia (<36° C)	Fluids	Lactated Ringer's	10-40 ml/kg/hr warmed to 37° C	Hypervolemia, hypoproteinemia, pulmonary edema
	H₂O-filled heating pad		Warmed to 38° C (warm slowly)	
Disseminated intravascular coagulation (DIC)	Correct hypotension	Lactated Ringer's	10-40 mg/kg/hr IV	Hypervolemia, hypoproteinemia, pulmonary edema
	Correct hypoxemia	Nasal catheter Ventilation	2-4 L/min V_T = 14 mg/kg	Decreased venous return, respiratory alkalosis
	Correct acidosis	Sodium bicarbonate	0.5-1.0 mg/kg IV	Bleeding
	Heparin		Dog: 500 U/kg tid s.c. Cat: 250-400 U/kg tid s.c.	
Cellular ischemia	Fluids	Lactated Ringer's	10-40 ml/kg/hr IV	Hypervolemia, hypoproteinemia, pulmonary edema
	Oxygen	Nasal catheter	2-4 L/min	
	Dexamethasone sodium phosphate	Azium (Schering)	4-6 mg/kg IV	
	Prednisolone sodium succinate	Solu-Delta-Cortef (Upjohn)	>10 mg/kg IV	

*Questionable efficacy during severe low-flow states

in 6% dextran have recently been used to help restore and maintain cardio-vascular function

A. Hypertonic (7% and 25%) saline solutions and hypertonic saline (25%) mixed with dextran 70 (24%) solution are being used to treat hemorrhagic traumatic and endotoxic shock with remarkably good response

    1. 3-4 ml/kg of 7% saline produces a beneficial hemodynamic response

III. Antibiotics: Blood cultures and cultures of relevant body fluids or exudates should be taken before the administration of antimicrobial therapy but are often uninformative

IV. Surgical intervention: Many patients with shock may have an abscess or other local situation where surgical drainage and excision are required. Immediate surgical intervention is of paramount importance. The patient will continue to deteriorate unless the focus is removed or drained

CHAPTER TWENTY-SEVEN

Euthanasia

"Sweet is true love though given in vain,
and sweet is death who puts an end to pain."
ALFRED LORD TENNYSON

OVERVIEW

Euthanasia is an important pharmacologic and economic issue concerning the prolongation of animal pain and suffering. Almost all drugs used for chemical restraint and anesthesia have the capability of producing death, provided the dose of drug administered is adequate. These drugs offer the advantage of producing total unconsciousness before cardiopulmonary arrest and the elimination of brain electrical activity. This section does not presume to identify what technique should be considered the best method of euthanasia but details the various techniques applied to produce euthanasia.

GENERAL CONSIDERATIONS

I. Euthanasia is the act of inducing painless death in animals. Death may be defined as permanent abolition of CNS function
   A. Euthanasia often requires the ability to physically restrain the animal
   B. In many species, capture and immobilization for euthanasia may cause a variety of aesthetically unpleasant responses
      1. Vocalization
      2. Avoidance or aggressive behavior
      3. Immobility ("frozen with fear")
      4. Urination and defecation
      5. Sweating, salivation
      6. Skeletal muscle tremors, spasms, or shivering

TABLE 27 - 1

METHODS FOR PRODUCING EUTHANASIA

Agent	Site of action	Advantages	Disadvantages	General comments
Hypoxic agents				
Carbon monoxide (CO)	Carbon monoxide combines with hemoglobin, preventing combination with O_2	Unconsciousness occurs rapidly; inexpensive	Persistence of motor activity after unconsciousness until death	Acceptable
Muscle relaxants	Paralysis of respiratory muscles by depolarizing or nondepolarizing neuromuscular blockade	Inexpensive	Animal remains conscious until death occurs from hypoxia; no analgesia	Unacceptable
Depolarizing				
Succinylcholine				
Decamethonium				
Nondepolarizing				
Curare				
Gallamine				
Pancuronium				
Nitrogen inhalation	Reduced partial pressure of oxygen (Pa O_2)	Unconsciousness; inexpensive	Motor activity remains until death	Acceptable
Electrocution (current through brain)	Spastic paralysis of respiratory muscles and fibrillation of heart	Inexpensive	Slow unconsciousness; pain from muscle spasms	Acceptable(?)

Direct central nervous system depression

Anesthetic gases*

Agent	Mode of action	Advantages	Disadvantages	Recommendation
Ether Chloroform Methoxyflurane Enflurane Halothane	Direct depression of cerebral cortex; death due to respiratory and cardiovascular failure	Unconsciousness; analgesia; no motor activity	Potential pollution of environment; potentially expensive	Acceptable
Barbituric acid derivatives	Direct depression of cerebral cortex; respiratory and cardiovascular failure	Unconsciousness; inexpensive	Transient excitement	Acceptable
Chloral hydrate and chloral hydrate combinations	Direct depression of cerebral cortex; respiratory and cardiovascular failure	Unconsciousness; inexpensive	Transient anxiety	Acceptable
T-61	Direct depression of cerebral cortex; respiratory and cardiovascular failure	Unconsciousness	Transient excitement and motor activity	Acceptable

Physical or mechanical agents

Agent	Mode of action	Advantages	Disadvantages	Recommendation
Electrocution (current through brain)	Direct depression of brain; death due to hypoxia	Inexpensive; immediate unconsciousness	Violent muscle contractions	Acceptable(?)
Gunshot or captive bolt	Direct concussion of brain	Inexpensive; immediate unconsciousness	Motor activity may continue until death	Acceptable
Decapitation	Elimination of brain blood supply and central nervous system input	Inexpensive; immediate	Aesthetically unpleasant	Acceptable for rodents and some fowl

*Inhalation or gaseous anesthetic agents, although effective, are not only expensive, but if adequate precautions are not taken, produce a hazard to personnel due to atmospheric pollution. To avoid pollution, scavenging devices are recommended. Because of the high percentage of concentrations and high gas flow rates of inhalation anesthetic agents necessary to produce death, their use is not recommended in large animals. Modified from J Am Vet Med Assoc Panel on Euthanasia. J Am Vet Med Assoc 188: 252-268, 1988.

C. Selection of a method of euthanasia is dependent on:
 1. Species of animal
 2. Size and weight
 3. Type of physical restraint necessary
 4. Personnel (skill of and risk to)
 5. Number of animals to be euthanatized
 6. Economic factors
 7. Facilities available
D. Tranquilizers or other depressant drugs are recommended prior to administration of euthanatizing drugs in excitable or vicious animals
E. Pain perception requires a functional cerebral cortex. An unconscious animal does not experience pain
 1. Pain-provoking stimuli in an unconscious animal may evoke a reflex motor or sympathetic response

AVAILABLE METHODS

I. Euthanatizing agents include mechanical, chemical, electrical, and gaseous methods of producing death
II. Euthanatizing agents produce death by three mechanisms
A. Hypoxia, direct or indirect
B. Depression of the central nervous system
C. Physical damage or concussion of the brain

EVALUATION CRITERIA

I. Criteria for evaluation of methods of euthanasia are important to the development of acceptable euthanatizing methods and include:
A. Production of death without pain
B. Restraining capabilities of the method used; ability to minimize physical and psychological stress
C. Time required to produce:
 1. Loss of consciousness
 2. Death
D. Reliability
E. Safety to personnel
F. Emotional effect on observers
G. Economic considerations
H. Compatibility with histopathologic evaluation
I. Equipment or drug availability and abuse potential
II. Several of the more common methods used for producing euthanasia, their advantages and disadvantages, and their acceptability are listed in Table 27-1

DRUGS

I. Strychnine, magnesium sulfate, and nicotine are intravenous drugs commonly suggested for use as euthanasia agents. Their individual use as the sole euthanatizing agent is *absolutely* unwarranted. Like the neuromuscular blocking drugs, these drugs:

A. Do not produce unconsciousness
B. Do not produce analgesia
C. Have no anesthetic effect
D. Lead to specific problems
    1. Strychnine produces violent muscle contractions associated with extreme pain
    2. Magnesium sulfate causes death due to asphyxia
    3. Nicotine produces convulsions prior to death and is extremely hazardous to personnel

II. The most common drugs used for euthanasia of dogs, cats, horses, and cattle are:

A. Pentobarbital sodium for euthanasia
    1. 1 ml/10 lb
B. Chloral hydrate
    1. To effect, 0.5-1.0 ml/lb of a 7% solution
C. T-61
    1. 0.14 mg/lb

Listing of Commonly Used Drugs and Apparatus and Their Manufacturers

DRUGS

AERRANE (isoflurane)
Anaquest
2005 West Beltline Highway
Madison, WI 53713-2318

AGEUM-DEXAMETHASON
Sorensen Res. Co.
P.O. Box 15588
2511 S.W. Temple
Salt Lake City, UT 84115

AMIDATE (etomidate)
Abbott Laboratories
North Chicago, IL 60064

AMINOPHYLLINE
Invenex Laboratories
Div. of LyphoMed, Inc.
Melrose Park, IL 60160

AMINOPHYLLIN INJ.
(aminophylline inj. USP)
Searle Pharmaceuticals, Inc.
Chicago, IL 60680

ATIVAN (lorazepam)
Wyeth Laboratories, Inc.
Philadelphia, PA 19101

ATROPINE
Elkins-Sinn, Inc.
Cherry Hill, NJ 08034

ATROPINE SULFATE INJ.
Elkins-Sinn, Inc.
Cherry Hill, NJ 08034

AZIUSM (dexamethasone)
Schering Veterinary
Schering Corp.
Kenilworth, NJ 07033

BENADRYL (diphenhydramine
hydrochloride inj. USP)
Parke-Davis
Div. of Warner-Lambert Co.
Morris Plains, NJ 07950

BEUTHANASIA-D SPECIAL
Burns-Biotec Lab., Inc.
Omaha, NE 68103

BIO-TAL (thiamylal sodium)
Bio Ceutic Division
Boehringer Ingelheim Animal
Health Inc.
St. Joseph, MO 64502

BRETYLOL (bretylium sodium)
Arnar-Stone Del Caribe, Inc.
Aguadilla, PR 00604

BREVITAL SODIUM INJ.
(methohexital sodium)
Eli Lilly and Co.
Indianapolis, IN 46285

BREVANE (methohexital)
Corn State Labs., Inc.
Omaha, NE 68101

BUMEX (bumetanide)
Roche Laboratories
Div. of Hoffman-LaRoche, Inc.
340 Kingsland Street
Nutley, NJ 07110

CALCIUM CHLORIDE
LyphoMed, Inc.
Melrose Park, IL 60160

CALCIUM GLUCONATE INJ, USP 10%
Elkins-Sinn, Inc.
Cherry Hill, NY 08034

CARBOCAINE V (mepivacaine
hydrochloride 2%)
Winthrop Veterinary
Sterling Animal Health Products
Div. of Sterling Drug Inc.
New York, NY 10016

CHLOROPENT (chloral hydrate
magnesium sulfate pentobarbital)
Fort Dodge
800 Fifth St., N.W.
Fort Dodge, IA 50501

DANTROLENE (dantrium)
Norwich-Eaton Pharmaceuticals
1327 Eaton Avenue
Norwich, NY 13815

DEMEROL (mepiridine hydrochloride)
Winthrop Laboratories
90 Park Avenue
New York, NY 10016

DOBUTREX (dobutamine
hydrochloride)
Eli Lilly & Co.
Indianapolis, IN 46285

DOPRAM V (doxapram hydrochloride)
Elkins-Sinn, Inc.
Cherry Hill, NJ 08034

DURATEARS
Alcon Laboratories, Inc.
Fort Worth, TX 76134

ELANONE-V Inj. (lenperone
hydrochloride inj.)
Animal Health Group
A.H. Robins Co.
Richmond, VA 23220

ELTRAD IV
Professional Veterinary Laboratories
Minneapolis, MN 55437

EPHEDRINE
Eli Lilly and Co.
307 E. McCarty
P.O. Box 618
Indianapolis, IN 46206

EPHEDRINE SULFATE INJ. USP
Eli Lilly and Co.
Indianapolis, IN 46285

EPINEPHRINE
Anthony Products
Arcadia, CA 91006

EPINEPHRINE 1:1000
VEDCO Inc.
Overland Park, KS 66204

ETHRANE (enflurane)
  Ohio Medical Products
  P.O. Box 1319
  3030 Airco Drive
  Madison, WI 53701
  (608-221-1551)
EUTHOL
  Pitman-Moore, Inc.
  Washington Crossing, NJ 08560
FLAXEDIL (gallamine triethiodide)
  Davis and Geck
  American Cyanamid Company
  Pearl River, NY 10965
GUAIFENESIN USP POWDER
  Life Science Products
  P.O. Box 8111
  St. Joseph, MO 64506
GUAILAXIN
  A.H. Robins
  1407 Cummings Drive
  Richmond, VA 23220
GLYCERYL GUAIACOLATE
  Summitt Hill Labs
  P.O. Box 1
  Avalon, NJ 08202
HALOTHANE (fluothane)
  Astra Pharmaceutical Products
  7 Neponset Street
  Worcester, MA 01606
HALOTHANE
  Halocarbon Lab., Inc.
  82 Burlews Court
  Hackensack, NJ 07601
INDERAL INJ. (propranolol
hydrochloride)
  Ayerst Laboratories, Inc.
  New York, NY 10017
INOTROPIN (dopamine HCl)
  Arnar-Stone Labs., Inc.
  601 E. Kensington Road
  Mt. Prospect, IL 60056
INNOVAR-VET (fentanyl-droperidol)
  Pitman-Moore, Inc.
  Washington Crossing, NJ 08560

ISUPREL (isoproterenol)
  Sterling Drug, Inc.
  New York, NY 10016
KETASET (ketamine HCl)
  Bristol Labs
  Div. of Bristol-Myers Co.
  P.O. Box 657
  Syracuse, NY 13201
LANOXIN (digoxin inj.)
  Burroughs Wellcome Co.
  Research Park, NC 27709
LASIX (furosemide)
  Taylor Pharmaceuticals
  Decatur, IL 62525
LEVOPHED BITARTRATE
(norepinephrine bitartrate inj. USP)
  Sterling Drug, Inc.
  New York, NY 10016
LIDOCAINE HCL 2%
  VEDCO, Inc.
  Overland, KS 66204
  Mfd. by:
  Anthony Products
  Arcadia, CA 91006
LORFAN (levallorphan tartrate)
  Roche Laboratories
  Div. of Hoffman LaRoche, Inc.
  340 Kingsland Street
  Nutley, NJ 07110
MANNITAL HEXANITRATE
  Travenol Labs., Inc.
  Deerfield, IL 60015
MANNITOL 20%
  Anthony Products
  Arcadia, CA 91006
MARCAINE HCl 0.25% WITH
EPINEPHRINE 1:200,000
(bupivacaine HCl and epinephrine)
  Sterling Drug, Inc.
  New York, NY 10016
METOPHANE (methoxyflurane)
  Pitman-Moore, Inc.
  Washington Crossing, NJ 08560

MORPHINE
Elkins-Sinn, Inc.
Cherry Hill, NJ 08034

NALLINE (nalorphine)
Merck, Sharpe & Dohme
Div. of Merch & Co., Inc.
West Point, PA 19486

NALLINE HYDROCHLORIDE
(nalorphine hydrochloride)
Merck Animal Health Div.
Merch & Co., Inc.
Rahway, NJ 07065

NARCAN (naloxone hydrochloride)
Pitman-Moore, Inc.
Washington Crossing, NJ 08560

NEMBUTAL (pentobarbital)
Abbott Laboratories
Abbott Park
North Chicago, IL 60064

NESACAINE 2% INJ. (chloraprocaine
hydrochloride)
Pennwalt Prescription Products
Pharmaceutical Division
Pennwalt Corporation
Rochester, NY 14623

NUBAIN (nalbuphine hydrochloride)
Du Pont Pharmaceuticals, Inc.
P.O. Box 363
Manati, PR 00701

NUMORPHAN (oxymorphone)
Du Pont Pharmaceuticals, Inc.
Manati, PR 00701

PAVULON (pancuronium bromide)
Organon Inc.
West Orange, NJ 07052

Pentothal (thiopental)
Abbott Laboratories
Abbott Park
North Chicago, IL 60064

POTASSIUM CHLORIDE
Travenol Labs., Inc.
Deerfield, IL 60015

PRISCOLINE HCl
(tolazoline HCl USP)
CIBA Pharmaceutical Co.
Div. CIBA-GEIGY Corp.
Summit, NJ 07901
Mfd. by:
Taylor Pharmacol Co.
Decatur, IL 62525

PROMACE (acepromazine maleate)
Fort Dodge Laboratories, Inc.
800 Fifth Street
Fort Dodge, IA 50501

PRONESTYL (procainamide)
E.R. Squibb and Sons, Inc.
Princeton, NJ 08540

PROSTIGMINE (neostigmine)
Roche Laboratories
Div. of Hoffman-LaRoche, Inc.
340 Kingsland Street
Nutley, NJ 07110

PROTAMINE SULFATE
Eli Lilly and Co.
Indianapolis, IN 46285

QUINIDINE GLUCONATE
Eli Lilly & Co.
307 E. McCarty
P.O. Box 618
Indianapolis, IN 46206

REGONOL PYRIDOSTIGMINE
Organon, Inc.
W. Orange, NJ 07052

ROBINUL-V (glycopyrrolate)
A.H. Robins
1407 Cummings Drive
Richmond, VA 23220

ROMPUN (xylazine)
Haver Lockhart
Bayvet Division
Miles Laboratories, Inc.
Shawnee, KS 66201

SODIUM BICARBONATE INJ.
Andro Pharmaceutical
Arcadia, CA 91006

SODIUM PENTOBARBITOL INJ.
(65 mg/ml)
   Anthony Products Co.
   Arcadia, CA 91006

SOLU-DELTA-CORTEF
(prednisolone sodium)
   Upjohn Co.
   7000 Portage Road
   Kalamazoo, MI 49001

SOLU-DELTA-CORTEF
(100 mg-500 mg)
(prednisolone sodium succinate)
   The Upjohn Co.
   7000 Portage Road
   Kalamazoo, MI 49001

SPARINE (promazine)
   Wyeth Laboratories
   Box 8299
   Philadelphia, PA 19105

STADOL (butorphenol)
   Bristol Laboratories
   Div. of Bristol-Myers Co.
   P.O. Box 657
   Syracuse, NY 13201

STIGLYN 1 = 500 (neostigmine
methylsulfate inj.)
   Pitman-Moore
   Washington Crossing, NJ 08560

STRESNIL (azaperone)
   Taylor Pharmacol Company
   Decatur, IL 62525

SUCOSTRIN (succinylcholine chloride)
   E.R. Squibb & Sons
   P.O. Box 4000
   Princeton, NJ 08540

SUBLIMAZE (fentanyl)
   McNeil Laboratories
   Camphill Road
   Fort Washington, PA 19034

SUFENTA (sufentanil citrate)
   Janssen Pharmaceutica, Inc.
   Piscataway, NJ 08854

SURITAL (thiamylal)
   Winthrop Laboratories
   90 Park Avenue
   New York, NY 10016

TALWIN (pentazocine)
   Winthrop Laboratories
   90 Park Avenue
   New York, NY 10016

TELAZOL (tiletamine-zolazepam)
   A.H. Robins
   1407 Cummings Dr.
   Richmond, VA 23220

TORBUGESIC AND TORBUTROL
(butorphanol tartrate)
   Veterinary Products
   Bristol Laboratories
   Div. of Bristol-Myers Co.
   Syracuse, NY 13221-4755

TRACRIUM (atracurium besylate)
   Burroughs Wellcome Co.
   Research Triangle Park, NC 27709

VALIUM (diazepam)
   Hoffman-LaRoche, Inc.
   340 Kingsland Street
   Nutley, NJ 07110

VECURONIUM BROMIDE (norcuron)
   Organon, Inc.
   W. Orange, NJ 07052

VERSED (midazolam HCl)
   Hoffman-LaRoche, Inc.
   340 Kingsland Street
   Nutley, NJ 07110

VETALAR (ketamine HCl)
   Parke-Davis & Co.
   Joseph Campau at the River
   Detroit, MI 48232

WYAMINE SULFATE
(mephentermine sulfate)
   Wyeth Laboratories, Inc.
   Philadelphia, PA 19101

XYLOCAINE (lidocaine)
Parke-Davis & Co.
Joseph Campau at the River
Detroit, MI 48232

YOHIMBINE HCl
Mfd. by:
Bowman Pharmaceutical
Canton, Ohio 44702
Dist. by:
Consolidated Midland Corporation
Brewster, NY 10509

APPARATUS

VAPORIZERS

Halothane:

Fluotec
Fraswer-Sweatman, Inc.
5490 Broadway
Lancaster, NY 14086
(716-684-0564)

Fluomatic
Foregger Co., Inc.
680 Old Willets Path
Smithtown, NY 11787

Vapor
North American Drager
P.O. Box 121
Telford, PA 18969

Methoxyflurane:

Pentec
Fraser-Sweatman, Inc.
5490 Broadway
Lancaster, NY 14086
(716-684-0564)

Vapor
North American Drager
P.O. Box 121
Telford, PA 18969

Ohio Ether 8
Ohio Medical Products
P.O. Box 1319
3030 Airco Drive
Madison, WI 53701
(608-221-1551)

Snyder
Snyder Laboratories
1458 Fifth Street
P.O. Box 508
New Philadelphia, OH 44663

Ehtrane
Fraser-Harlake
145 Mid County Drive
Orchard Park, NY 14127

Forane
Fortec
Fraser-Harlake
145 Mid County Drive
Orchard Park, NY 14127

APPARATUS

Bissonnette Ayers T
Fraser-Sweatman, Inc.
5490 Broadway
Lancaster, NY 14086
(716-684-0564)

Norman Mask Elbow
Dupaco, Inc.
Box 98
San Marcos, CA 92069

Life Pac Pressure Infusion Cuff
Technologies, Inc.
Houston, TX 77063

Kuhn System
North American Drager
P.O. Box 121
Telford, PA 18969

Esophageal Stethoscope
  Portex, Inc.
  42 Industrial Way
  Wilmington, MA 01887

Infusion Pump Model AS5D
  Travenol Laboratories, Inc.
  Auto Syringe Division
  Londonderry Turnpike
  Hooksett, New Hampshire 03104

Intravenous Catheters
  Sorensen Lab.
  Abbott Lab.
  North Chicago, IL 60064

Angiocath
  Deseret Medical, Inc.
  Becton Dickinson and Company
  Sandy, Utah 84070

Surflo Catheters
  Terumo Corp.
  Tokyo, Japan

Endotracheal Tubes
  Dow-Corning Corp.
  Silastic Endotracheal Tube
  (w/disc-cuff)
  Medical Products Div.
  Midland, MI 48640

Bivona Endotracheal Tubes
  Bivona, Inc.
  5700 W. 23rd Avenue
  Gary, Indiana 46406

Portex Endotracheal Tubes
  Portex, Inc.
  42 Industrial Way
  Wilmington, MA 01887

Y-type Blood-Solution
Administration Jet
  Travenol Lab., Inc.
  Deerfield, IL 60015

Buretrol In-line Burette
  Travenol Lab., Inc.
  Deerfield, IL 60015

Blood Warmer Coil with
Extension Set
  Fenwal Laboratories, Inc.
  Div. of Travenol Lab., Inc.
  Deerfield, IL 60015

Link Sales Co.
2426 S. 73rd Street
Milwaukee, WI 53219
(414-541-1100)

Ohio Medical Products
P.O. Box 1319
3030 Airco Drive
Madison, WI 53701
(608-221-1551)
(800-582-2057)

Foregger Co., Inc.
680 Old Willets Path
Smithtown, NY 11787

Snyder Laboratories
1458 Fifth Street
P.O. Box 508
New Philadelphia, OH 44663

Sorensen Research Co.
4455 Atherton Drive
Salt Lake City, UT 84123
(800-522-2688)

ANESTHETIC MACHINES

Foregger Compact
  Foregger Co., Inc.
  680 Old Willets Path
  Smithtown, NY 11787

Dupaco Compact 78
  Dupaco, Inc.
  Box 98
  San Marcos, Ca 92069

Fraser-Sweatman VMS
  Fraser-Sweatman, Inc.
  5490 Broadway
  Lancaster, NY 14086
  (716-662-6650)

Narkomed
  North American Drager
  P.O. Box 121
  Telford, PA 18969
  (215-723-9824)

Pitman-Moore 980
  Pitman-Moore, Inc.
  Washington Crossing, NJ 08560

Stephens Anesthesia Machine
  Henry Schein Inc.
  5 Harbor Park Drive
  Port Washington, NY 11050

Ohio Medical
  Ohio Medical Products
  P.O. Box 1319
  3030 Airco Drive
  Madison, WI 53701
  (608-221-1551)

Snyder L.A.
  Synder Laboratories
  1458 Fifth Street
  P.O. Box 508
  New Philadelphia, OH 44663

VENTILATORS

Pitman-Moore
  Pitman-Moore, Inc.
  Washington Crossing, NJ 08560

Bird
  Bird Corporation
  Palm Springs, CA 42262
  (714-327-1571)

Metomatic Veterinary Ventilator
  Ohio Medical Products
  P.O. Box 1319
  3030 Airco Drive
  Madison, WI 53701

N.A. Drager
  North American Drager
  P.O. Box 121
  Telford, PA 18969

Model 320Y Veterinary Ventilator
  Gould
  Cardiopulmonary Products Division
  Dayton, OH 45449

MONITORING EQUIPMENT

Bentley-Trantec Pressure Transducer
  Bentley Trantec, Inc.
  17502 Armstrong Avenue
  Irvine, CA 92714

Datascope 850 Monitor & Recorder
  Datascope Corp.
  580 Winter Avenue
  Paramus, NJ 07652

Datascope P-2 Pressure Module
  Datascope Corp.
  580 Winter Avenue
  Paramus, NJ 07652

Datascope P$_3$ Pressure Module
  Datascope Corp.
  Paramus, NJ 07652

Ultrasound Blood Pressure Monitoring
Equipment
Doppler Model 811
  Parks Medical Electronic, Inc.
  P.O. Box 5669
  Aloha, OR 97006

Neonatal Blood Pressure Cuff
  Sterling International, Inc.
  P.O. Box 23565
  Milwaukee, WI 53223

DEFRIBRILLATORS

Electrodyne DS-95-M, D-84-M
Internal-External DC Defribillator
  Electrodyne Company, Inc.
  Norwood, MA 02062

Datascope M/D2J
  Datascope Corp.
  Paramus, NJ 07652

Physical Principles
of Anesthesia

I. Laws

  A. Boyle's law:

$$\text{Volume} = \frac{k}{\text{Pressure}} \qquad V \times P = k$$

$$P_1 V_1 = P_2 V_2$$

  B. Charles' law:

$$V = k + T \qquad T = {}^\circ K$$

$$\frac{V_1}{V_2} = \frac{T_1}{T_2}$$

  C. Gay-Lussac's law:

$$P = k \times T \qquad T = {}^\circ K$$

$$\frac{P_1}{P_2} = \frac{T_1}{T_2}$$

  From above:

$$\frac{P_1 V_1}{T_1} = \frac{P_2 V_2}{T_2}$$

  D. Gas law:

$$\frac{PV}{T} = n \frac{(1 \text{ atm})(22.41)}{273K}$$

$$PV = nRT \qquad R = 0.08206 \qquad 1 \text{ atm}/{}^\circ K$$

E. Henry's law:

$$V = \alpha P \qquad \begin{aligned} V &= \text{ volume of gas dissolved} \\ \alpha &= \text{ solubility coefficient} \\ P &= \text{ partial pressure} \end{aligned}$$

Note: The solubility of a gas or vapor in a liquid (α) decreases as the temperature increases

F. Law of partial pressure (Dalton's law): Each gas in a mixture exerts the same pressure as it would exert if it alone occupied the same volume at the same temperature. Since pressure measurements cannot distinguish different molecules in a mixed sample, the contribution to total pressure made by a given constituent is in proportion to the number of molecules of that constituent

G. Graham's law: The velocity or rate of diffusion is inversely proportional to the square root of the density

II. Terms

A. Vapor pressure
   1. Tendency for a liquid to evaporate
   2. When a liquid and its vapor are in equilibrium, the partial pressure that the vapor exerts

B. Heat of vaporization: the amount of heat required for a liquid to evaporate

C. Volumes of a vapor:

$$\frac{\text{Vapor pressure}}{\text{Total pressure}} \times 100 = \text{Vol \%}$$

D. Boiling point of a liquid: that temperature at which its vapor pressure is equal to the prevailing atmospheric pressure; generally stated for 760 torr

E. Critical temperature: when a liquid is confined in a strong container, that temperature at which the contents of the container will consist of vapor only

F. Critical pressure: when a liquid is confined in a strong container, that pressure that exists when the container has reached its critical temperature. *Note*: Liquid volumes may be converted to weight by: Volume (ml) $\times$ Density (g/ml) = Grams of liquid

G. Latent heat of vaporization: the amount of heat necessary to evaporate a quantity of liquid to its vapor state without any change in temperature; expressed in calories/g liquid. This heat is stored in the vapor

III. Specific partition coefficients

A. The solubility coefficient may be expressed as:
   1. Bunsen's absorption coefficient: amount of gas (volume) at STP that will dissolve in one volume of liquid when the partial pressure of the gas above the liquid is 1 atm
   2. Ostwald's solubility coefficient: the volume of gas absorbed by a unit volume of liquid when the partial pressure of the gas is 1 atm, the volume of gas being expressed at the temperature of the experiment

3. The partition coefficient
   a. May be expressed as the ratio of concentration of a substance in the gas phase and in the liquid phase (example: milligrams per milliliter). This also varies with temperature
   b. Partition coefficients are also used to relate the ratios of concentrations in any two phases that are in equilibrium
      (1) Liquid-liquid (oil-water)
      (2) Liquid-solid
      (3) Gas-solid

INDEX